Progress in Proctology

Proceedings of the 3rd International Congress
of Hedrologicum Conlegium

October 1968, Erlangen-Nuremberg, Germany

Editor: J. Hoferichter

Springer-Verlag Berlin Heidelberg New York 1969

ISBN-13: 978-3-642-87961-6 e-ISBN-13: 978-3-642-87959-3
DOI: 10.1007/ 978-3-642-87959-3

Softcover reprint of the hardcover 1st edition 1969

Title-No. 1601

Preface

"Hedrology" – a term coined by G. B. E. Simonetti (Milan) – is the oldest of all surgical specialities. It was re-introduced as Proctology by European surgeons at the turn of the century. Excellent work was performed by the surgeons Lisfrank, Dieffenbach, Velpeau, Volkmann, Kraske, von Heineke, Quenu, Rehn and Goetze.

Today this specialty includes the research, recognition and treatment of disorders of the entire colon, rectum and anus. Ever since the days of W. von Heineke (1868–1901), this specialty has been cultivated with special care at the Chirurgische Universitätsklinik Erlangen; scientific investigation has progressed and the operative technique has been improved.

Experts from 22 countries met here at the Third International Congress in order to exchange experience and to learn from the successes and failures of their colleagues.

These opinions and this knowledge have been summarized in the congress report. Thus it presents a survey of today's problems in proctology.

G. Hegemann
President of the
3rd International Congress

Contents

Contributors

ALQUIER, Y., Dr., Rue de la Petite Loge, Montpellier, France

ALFÖLDY, Á., Dr., Hospital Joannes and Ambulance, Budapest, Hungary

ALTARAS, J., Dr., Privatdozent für Röntgenologie, Wilhelm-Conrad-Röntgen-klinik, Giessen, Germany

ARAKAWA, K., M.D., Arakawa Surgical Clinic, Tokyo, Japan

ARNOLD, K., Dr., Chirurgische Klinik der Universität, Erlangen, Germany

BANCU, E., Dr., I. Surgical Clinic of University of Tirgu-Mureş, Tirgu-Mureş, Roumania

BARADNAY, GY., Dr., I. Surgical Clinic of University, Medical School, Szeged, Hungary

BARTH, G., Dr., Dr., Professor für Röntgenologie, Wilhelm-Conrad-Röntgen-klinik, Giessen, Germany

BERNHOFT, W. H., M.D., Assistant Clinical Professor, Department of Surgery, Division of Proctology, State University of New York, Buffalo, N.Y., USA

BONOMO, M., Dr., Istituto di Clinica Medica, Università di Bari, Bari, Italy

BRUERE-DAWSON, C. A., Dr., Rue de la Petite Loge, Montpellier, France

BUKHTEYEV, V. V., Dr., Gorky Street 154, fl. 14., Donetsk, 55, USSR

CAPURSO, A., Dr., Istituto di Clinica Medica, Università di Bari, Bari, Italy

CAYRON, G., Dr., Hôpitaux de Paris Membre de la Société Française de Procto-logie, Rouen, France

COLE, T. P., M.B., F.R.C.S., Department of Surgery, Woodend General Hospital, Aberdeen, Great Britain

COMAN, N., M.D., Radiologic Institute, University of Tirgu-Mureş, Tirgu-Mureş, Roumania

D'ADDABBO, A., Dr., Professor of Medicine, Istituto di Clinica Medica, Università di Bari, Bari, Italy

DAUM, R., Dr., Privatdozent für Chirurgie, Kinderchirurgische Abteilung der Chirurgischen Klinik der Universität, Heidelberg, Germany

DAVY, A., Dr., 5, Rue d'Écosse, Rouen, France

DEGRELL, I., Dr., Dozent für Chirurgie, Megyei, Tanács Kórháza, Zrinyi Miklós u. 1. sz., Zaelaegerszeg, Hungary

DENECKE, K., Dr., Professor für Chirurgie, Städtische Krankenanstalten, Fürth, Germany

DEUCHER, F., Dr., Professor für Chirurgie, Chirurgische Klinik des Kantonsspitals Aarau, Aarau, Switzerland

DITTRICH, H., Dr., Privatdozent für Chirurgie, Chirurgische Klinik der Universi-tät, Erlangen, Germany

DOXIADIS, TH., M.D., Professor of Medicine, Evangelismos Medical Center, Athens Greece

Drobni, S., Dr., IV. Számú Esbészeti Klinika Sziv-ês Érsebeszet, Budapest, Hungary
Dudunkov, Z., Dr., Surgical Section, Oncological Institute "Darvenitza", Sofia, Bulgaria
Elster, K., Dr., Professor für Pathologie, Pathologisches Institut der Universität, Erlangen, Germany
v. d. Emde, J., Dr., Chirurgische Klinik der Universität, Erlangen, Germany
Ewen, S., M.D., Department of Surgery, Woodend General Hospital, Aberdeen, Great Britain
Feher, M., Dr., Hospital Joannes and Ambulance, Budapest, Hungary
Fornells, E., Dr., University School of Barcelona, Department of Proctology, Barcelona, Spain
Gaetani, G., Dr., Istituto di Clinica Chirurgica, Università di Bari, Bari, Italy
Gall, F., Dr., Professor für Chirurgie, Chirurgische Klinik der Universität, Erlangen, Germany
Garrigues, J. M., Dr., Rue de la Petite Loge, Montpellier, France
Georgiadis, N. J., M.D., Associated Professor of Surgery, 3, Koumbari Street, Athens, Greece
Giannacos, N., M.D., Assistant Professor, Department of Radiology, St. Sophias Children Hospital, Athens, Greece
Grozescu, T., Dr., I. Surgical Clinic of University of Tirgu-Mureş, Tirgu-Mureş, Roumania
Gusinde, J., Dr., Chirurgische Klinik der Universität, Erlangen, Germany
Haas, P., Dr., Orvostov Ábbképzó Intézet, Sebészeti Transzéke, Budapest, Hungary
Hecker, W. Ch., Dr., Professor für Chirurgie, Kinderchirurgische Abteilung der Chirurgischen Klinik der Universität, Heidelberg, Germany
Hellbach, R., Dr., Städtische Krankenanstalten, Fürth, Germany
Hoferichter, J., Dr., Privatdozent für Chirurgie, Chirurgische Abteilung des Stadtkrankenhauses, Wolfsburg, Germany
Hopkinson, B. R., M.D., F.R.C.S., Queen Elizabeth Hospital, Edgbaston, Birmingham, Great Britain
Kalima, T., M.D., II. Surgical Clinic, University of Helsinki, Helsinki, Finland
Keminger, K., Dr., Universitätsdozent, I. Chirurgische Universitätsklinik, Wien, Austria
Kemmerer, G., Dr., Chirurgische Klinik der Universität, Erlangen, Germany
Keresztessy, Ad., Dr., I. Surgical Clinic of University of Tirgu-Mureş, Tirgu-Mureş, Roumania
Keresztessy, Am., Dr., I. Surgical Clinic of University of Tirgu-Mureş, Tirgu-Mureş, Roumania
Kirov, St., Dr., Surgical Section, Oncological Institute "Darvenitza", Sofia, Bulgaria
Krestev, B., Dr., Professor, Surgical Section, Oncological Institute "Darvenitza", Sofia, Bulgaria
Kyle, J., M.D., Department of Surgery, Woodend General Hospital, Aberdeen, Great Britain

KYRLE, P., Dr., Universitäts-Professor, Krankenanstalt Rudolfstiftung der Stadt Wien, II. Chirurgische Abteilung, Wien, Austria

LEITNER, R., Dr., Krankenanstalt Rudolfstiftung der Stadt Wien, II. Chirurgische Abteilung, Wien, Austria

LENTINI, J., Dr., University School of Barcelona, Department of Proctology, Barcelona, Spain

LEOUTSAKOS, B., M.D., King Paul Hospital, University of Athens, Athens, Greece

LEVY, E., M.D., 1749 Grand Concourse, Apt. 8, New York, N.Y., 10453, USA

LIGHTWOOD, R., M.D., Surgical Research Laboratories of the Queen Elizabeth Hospital, Birmingham, Great Britain

MAREL, U., Dr., 45, Rue d'Elbeuf, Rouen, France

MATYASHIN, I. M., Dr., Professor für Chirurgie, Lesja Ukrainka Boulevard, Kiew, USSR

MEIER-RUGE, W., Dr., Privatdozent, Pathologisches Institut der Universität, Basel, Switzerland

MONTAGUE, J. F., M.D., 104 East 40th Street, New York, N.Y., 10016, USA

MORAN, T. F., M.D., Medical Arts Building, 327 North Washington Avenue, Scranton, Pa., USA

MORGER, R., Dr., FMH Chirurgie, Kinderchirurgie, Ostschweizerisches Säuglings- und Kinderspital, St. Gallen, Switzerland

MOSKOUTIS, N., M.D., Consultant Gastroenterologist, Evangelismos Medical Center, Athens, Greece

MULLER, CH. A., Dr., Spécialiste F.M.H. Chirurgie, Lausanne, Switzerland

NARASAKA, T., M.D., Department of Internal Medicine, Tohoku University, School of Medicine, Sendai, Japan

NICOLAIDIS, C., M.D., Consultant Gastroenterologist, Department of Clinical Therapeutics, University of Athens, Athens, Greece

NIEMIRO, B. J., M.D., Pleasant Street 575, Holyoke, Mass. 01040, USA

NÖTHIGER, F., Dr., Chirurgische Klinik des Kantonsspital Aarau, Aarau, Switzerland

ORTIZ, R., Dr., University School of Barcelona, Department of Proctology, Barcelona, Spain

OTTENJANN, R., Dr., Privatdozent für Medizin, Medizinische Klinik der Universität, Erlangen, Germany

PALEOLOGOS, T., M.D., Evangelismos Medical Center, Athens, Greece

PÁPAI, Z., Dr., Professor, I. Surgical Clinic of University of Tirgu-Mureş, Tirgu-Mureş, Roumania

PAPILLON, J., Dr., Professeur a la Faculté Radiologiste de Hôpitaux, 12, Quai Général-sarrail, Lyon, France

PARKS, A. G., M.Ch., F.R.C.S., St. Mark's Hospital, London, Great Britain

PELTOKALLIO, P., M.D., II. Surgical Clinic, University of Helsinki, Helsinki, Finland

PERTALLA, Y., M.D., II. Surgical Clinic, University of Helsinki, Helsinki, Finland

PETRI, G., Dr., Professor of Surgery, I. Surgical Clinic, University Medical School, Szeged, Hungary

PHOCAS, EL., M.D., I. Medical Clinic, University of Athens, School of Medicine, Athens, Greece

Pupp, A., Dr., I. Surgical Clinic, University of Tirgu-Mureş, Tirgu-Mureş, Roumania
Rehbein, F., Dr., Professor für Chirurgie, Kinderchirurgische Klinik, Bremen, Germany
Reifferscheid, M., Dr., Professor für Chirurgie, Abteilung für Allgemeine Chirurgie der Medizinischen Fakultät an der Rheinisch-Westfälischen Technischen Hochschule, Aachen, Germany
Romualdi, P., Dr., Professor, Ospedale del Bambino, Gesù, Roma, Italy
Rubino, M., Dr., Istituto di Clinica Chirurgica, Università di Bari, Bari, Italy
Samenius, B., M.D., Department of Surgery I, Sahlgrenska Sjukhuset, Gothenburg, Sweden
Schaudig, H., Dr., Privatdozent für Chirurgie, Chirurgische Klinik des Kreiskrankenhauses, Bad Mergentheim, Germany
Schier, J., Dr., Chirurgische Klinik der Universität, Mainz, Germany
Schwartz, R., Dr., 172 Bd. Haussmann, Paris, France
Schwemmle, K., Dr., Chirurgische Klinik der Universität, Erlangen, Germany
Simonetti, G. B. E., Dr., Via S. Raffaele 3, Milano, Italy
Southwood, W. F. W., M.D., Upton House, Bathwick Hill, Bath, Somerset, Great Britain
Svinhufvud, U., M.D., II. Surgical Clinic, University of Helsinki, Helsinki, Finland
Takebe, T., M.D., Department of Internal Medicine, Tohoku University, School of Medicine, Sendai, Japan
Thiele, G. H., M.D., Plaza Time Building, 411 Nichols Road, Kansas City, Missouri 64112, USA
Thompson, H. R., Mr., F.R.C.S., 14, Devonshire Place, London W. 1, Great Britain
Trampaklos, A. I., M.D., General State Hospital Agia Olga, II. Surgical Division, Athens, Greece
Tsilividis, S., M.D., General State Hospital Agia Olga, II. Surgical Division, Athens, Greece
Varró, V., Dr., I. Surgical Clinic of University, Medical School, Szeged, Hungary
Watanabe, H., M.D., Department of Internal Medicine, Tohoku University, School of Medicine, Sendai, Japan
Widmer, A., Dr., Chirurgische Klinik des Kantonsspital, Aarau, Aarau, Switzerland
Wilensky, T., M.D., 701 North Logan Street, East Lansing, Mich. 48915, USA
Yamagata, S., M.D., Professor of Medicine, Department of Medicine, Tohoku University, School of Medicine, Sendai, Japan
Yiotsas, Z., M.D., Evangelismos Medical Center, Athens, Greece
Zambouras, D. A., M.D., General State Hospital Agia Olga, II. Surgical Division, Athens, Greece

The Future of Proctology

J. F. Montague, New York, USA

It is claimed that the past often foretells the future and in consequence I shall dwell a few minutes upon the history of proctology as a specialty.

Specialism of all kinds has been induced by the recent truly tremendous expansion in knowledge, by the improvements in communications and in some degree by the unparalelled population explosion. Those of you who have been so fortunate to practice medicine over the last few decades are, I am sure, often uncomfortably aware of the difficulty as well as the necessity of keeping up with this great increase in knowledge and improvements of techniques in our specialty. Since there appears to be no likelihood of imminent abatement in this forward surge of knowledge, technique or population, it seems reasonable to assume that specialism will become an ever increasing necessity in matters dealing with medicine and surgery.

The great tendency throughout the world toward concentrated populations in ever expanding cities, also favors the development of specialism since it makes it economically possible for a doctor to confine his attention to one particular field of medicine. As an observer and active practitioner in the specialty of proctology for nearly half a century, it is my belief that the specialty has grown, not only because of the inexorable trend toward specialization in general, but to an even greater degree because the active workers in proctology have made it a more valuable area of medical practice, in so far as the public welfare is concerned. It is incumbent upon us to make it more worthy in the years to come.

It appears to me that this may be accomplished in the future by activities in certain areas. Continued studies in an effort to accurately define the bacterial flora existing in the colon and terminal bowel is certainly greatly to be desired. The role that intestinal flora play in both health and disease certainly should be a fertile field for investigation. Perhaps the most urgent feature of any investigation is to determine both the bacteriology and pathology involved in ulcerative colitis and ulcerative proctitis.

As a corollary to such an investigation, increased knowledge of the physiology of the colon and terminal bowel should be sought. There are still some defects in our knowledge of the mechanics of constipation prolapsus and Hirschsprung's disease. The intricacies of the neural apparatus of the colon and terminal bowel need clarification. A study of the lymphatics would be useful.

Finally, I do believe that in the future, the rectal and colonic mucosa will be to a fuller extent recognized and used as an avenue for medication of systemic disease. While this has been done to a limited degree for the production of general anesthesia by the use of Avertin and for the administration of some medicines, I personally feel that the great opportunities offered have been neglected, in consideration of the fact that by using the rectal avenue of medication, the stomach and the upper intestinal tract can be spared the disturbing effects of medication, it is hard to understand why the method is not more generally used.

To conclude the list of desirable areas of future expansion of proctology as a specialty, I add the following: principles of medical communication should, in my opinion, be one of the vital and potentially productive areas for our future endeavors.

During the past few decades, specialists in colonic and rectal surgery, by their competent activity, have amassed a huge fund of knowledge and skill in the understanding and successful treatment of diseases of the colon and rectum. This reservoir of knowledge can be made to redound to the benefit of all mankind if it is made available to the medical profession at large. This act would greatly increase the stature of the specialty and justify the esteem in which it is now held by medical personnel throughout the world.

A bell that is rung in a vacuum emits no sound; it is only when its vibrations are conducted by atmospheric waves that we can hear it ring. So, too, all knowledge must be disseminated to be effective. Such communication must be precise, well organized and expressed in understandable language.

Clinical observations require accurate reporting; clinical trials need competent interpretations; refined surgical techniques are worthy of study, testing and dispassionate evaluation. The mountain of data acquired in this truly scientific manner should be reported by presentation to local medical societies, to state societies and, of course, to proctologic societies. In the case of extended research, monographs should be forthcoming. From those, with long therm experience, textbooks will emanate – as they should. All this is legitimate, worthwhile medical communication, so obvious, perhaps, as to be taken for granted. Let it not be neglected! Nor should the practitioners of proctology overlook the fact that the general practitioner, the general surgeon and the lay public, too, need to be reminded constantly of the special skills which are the heritage of proctologists of today. Communicate!

In the not too distant past, the physician or surgeon who wrote articles for the medical journals or who, better still, wrote a textbook might have found himself the target of professional criticism. Even when such writings were directed to his professional colleagues, cynical and often sneering remarks were made as to the volume of writings. Thus, many capable and well-intentioned young men in the field of medicine were discouraged in their attempts to promote intelligent discussion of the problems which always exist in the clinical practice of medicine.

Still greater furor of criticism erupted when any physician attempted to write a book which sought to inform the laity concerning the nature of illness and the sensible method to pursue in obtaining proper care of ailments. These frenetic critics completely overlooked the fact that if ethical physicians neglected their duty as teachers of public health, the gaping need almost certainly would be filled by some charlatan with a facile pen. Who then, can reasonably question the value of dignified, competent and skillful communication in the field of medical affairs.

As one whom the passing of time and a kindly providence has made an elder of proctology, the spectacle of these great changes in medical thought prompts me to bring their great value to the attention of those presently active in the specialty

I have practiced for more than 50 years. It seems obvious that the worthy specialty that has been created can add much to the sum total of surgical knowledge and skill and that still brighter new chapters in proctology can be written.

Just as virtue is its own reward, so too is education. All medicine will benefit, and the specialty too. The reward will be a broader recognition and appreciation of the earnest endeavors and, at times, brilliant accomplishments of the earlier workers in surgery of the colon and rectum.

Let then the bell ring forth. Give proctology an atmosphere of scholarly expression through which to distribute the newer funds of knowledge and the lately acquired arts. Do so and earn the esteem of the noble profession of medicine and the gratitude of all mankind.

I. Injuries of the Colon and Rectum

Injuries of the Colon and Rectum

J. Hoferichter, Erlangen, Germany

The prognosis of intra-abdominal organ injuries is unfavourable [21], particularely injuries to the large intestine with a reported mortality rate of roughly 30% [14, 45] (Table 1).

Table 1. *Mortality from injuries of the colon*

	No. injured	† (%)
Tucker (1954)	42	14,3
Gremmel (1960)	12	58
Roof et al. (1961)	217	13
Patton (1961)	58	9
Reifferscheid* (1962)	1722	30
Razemon et al. (1966)	14	14

* Collected statistics.

This poor prognosis is largely due to the fact that even during operation, the extent of the injury is difficult to establish. The edges of the wound can be damaged by pressure or by disturbances in the blood circulation, resulting in a secondary necrosis of the intestinal wall. In addition, a coliperitonitis may take place and, in cases of retroperitoneal injuries, a possible gas gangrene [22].

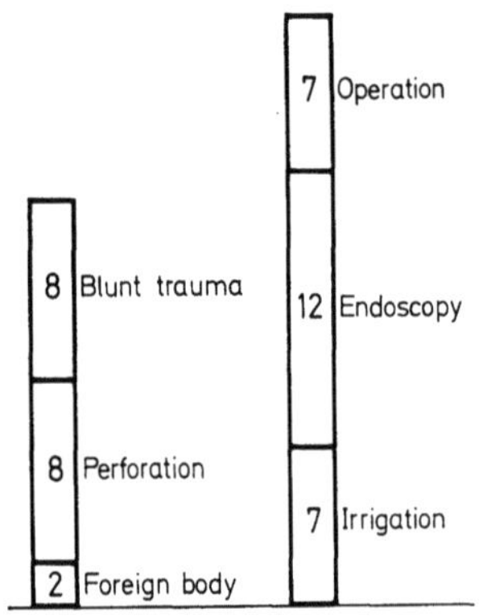

Fig. 1. Causes of 44 injuries to colon and rectum

For many surgeons, the poor results of surgical treatment are even today the reason why therapeutic principles are still adhered to which have long been abandoned in routine surgery of the colon. As a result of our own experience we cannot share this pessimism. We are rather of the opinion that civilian injuries to the colon – with few exceptions – can be treated by primary suture or resection without proximal colostomy.

Injuries to the large intestine are seldom met, with the exception of war injuries and those incurred in the slums of big cities. In the past 12 years, we encountered 44 cases of injury to the intestine. Of these, 8 were the result of blunt abdominal trauma and 36 the results of perforations due to foreign bodies or instruments (Fig. 1).

The colon occupies a large space within the abdominal cavity. Despite this fact, however, it is involved correspondingly often only in cases of open – perforated – injuries. Comprehensive collective statistics – dealing almost exclusively with war or civilian shot and stab wounds – show that in cases of open abdominal injuries, the large intestine is involved in almost 40% [45] (Table 2).

Table 2. *Frequency of injuries of the colon due to perforating abdominal trauma*

	Total Number of Injuries	Percentage of Colon Injuries %
Sec. aux. surg. Group* (1945)	3157	35,1
R. B. ALLEN et al. (1957)	67	19,5
REIFFERSCHEID* (1962)	3254	37,7

* Collected Statistics.

Blunt Injuries

The colon is largely protected from blunt injuries by the bony thorax and the pelvis. For this reason and despite the fact that it has a wide lumen, continuously filled with gas and excreta, a thin wall and that it is provided in part with a poor blood supply, the colon can be injured only with difficulty [21] (Table 3).

Table 3. *Frequency of injuries due to blunt abdominal trauma*

	Total Number of Injuries	Percentage of Colon Injuries %
SPATH (1955)	121	1,7
C. E. WELCH (1957)	200	5
R. B. ALLEN et al. (1967)	297	1,5
MARTIN (1960)	271	2,9
K. J. WELCH (1962)	181	0,6
HOFERICHTER (1967)	54	5

Of some practical significance is a division of injuries in accordance with the mode of occurrance; contused, ruptured and tear injuries [14]. Contused injuries manifest wide wall damage near the point of rupture and, for this reason, require extensive oversewing or resection.

Only three out of eight injuries resulting from a blunt trauma included a primary colon perforation. In the other cases, the colon was injured secondarily by the consequences of the contusion or by damage to the blood vessels. All patients were treated by oversewing or primary resection. Three deaths resulted from gangrene of the small intestine, necrosis of the pancreas and cardiac failure. They did not result directly from the injury to the colon.

The perforation of a hollow organ in the abdomen leads to peritonitis. Because of the contractions of the appropriate segment of the intestine, this develops relatively late however. This delays its discovery and worsens the prognosis. The evaluation of all the signs and symptoms may be effected only with reference to the indication for an operation. In most cases radiography is of no value. With the simultaneous rupture of the diaphragm, free air enters into the thorax. A negative X-ray finding must never be allowed to influence an indicated laparotomy [40].

These diagnostic difficulties are particularly great when the abdominal trauma is overshadowed by other injuries, such as injuries to the skull. In such a case, abdominal symptoms are recognized, if at all, only after the patient has recovered consciousness [21] (Fig. 2).

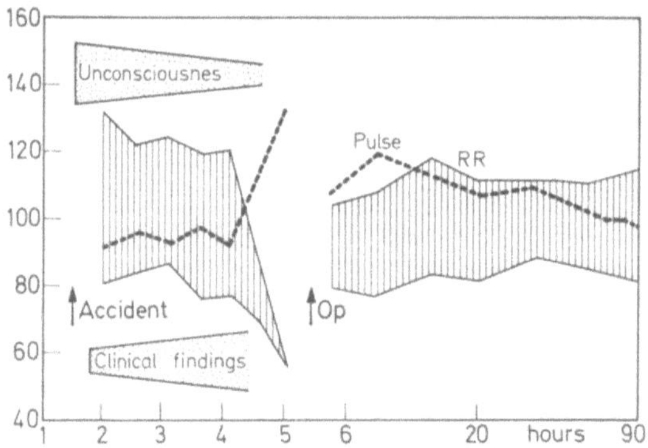

Fig. 2. Colon injury masked by head injury: abdominal symptoms appeared only after consciousness returned. Operation is often delayed for this reason

Also difficult to recognize are perforations of retroperitoneal sections of the intestine in which peritonitis does not develop until a very late stage, if at all [22, 57]. For this reason, the retroperitoneal sections of the colon must always be freely exposed, during laparotomy, if no intraperitoneal perforation is discovered [22].

Perforating Wounds

With the exception of war injuries – perforating injuries of the colon occur – in quantity only in certain areas such as the slums of large cities [25, 41, 43, 46]. We have seen only one shot wound of the caecum as well as two late stenoses.

Foreign Body Injury

The large intestine can also be injured by intraluminal foreign bodies [53]. A wide range of questionable literature exists on foreign bodies introduced via the rectum [11, 29, 31, 32, 42, 44, 56]. Generally their removal is easy on account of the usually relaxed tone of the anal sphincter, but perforations may also occur.

Swallowed objects may also lead to perforations of the large intestine. Such perforations usually occur gradually and are in general accompanied by abscesses. A rare but typical example is the perforation of a sigmoid diverticulum by a swallowed chicken bone [16]. The accompanying symptoms – as found by left side colon disease – are displaced to the right side and sometimes misinterpreted as an appendicitis [7, 50]. This is one more reason to examine thoroughly and carefully the entire intestine, after the removal of a non-infected appendix.

Impalement Injuries

In cases of impalement injuries, the extraperitoneal rectum and the anal closure mechanism are often also involved. The intestine can be injured from the outside or endoluminally. Each of the five cases of impalement was the result of an – usually agricultural – accident. In each case it was possible to carry out a primary reconstruction of the sphincter. Only in cases of an extensive subperitoneal disruption of the rectum is a proximal colostomy nowadays obligatory.

Intraperitoneal damage after impalement is extremely difficult to recognize [13]. This experience is more than 2.000 years old. The death penalty was carried out in China by impalement. In the Middle Ages, too, in Europe this form of execution was carried out to respectable persons in order to avoid visible signs of wounds. Edward II of England was murdered in this way in 1327 [9].

Instrumental Perforations

Today we are reminded of this unprofessional use of medical experience by the instrumental perforations caused in increasing number [55]. More than half of the injuries to colon and rectum observed by us were injured operatively during instrumental manipulations. This corresponds largely to the experience gained by others (Fig. 1). Particularly liable to injury is the large intestine of the new-born [8, 37, 40]. The wall is extremely thin and the distance of the peritoneal duplicature from the anus is less than 3 cm [8].

Surgical Injuries

During operations within the small pelvis or on the retroperitoneal organs, the colon can be unintentionally damaged.

As a result of the close proximity to the colon and to the female genital organs, approximately one incidental injury to the colon occurs in about 240 abdominal or 310 vaginal gynaecological interventions [12]. It is even more frequent in cases of tumour cystectomy in the male. We have seen four examples of such injuries but they also occurred following nephrectomy and hemicolectomy.

All these perforations were immediately seen and treated surgically. Only a single case of sigmoid perforation – which occurred in another hospital during the operation on a perforated appendix – remained undiscovered and led to peritonitis of the floor of the pelvis. This injury had to be treated secondarily. We were able to do without a proximal colostomy (Table 4).

Table 4. *Colon injuries due to instrumentation*

		Closure	Resection	Prox. Colostomy	Mortality
During Operation	7	6	1	1	—
Laparoscopy	2	1	—	—	1
Cystoscopy	3	3	—	1	1
Rectoscopy	7	5	1	1	2
Enema	3	2	1	1	1
Barium Enema	4	3	1	1	1
	26	Surgical Clinic of the University Erlangen-Nuremberg 1956–1968			

From these observations, certain consequences may be drawn for all abdominal operations in which there is danger of damage to the colon; the large intestine should be thoroughly cleaned before the operation in order to minimize the results of a possible injury.

Injuries During Endoscopy

The dangers associated with endoscopic examinations are known and can be gauged exactly. The percentage of complications is negligible when it is compared to the usefulness which we or our patients observe daily as the results of these examinations (Table 5).

Table 5. *Mortality of colon injuries*

Perforations due to Instrumentation	Injuries	Mortality %
HAMIT* (1955)	68	78
THORBJARNARSON (1962)	18	22
FONKALSRUD (1965)	10	30
Injuries due to Rectoscopy		
CROHN et al. (1936)	30	53
MENEGEAUX (1938)	12	58
ANDRESEN* (1947)	94	47
ANDRESEN (1947)	46	41
Injuries due to Contrast Medium		
ZHEUTLIN et al. (1952)	53	47

* Collected Statistics.

Proctoscopy

The frequency rate of damage to the colon during proctoscopy is estimated at 1:20,000 [13]. The diseased intestine is particularly vulnerable [13], but despite this fact the majority of perforations occurs in completely healthy sections of the intestine [1, 17].

This injury is usually discovered during the time of the examination [51]. If this is not the case, peritonitis of the pelvic floor develops. The mortality rate due to the results of the injury increases by more than 100% if surgical intervention is delayed more than 12 hours [1].

Of seven perforations observed during proctoscopy, five involved perfectly normal sections of the intestine. In two cases, the damage occurred in the vicinity of a malignant growth. These patients came to us at a late stage and expired later as a result of the original disease (Table 4).

As the intestine is always particularly thoroughly cleared before the examination, only slight contamination of the abdominal cavity with excretions occurred in the event of perforation [55]. For this reason, a proximal colostomy can always be dispensed with if the surgical treatment is performed in good time.

Cystoscopy – Laparoscopy

In laparoscopy and cystoscopy the injury to the wall occurs from the exterior. It involves an unprepared, excreta-filled intestine and the consequences are correspondingly more serious.

Of five cases, one was a moribund, 71-years-old woman who came to us 14 days after the perforation with a faecal peritonitis. She died half an hour after admission without being operated on. In another case, in which the injury had been incurred 16 days previously, a diagnosis of peritonitis of the pelvic floor was made. This patient survived (Table 4).

Thermometer Injuries

Injury to the subperitoneal section of the rectum can also be effected by means of a glass thermometer introduced rectally [15]. This type of injury is particularly common in small children. In the majority of cases, there is no perforation but merely bleeding from a laceration of the wall.

Injuries Incurred During Enemas

The most frequent cause of iatrogenic injuries to the colon and rectum are manipulations carried out during irrigations. The perforation is usually caused by the tip of the intestinal tube introduced through the rectum. This was the case in all the injuries observed by us.

Rupture as a result of the pressure of the enema probably occurs only in a diseased intestine. The normal colon withstands an internal pressure of 500 to 600 mmHg (mercury) [18]. However, in individual cases, colon rupture has also been observed to occur under low pressures [4, 26]. The pressure required to cause a rupture is lower in senile persons than in juveniles [4]. By way of illustration, the defecation pressure is as high as 200 mmHg. With temporary colonic spasm a pressure of up to 170 mmHg has been measured in the colon [2]. However, when enemas are administered, the intraluminal pressure averages no more than some 22 mmHg (38]. Consequently, the pressure associated with enemas can hardly lead to injuries.

The pressure required for rupture, increases – in accordance with La Place's law – continuously with the diminution of the lumen from the caecum to the rectum, provided that the iliocaecal valve is funktioning properly [47, 51].

Bursting ruptures – like the diastatic ruptures of the colon or the so-called spontaneous ruptures [48] – are due to the wide lumen and the thin wall, which is found almost exclusively in the caecum or in the ascending part of the colon. In every case, however, a weakness or disease of the intestinal wall can be demonstrated [48]. Bursting of deeper sections of the colon is only possible when accompanied by a circumscribed weakness in the wall. A typical contributory factor is a previous biopsy of the intestinal wall.

Spontaneous perforations during defecation are probably just as rare as those after minimal traumas [20, 27, 36, 53]. The introduction of foreign bodies in such cases is naturally not disclosed by the patient.

In extremely rare cases a rupture of the colon is possible even when unaccompanied by organic damage to the wall. Thus, for example, rupture preceded by ischaemic necrosis of the wall can occur as a result of an overextension of colon sections through blockade of the ganglia in the Ogilvie syndrome, or after the use of ganglionic blocking agents [39]. Of interest is the recently reported rupture of the colon after the implantation of a cardiac pacemaker [24].

As a rule, perforations made by instruments are discovered during the examination itself. If this is not the case, the discovery of the consequences is very difficult.

From the linea dentata there is no sensitivity in the mucosa of the rectum. For this reason the majority of these injuries occur without any accompanying pain. This is particularly true for children and old people, but also for perforations which go through a colostoma. On account of the lack of symptoms, it is often difficult to convince the patient of the necessity of a laparotomy.

Complications of the Barium Enema

Owing to the toxicity of the dissolved substances in the enema solution, additional damage can occur [19, 51, 61]. The significance and consequences of this typical complication in contrast medium examinations are still being debated, although it can be reckoned with once in every 5,000 examinations [28]. Ever since we have taken, as a matter of principle, to supervising the introduction of the intestinal tube and the contrast medium by means of image-intensifier television, we have seen no more injuries of this nature.

Intraperitoneal barium causes peritonitis with massive adhesions. This contamination of the abdominal cavity with barium and excreta together, is considered to be particularly deleterious [6]. The toxicity of barium, however, seems to be low as contrast medium incapable of being removed at the operation can be shown to be present for weeks or months without further consequences for the patient.

The tannic acid contained in the contrast media has a particularly toxic effect [30, 35]. For this reason, no tannic acid-containing contrast media have been made or used in Germany for a number of years.

Serious local consequences are associated with the intramural spreading after injury to the mucosa alone [51, 52]. Here, the rectum usually cannot be saved. Fatal systemic consequences are associated with the penetration of the contrast medium into the submucous veins [51].

Colostomy Perforations

Perforations as a result of manipulations to the colostoma have a particularly poor prognosis. These occur especially when the section of the intestine leading to the opening is fixed by a short mesenterium, an incisional hernia, the recurrence of a tumor or a peritoneal carcinosis.

As a rule, it is the advanced basic disease (carcinosis) which proves to be fatal. The majority of the reported perforations in anus praeter ended with the death of the patient [51]. We have confirmed these findings.

Posttraumatic Stenosis

Subsequent to a primary injury of the colon wall not involving a perforation, there develops in the course of a number of years or even decades, a cicatricial stenosis originating from shrinking processes in the scar tissue [34]. These typical effects of splinter wounds contracted during the last war are now manifesting themselves – 25 years later – in the clinical picture of a recurrent subileus.

In the case of small splinters, a carcinoma cannot be excluded with certainty by radiography or even at operation (Fig. 3). The diagnosis can be made only after thorough examination of the resected sample.

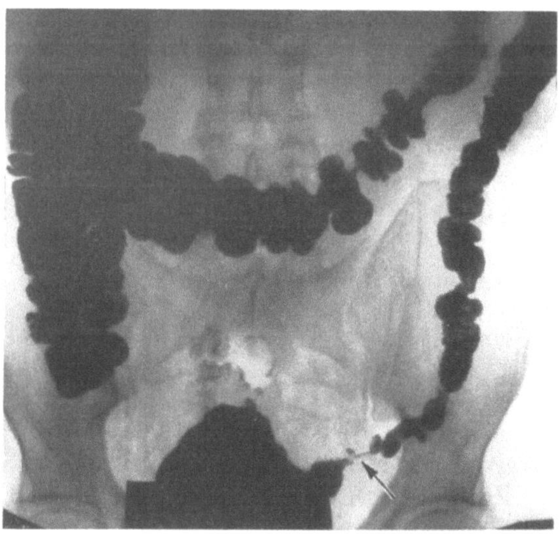

Fig. 3. Cicatricing stenosis of the colon simultating a colon carcinoma 20 years after injury through a metal sliver

Therapy

Injuries of the colon can heal spontaneously [10, 58]. In numerous animals, this is the rule rather than exception. Carps survive the bites of a heron by developing an anus praeter [60]. As a rule, however, a coliperitonitis develops, which, leads to death if left untreated. In the case of retroperitoneal injuries, there is the additional danger of gas gangrene.

For this reason, an operation is indicated whenever an injury to the colon is demonstrated or suspected. The surgical technique of the intervention is, however, still a matter for discussion. Injuries of the colon often represent, for the physician, an individual, dramatic event [3]. For this reason, we must have recourse to the experiences of others. Here it can be seen that with colon injuries the operation technique introduced by Mikulicz in 1903 and improved by Rankin in 1930 is still recommended today as the "Fastest intervention" [59]. The primary suture is however, secured by the abdominal wall or a proximal colostomy [23, 25, 54, 59].

This procedure has proved itself in two world wars as well as in Korea and Vietnam. Civilian injuries have, in comparison, considerably less extensive contusions of the soft parts [43], are seldom multiple and are treated operatively at an earlier stage. For this reason, it seems justified to extend the considerations applying to general surgery of the colon to include the injuries as well [13, 33].

General measures such as nasogastric tube, urethral catheter, infusion- and drug-therapy, tetanus prophylaxis, and at least in the case of retroperitoneal injuries, gas gangrene prophylaxis need no further comments [46].

A rupture of the colon unaccompanied by demonstrable damage to the neighbouring wall sections or to the blood vessels is oversewn without proximal colostomy [33]. Extensive injuries, with wide contused edges and simultaneous damage to the mesenteric vessels make a primary resection compulsory. Proximal leading-off of the faeces on principle can be considered only in cases of extensive subperitoneal injury to the rectum [58].

Only in the case of an extremely poor general condition [49], extensive trauma with multiple intraabdominal organ or colon damage [41, 49] as well as in the case of considerable delay in the surgical treatment should the following considerations [25] – especially when the surgeon is inexperienced – be taken into account:

in connection with the transverse colon and the sigmoid flexure, the presentation after Mikulicz,

in connection with the right flexure and the left colon, oversewing and proximal colostomy,

in connection with the right colon, the securing of the suture by a drain colostomy or ileotransversostomy [5].

Results

In the last 12 years we have treated 44 cases of injury to the colon using this consideration as a basis. During this period we have lost only three patients as a result of the effects of the colon injury itself. One of these patients was admitted in a moribund state with faecal peritonitis and died without being operated on. Five other patients died of injuries to other organs or from the original disease (Table 6).

Table 6. *Operative therapy in 44 colon injuries*

		Mortality due to Colon Injuries	Other Diseases or Injuries	
Not operated	2	1	1	Cardiac Arrest
Exteriorization	1		1	Carcinosis
Prim. Closure	25	1		
Resection	7	1	2	Gangrene of the Small Intest. Tumor Cachexia
Prim. Closure + Prox. Colostomy	9		1	Necrosis of the Pancreas
	44	3	5	

Surgical Clinic of the University Erlangen-Nuremberg 1956–1968.

The treatment of choice in colon injuries is therefore in accordance with the principles of colon surgery applicable today. These are primary oversewing or resection without proximal colostomy and thus the avoidance of unnecessary and, in the case of the colon, dangerous follow-up operations.

In this way, the dangers connected with civilian injuries to the colon which were at one time considerable, can be reduced to a minimum.

Bibliography

1. Andersen, A. F. R.: Perforations from Proctoscopy. Gastroenterology **9**, 32 (1947).
2. Best, C. H., and N. B. Taylor: Physiological Main of Medical Practica. Baltimore: Edison Williams & Wilkins Co. 1945.
3. Blaha, H.: Dickdarmperforationen. Chirurg **36**, 267 (1965).
4. Burt, C. A. V.: Pneumatic Rupture of Intestinal Canal. Arch. Surg. **22**, 875 (1931).
5. Byrne, J. J.: Advances in Diagnosis and Treatment of the Acute Abdomen. Surg. Clin. N. Amer. **39**, 1357 (1959).
6. Cochran, D. Q., C. H. Almond, and W. A. Shucart: An Experimental Study of the Effects of Barium and Intestinal Contents in the Peritoneal Cavity. Amer. J. Roentgenol. **89**, 883 (1963).
7. Fischer, A. W.: Fremdkörper und Parasiten des Darmkanals. Handbuch der praktischen Chirurgie, Band 3, 6. Auflage, Stuttgart 1929.
8. Fonkalsrud, E. W., and H. W. Clatworthy, Jr.: Accidental Perforation of the Colon and Rectum in Newborn Infants. New Engl. J. Med. **272**, 1097 (1965).
9. Furste, W., and H. Knoernschild: Perforations of the Distal Large Intestine Produced by Intraluminal Traumas. Amer. J. Surg. **99**, 665 (1960).
10. Gencic, M., and V. Glidzic: Traumatic Lesions of the Rectum. Lyon chir. **62**, 676 (1966).
11. Gillespie, W. F.: A Vaseline Bottle in the Rectum. Canad. med. Ass. J. **31**, 302 (1934).
12. Given, F. T., Jr., L. Old, Jr., and W. L. Lehew: Colon and Rectal Injuries in Gynecological Surgery. Virginia med. Mth. **93**, 320 (1966).
13. Goligher, J. C.: Injuries of the Rectum and Colon. Surgery of the Anus, Rectum and Colon. London: Cassell 1961.
14. Gremmel, H., und R. M. Konrad: Die Dickdarmperforationen. Zbl. Chir. **85**, 581 (1960).
15. Gumrich, H.: Mastdarmverletzungen durch Thermometer. Med. Welt **2**, 140 (1968).
16. Gunn, A.: Intestinal Perforation Due to Swallowed Fish or Meat Bone. Lancet **1**, 125 (1966).
17. Haas, P.: Die Komplikationen der Proktoskopie. Zbl. Chir. **92**, 2608 (1967).

18. HAMIT, H. F.: Perforation of the Colon After Barium Enema and Air Contrast Studies. Amer. Surg. **21**, 1226 (1955).
19. HARTMANN, A. W., and W. J. HILLS: Rupture of Colon in Infants During Barium Enema. Ann. Surg. **145**, 712 (1957).
20. HILL, M. C., W. P. BIEBER, R. L. KOCH, and W. COULSON: Extraperitoneal Perforations of the Gastrointestinal Tract. Amer. J. Roentgenol. **101**, 315 (1967).
21. HOFERICHTER, J.: Praktische Probleme beim Abdominaltrauma. Bruns' Beitr. klin. Chir. **214**, 58 (1967).
22. — Diagnostische Probleme bei retroperitonealen Darmrupturen. Münch. med. Wschr. **109**, 346 (1967).
23. HOLLE, F.: Stumpfe Bauchverletzungen. Med. Klinik **58**, 293 (1963).
24. HOLLINGS, R. M.: Spontaneous Perforation of the Caecum and a Cardiac Pacemaker. Aust. N. Z. J. Surg. **35**, 136 (1965).
25. ISAACSON, J. E., JR., R. L. BUCK, and H. R. KAHLE: Changing Concepts of Treatment of Traumatic Injuries of the Colon. Dis. Colon & Rectum **4**, 168 (1961).
26. KLEINSASSER, L. J., and H. WARSHAW: Perforation of Sigmoid Colon During Barium Enema. Ann. Surg. **135**, 560 (1952).
27. LAWLER, R. H.: Acute Perforation of Abdominal Viscus. Proc. Hedrologicum Conlegium, Tokyo 1965.
28. LORINC, P., and F. BRAHAME: Perforation of the Colon During Examination by the Double Contrast Method. Gastroenterology **37**, 770 (1959).
29. LOWICKI, E. M.: Accidental Introduction of Giant Foreign Body into the Rectum. Ann. Surg. **163**, 395 (1966).
30. LUCKE, H. H., K. E. HODGE, and N. L. PATT: Fatal Liver Damage After Barium Enemas Containing Tannic Acid. Canad. med. Ass. J. **89**, 1111 (1963).
31. MACHT, S. H.: Foreign Body in Rectum. Radiology **42**, 500 (1944).
32. MAC LEOD, F. H.: Removal of Foreign Bodies in Rectum. Canad. med. Ass. J. **57**, 488 (1947).
33. MADDEN, J. L.: Treatment of Perforated Lesions of the Colon by Primary Resection and Anastomosis. Dis. Colon & Rectum **9**, 413 (1966).
34. MAYS, E. T., and R. J. NOER: Colonic Stenosis After Trauma. J. Trauma **6**, 316 (1966).
35. MC ALLISTER, W. H., M. S. ANDERSON, G. R. BLOOMBERG, and A. R. MARGULES: Lethal Effects of Tannic Acid in the BARIUM Enema. Radiology **80**, 765 (1963).
36. MINKARI, T., and C. TURAN: Rectosigmoidal Rupture Caused by Effort During Defecation and Acute Evisceration of Several Loops of the Small Intestine Through the Anus. Ann. Surg. **154**, 967 (1961).
37. MOTHES, W., u. W. CH. HECKER: Iatrogene Perforationen im Verdauungstrakt bei Kindern. Münch. med. Wschr. **109**, 643 (1967).
38. NOVEROSKE, R.: Intracolonic Pressures Durang Barium Enema Examination. Amer. J. Roentgenol. **91**, 852 (1964).
39. OGILVIE, H.: Large-intestine Colic Due to Sympathetic Deprivation, New Clinical Syndrome. Brit. med. J. **2**, 671 (1948).
40. PARKER, J. J., and V. G. MIKITY: Radiographic Diagnosis of Intestinal Perforation in Early Infancy. Calif. Med. **104**, 35 (1966).
41. PATTON, T. B., and C. LYONS: The Treatment of Traumatic Injuries of the Colon. J. Trauma **1**, 298 (1961).
42. PRETTY, H. G.: An Ink Bottle in the Rectum. Canad. med. Ass. J. **31**, 302 (1934).
43. RAZEMON, P., C. GAUTIER, and J. DHAINAUT: Results of Treatment of Wounds of the Colon. Lille chir. **21**, 189 (1966).
44. REBELL, F. G.: The Problem of Foreign Bodies in the Colon and Rectum. Amer. J. Surg. **76**, 678 (1948).
45. REIFFERSCHEID, M.: Die allgemeinen traumatischen Verletzungen von Kolon und Rektum. Darmchirurgie. Stuttgart: Thieme-Verlag 1962.
46. ROOF, W. R., G. C. MORRIS, JR., and M. E. DEBAKEY: Management of Civilian Colon Injuries. Dis. Colon & Rectum **4**, 115 (1961).
47. ROSI, P. A., M. E. LICHTENSTEIN, L. S. TARLOW, and C. PORTES: Panel Discussion on the Colon. Amer. J. Gastroent. **40**, 41 (1963).

48. Rühl, R.: Zur Pathogenese der diastatischen Colonperforation. Chirurg. **37**, 368 (1966).
49. Sanders, R. J.: The Management of Colon Injuries. Surg. Clin. N. Amer. **43**, 457 (1963).
50. Schröder, K.: Zökumperforation durch einen Fremdkörper unter Appendizitis-Symptomatologie. Zbl. Chir. **93**, 626 (1968).
51. Seaman, W. B., and J. Wells: Complications of the Barium Enema. Gastroenterology **48**, 728 (1965).
52. Sector, G. W., and N. Susman: The Roentgen Recognition of Intramural Perforation Following Barium Enema Examination in Obstructing Lesions of the Sigmoid. Amer. J. Roentgenol. **89**, 776 (1963).
53. Seling, A.: Klinik der Rektumfremdkörper. Chir. Praxis **11**, 239 (1967).
54. Stucke, K.: Stumpfe Bauchtraumen. Med. Klinik **58**, 620 (1963).
55. Thorbjarnarson, B.: Iatrogenic and Related Perforations of the Large Bowel. Arch. Surg. **84**, 608 (1962).
56. Tsuji, K., and I. Tsuji: A Case of Foreign Bodies in Rectum. Proc. Hedrologicum Conlegium, Tokyo (1965).
57. Voigtlaender, H.: Berstung des Rectosigmoids durch stumpfe Gewalt. Mschr. Unfallhk. **67**, 347 (1964).
58. Weckesser, E. C., and T. C. Putman: Perforating Injuries of the Rectum and Sigmoid Colon. J. Trauma **2**, 474 (1962).
59. Williams, R. D., and A. A. Yurko: Controversial Aspects of Diagnosis and Management of Blunt Abdominal Trauma. Amer. J. Surg. **111**, 477 (1966).
60. Wunder, W.: Darmoperationen beim Karpfen. Z. ges. exp. Med. **141**, 219 (1966).
61. Zheutlin, N., E. C. Lasser, and L. G. Rigler: Clinical Studies on Effect of Barium in the Peritoneal Cavity Following Rupture of the Colon. Surgery **32**, 967 (1952).

Complications of Proctoscopy and Irrigoscopy

P. A. HAAS, Budapest, Hungary

One of the most tragic experiences in medical practice is the case where dangerous and perhaps fatal injuries arise from an examination. Fortunately, injuries resulting from proctoscopy and contrast enema are rare, but not as rare as the literature would seem to indicate. Circulars sent to reputable surgeons as well as our own practice revealed 43 cases of injuries from proctoscopy, and 3 from contrast enemas. Complications such as perianal thrombosis, fissure in ano etc. which are unpleasant but not dangerous for the patient are excluded. We distinguish 4 groups of injuries:

1. Perforation into the abdominal cavity,
2. Retro- or subperitoneal perforation,
3. Hemorrhage which does not stop by itself,
4. Extreme meteorism.

Predisposing factors for these injuries are cancer, ulcerative colitis, irregular curvatures of the rectum, adhesions in the pelvis as a result of inflammation. However, 13 out of 46 cases happened to patients with normal intestines. This points to the real cause of the complications, i. e. technical faults in examination. In 16 cases, complications were caused by wrongly performed biopsy, in some instances, by insufflation of air after biopsy, in one case by the too rapid inflow of barium enema. In the remaining cases the rough insertion of a proctoscope or an enema tube was responsible for the injury.

The greatest danger of perforation into the abdominal cavity is rapidly developing peritonitis. Out of 14 patients who underwent surgery within an hour, 4 died of peritonitis.

The most characteristic sign of retro- or subperitoneal perforation is retroperitoneal emphysema followed by a phlegmon. Hemorrhage is not a rare complication either and it may lead to serious consequences. As a rule, extreme meteorism is not dangerous in itself but the perforation of a remote part of the colon may occur.

In some cases, the injury can be recognized during the examination: fissures can be observed through the proctoscope or the serosa of the intestines appears. In all the three cases of injury caused by contrast enema, the radiologist recognized the injury immediately because the barium flowed out of the bowels. Yet, it is sometimes difficult to establish a diagnosis because at times pain is not felt until several hours after the examination. Thus, in 25 percent of the cases, patients underwent surgery more than 12 hours after the examination. Further proctoscopy for the sake of diagnosis is not recommended because the instrument used and the insufflation of air may increase both injury and infection. If a patient complains of abdominal pains, after proctoscopy, an x-ray examination of the abdomen must be performed in two planes without delay because this may reveal air under the diaphragm or retroperitoneal emphysema.

While some still adhere to conservative therapy, we do not recommend it. In the case of perforation into the abdominal cavity, laparotomy must be performed immediately. It is correct to apply sutures, if that is possible. In the case of tumor perforation, the tumor must be removed in the simplest possible way. If the suture of the opening is uncertain, a colostomy ought to be performed. But even in the case of successful suture, it is advisable to indroduce a tube through the anus above the site of the injury, to fix it to the skin, and to leave it there for 8 to 10 days.

Laparatomy is also advisable for handling cases of retroperitoneal injury. In cases of subperitoneal injury, the abscess arising around the area must be opened from the perineum. In cases of hemorrhage, if bleeding cannot be stopped by electrocoagulation or suture, it is advisable to perform a ligation of the two hypogastric arteries.

The prevention of injuries is extremely important. The proctoscope must be advanced delicately and under constant visual observation. Air must be used sparingly but the tube must be led into the open lumen only under visual control. Examination must be postponed if the patient is restless, the rectum is not clean or technical difficulties arise. We must not force the tube beyond a tumor. Biopsy must be the final phase of the examination and no air should be insufflated thereafter.

Injuries from barium contrast enema usually occur when there is a lack of cooperation between the doctor and aged, incontinent patients. A method for facilitating contrast enema has been elaborated by us. Under sterile conditions, in the operating room, in local anesthesia, we sew a tube into the anus with a double pursestring suture (Fig. 1, 2). After the examination, the tube is removed while the anesthesia is still effective. With proper technique, this procedure is entirely painless. The doctor himself introduces the tube under good lighting conditions

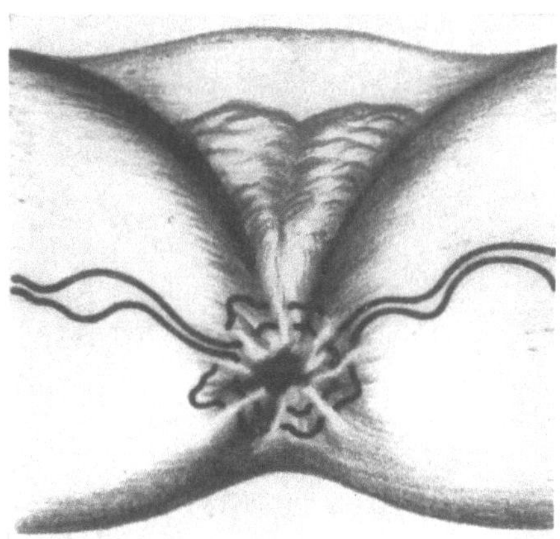

Fig. 1

The possibility of injury is thus eliminated. The examination itself is made easier: the attention of the radiologist is not distracted by the behavior of the patient, the colon can be filled centimeter by centimeter, while the rectum itself can be thoroughly examined. We have carried out irrigoscopic examinations with this procedure in hundreds of cases without complication, and on the part of the patient, the examination was not nearly as unpleasant, aside from the first slight prick of the needle, as irrigoscopy is usually carried out either with a tube or balloon catheter.

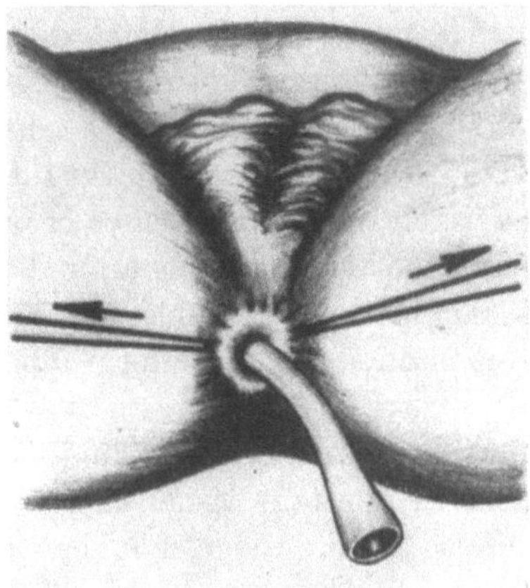

Fig. 2

Bibliography

ANDRESEN, A. F. R.: Gastroenterology **9**, 32 (1947).
BORGSTRÖM, S.: Acta chir. Scand. **104**, 465 (1953).
HAAS, P., and L. BARNA: Magy. Radiol. **11**, 173 (1967).
— Zbl. Chir. **92**, 2608 (1967).
NATHAN, M. H., and R. COHEN: Amer. J. Roentgenol. **84**, 1121 (1960).
NOVEROSKE, R. J.: Amer. J. Roentgenol. **96**, 326 (1966).

Barium Peritonitis

H. Dittrich, Erlangen, Germany

A radio-opaque enema with barium sulfate which perforates the colon and flows into the abdominal cavity leads to the death of the patient in 53 % of cases. This percentage was found in a total of 83 cases in the literature and 3 patients who where operated upon for the ominous results of this lesion in the Chirurgische Universitätsklinik Erlangen.

According to Loring, the frequency of this complication is 2 per 10,000 barium enemas. It seems very probable that only a small number of these cases is published (Seaman). The literature contains only a few isolated cases, but Zheutlin et al. were able to collect 53 cases through questionnaires sent to over 100 large radiology centres in the United States. The chief application of the barium enema is the radiologic diagnosis of colon diseases. It is used relatively rarely as a therapeutic measure for restoring colon invaginations, the so-called hydrostatic method of deinvagination (Nordentoft, Juillard).

The main causes of perforation (amplified by Zheutlin) are:

1. injury by the tip of the intestinal tube (Seaman)
2. injury by previous instrumentation e. g. proctosigmoidoscopy biopsy (Thorbjarnarson, Farger, Hemley, Kaucky and Beck)
3. injury by a previous cleansing enema
4. intestinal diseases
a) carcinoma (Scheidt, Zheutlin)
b) ulcerative colitis (Isaacs, Nissen)
c) diverticulitis (Kleinsasser, Le Roy)
d) fissures
e) invagination, volvulus
f) perforated appendicitis
g) mesenteric thrombosis
h) neonatal malformations of the rectum in new-borns (Mothes and Hecker, Standard)
5. increased hydrostatic pressure during the enema (Burt Seaman)
6. short mesentery in cases of colostomy (Davis, Grillo, Zheutlin).

The most frequent cause is the direct injury by a straight, inflexible rectal tube at the level of the peritoneal fold, 6–13 cm from the anal ring. Just as frequent is the perforation in the case of a colostomy with a short mesentery at the site of the stoma. A further partial cause in these direct perforations especially in cases where the intestinal wall is damaged, is the increased pressure of the enema.

BURT determined the bursting pressure in 87 intestinal segments and found that no intestinal wall could withstand a pressure over 318 mmHg. The amount of variation was very wide. The lowest perforation pressure was 50 mmHg. According to LORING the lowest perforation pressure is 21 mmHg. The data reported by DECARLO which coincides with that of BURT indicates that the converted critical pressure at the tip of the rectal tube is 246–285 g/cm². A pressure of 100 g/cm² at the tip of the intestinal tube is attained when 300 g of barium are suspended in 1 liter of water and the irrigation is carried out from a height of about 1 meter. Under these conditions perforation is avoidable.

Our 3 cases of barium enema perforations were due to the following causes:

1. 56-year-old man, abdominal sacral rectum amputation, postoperative ileus. Several enemas through the colostomy. Barium enema because of increasing abdominal complaints. During this procedure sudden severe pain, extravasation of barium into the abdominal cavity. Immediate laparotomy. Oversewing of penny-sized perforation at the flexure of the colon.

2. 3-year-old boy. Attempt to carry out a deinvagination of the descending colon through a barium enema. Perforation of the invagination because bursting pressure is attained. Referral to our clinic 3 hours later, immediate operation: resection of the splenic flexure of the colon, end-to-end anastomosis.

3. 52-year-old man, barium enema in order to exclude colon disease. Perforation by the rectal tube at a level of 8–13 cm. Immediate operation. Oversewing at the site of perforation.

At laparotomy all patients revealed severe encrusting of the visceral and parietal peritoneum by contrast medium. Larger particles could not be removed without injuring the serous membrane. The finer granules (about 0.3 mm in diameter) could not be completely removed. All three patients survived this complication. The first patient had several more subileus states. However, they could all be ameliorated by conservative means.

We believe that the decisive factor for survival after the operation in our patients was the brief time span between perforation and operation. This is in agreement with the literature which reports the best results with operative treatment within the first 3 hours (ZHEUTLIN). In cases of prolonged peritonitis, the abdominal cavity is rapidly contaminated and the barium suspension which irritates the peritoneum very intensely rapidly leads to an infectious, adhesive peritonitis. Death usually ensues on the third day. ISAACS and NISSEN found liver abscesses as well.

A special complication which was probably the cause of death was described in 5 of the 86 cases in the literature. At autopsy there was massive capillary pulmonary embolization (THREUMNER, ROMAN, ROSENBERG, ISAACS, GEIPEL). Factors which favor this mechanism are the injury to the submucous veins, the aspiration of the venous plexus and the presence of intraluminal pressure (THREUMNER). We have attempted to investigate these conditions in animal experiments. Instillations of 130 ml of barium suspension per 10 g into the abdominal cavity did not lead to demonstrable emboli. The same quantity of barium following a perforation of the rectum at a level of 8 cm led to slight, disseminated capillary embolization. If the colon burst under a pressure of 600 mmHg there is massive embolization in the lung which probably leads to death due to right heart failure.

II. Anal Fistulas

A Pictorial History of Surgical Treatment of "Fistula in Ano"

G. B. E. SIMONETTI, Milano, Italy

The history of Hedrology[1] coincides with the history of human civilization. The "fistula in ano" is one of the diseases which have affected mankind of all times; its description, expressed more or less clearly in the various periods, and its treatments (ligatures, incision, incision with previous ligature, two times incision, excision, actual and potential cautery), are elements constantly recurring in all texts of pathology which have reached us.

Egypt

IRJ's stele, discovered in 1926, records a court hedrologist who lived 2500 years before Christ. The treatment at that time was both surgical (as it is proved by the discovery of tools for incision) and medical. The Chester Beatty papyrus no. 6 (1200 B. C.) of the British Museum, which is considered to be a copy of far more ancient papyri, is a manual of practical Hedrology of the "shepherd of the anus" (phwjt), a figure of a specialist which will continue for centuries till the Alexandrine period, and even further.

India

SUSRUTA (4th Century B. C.?–1st Century A. D.?). This author relates the medical knowledge transmitted in inheritance from teacher to pupil, whose principles go back as far as the origin of Indian civilization (30th–40th Century B. C.?); he very well illustrates and deals with the various kinds of fistulas and their treatment by means of incision followed by cauterization. Special tools are used. Excision is condemned.

Greece

During HIPPOCRATES's time (460–365 B. C.) Hedrology is highly honoured: the treaty "De Fistulis"[2] has always presented great difficulties for the translators of

[1] Hedrology: neologism suggested by the Author and composed from the Greek words ἕδϱη (terminal bowel) and ϰόγοϱ (speech). I am indebted to Professor A. PAREDI PREFETTO of the Biblioteca Ambrisiana of Milano for his advice.

[2] 'Ιπποϰότουϱ πεϱί συϱίγγων.

all times, who have translated it in ways sometimes contradictory and even incomprehensible. I have made a personal study of the interpretation of the various treatments described in the text in an ionic dialect, printed by ALDO MANUZIO (1525), as well as in some other manuscripts. Abscesses and tubercles must be incised precociously. Non-communicating fistulae (sinus) must be incised, following a probe as a guide, and then cauterized by means of a dilution of copper flowers. Such cauterization alone, is carried out in deep third degree sinuses by means of injection with a bladder.

Some fistulae, which I assume can be identified with the tubercular ones, are treated by flax gauze imbibed with copper flowers dilution, introduced into the canal through the ulcerated internal opening visualized by means of a speculum (*Κατοπτήϱ*).

The ligature is applied with a flax thread interwoven with horse hair. Both the constriction and the separation are obtained by pulling and twisting the knot daily, without undoing it, over one week. A copper flowers cauterization follows.

MEGES (c. 20 B. C.), the last of the famous medical men of the isle of Cos, incised the fistula which reaches cartilage and bone (pilonidal sinus?). The ligature is obtained by means of a slip-knot and is extended to the sinus by introducing a thin rope with a gimlet or a pointed eye – tipped probe. This technique is not described in the Hippocratic collection but I believe that it was also used in that period, 3 or 4 centuries before, by the fact that a pointed-eye tipped probe existed among the tools of the Hippocratic period (Meyer-Steineg collection).

Greco-Roman Period

CELSUS (25 B. C.–50? A. D.) in his outstanding description which we can read in the Princeps edition (Florence 1478) performed the ligature after having accomplished a total excision of the superfical plane and the only incision which is interrupted in its central part is performed by following a probe. According to another interpretation, the excision should be made by means of two parallel cuts between which some small threads (linamenta) are placed in order to avoid bridge formation during the cicatrization.

The modern fistulotomy in 2 stages and fistulectomy are repetitions of CELSUS's treatment.

HELIODORUS (c. 1st Century A. D.) and ANTYLLOS (c. 150 A. D.) in Rome performed the incision by following a flat probe. The probe was introduced into the whole fistula, pulled out through the anal canal with the aid of the finger, and then turned downwards. In this way the incision of the shortest sphincteric segment is obtained, to reduce the danger of the loss of control. For a very deep fistula, a preliminary incision is performed in the most internal tract with a syringotome and then the operation is continued as described above. The sinuses with an internal orifice are pulled out by means of a hook and excised. The similarity to some modern techniques is evident.

GALEN (130–200 A. D.) treated fistulas with drainage and chemical cauterization.

LEONIDAS of Alexandria (c. 200 A. D.) and AETIOS of Amida (502–575 A. D.) performed the incision after previous ligature and pulling with a folded probe.

PAUL of Aegina (625–690 A. D.) used a bent bistoury and left the Hippocratic ligature for fearful patients.

Arabia

ABULCASIS (936–1010? A. D.) used cautery selected according to the size of the sinus, and he also incised the fistulas with the "spinaeformis scalpellus". He discouraged the treatment of deepest fistulas.

Europe

Salerno School. ROGER of Palermo (c. 1170) and ROLAND of Parma (c. 1250) preferred chemical cauterization (unguentum ruptorium) and sometimes used the ligature.

LANFRANCHI of Milan († 1306) who gave new strength to the Surgical Schools of Lyon and Paris, improved the Arab technique of cauterization.

Bologna School. This School is of fundamental importance in the XIII and XIV centuries for the progress of modern techniques. Outstanding are WILLIAM of Saliceto (1210–1277), HUGO BORGOGNONI of Lucca and his pupil THEODORIC of Cervia (1205-1298) and BRUNUS of Longoburgo (c. 1252).

To these two latter authors, well known as precursors of asepsis and anesthesia, we owe, the observation of the "fori prope anum" (anal crypts) which may cause apostemata and fistulas as a result of inflammation. This was stated four centuries before MORGAGNI! The method suggested is the incision with a curved bistoury with previous ligature of the parts to be incised, followed by excision of the callosities. With MONDINO DE LIUZZI (c. 1276–1326) most famous anatomist, BERTUCCIUS (Alberti) († 1347), teacher of GUY DE CHAULIAC (1300–1368), head of the French surgical school – who adopted the incision alone without excision –, and then with *Pietro of Argellata* († 1423) the comparative studies of syringo-therapy show a trend favourable to incision with previous ligature and pulling.

JOHN ARDERNE (1307–1390) in England performed the incision after the ligature and pulling of the fistula by means of special tools.

LEONARDO DA VINCI (1452–1519) studied sphincteric function (Fig. 1).

AMBROISE PARÉ (1517–1590) in France performed the classic ligature and incision. For sinuses, the ligature is performed by the introduction of a small metal tube and a sharp needle through the tube.

Padua School. PIETRO of Abano (1250–1316) used only potential cauterization. ANDREAS DELLA CROCE (1509–1575) used special curved syringotomes. This technique was improved by FABRICIUS of Acquapendente (1537–1619) who is in my opinion the outstanding hedrologist of the Renaissance. He used the incision with syringotomes both ball tipped and pointed, respectively for fistula and sinus. According to my personal study, the "bistouri à la royale" used by FÉLIX and BESSIÉRE in 1686 to treat the fistula of King Louis XIV was a modification of the syringotome of Fabricius. His technique was completed by DOMENICO MARCHETTI (1626–1688) another great scholar of the Padua School, who also fixed the limits of incision to maintain control, in a famous dispute he had with Riolan. JOHANN SCHULTES of Ulm (1595–1645) Fabricius's pupil, in his famous "Armamentarium Chirurgicum" followed the technique of Fabricius and modified it. He introduced the syringotome pulling it with a thread which had previously been put through an eye-tipped probe through the tract. During the operation the patient is in a kneeling position and leaning on his hands. ANDREAS VESALIUS (1514–1564) studied the function of the muscles of the ano-rectal tract, that G. B. MORGAGNI (1682–1772) illustrated under the anatomo-pathologic viewpoint. G. D. SANTORINI (1681–1737) gave a detailed picture of the musculature illustrating it with splendid tables that are fundamental in the study of the anatomic syringotomy. PERCIVAL POTT (1713–1788) in London, fixed the ball tipped syringotome of Fabricius to a handle and used such a modified bistoury both for fistula and sinus.

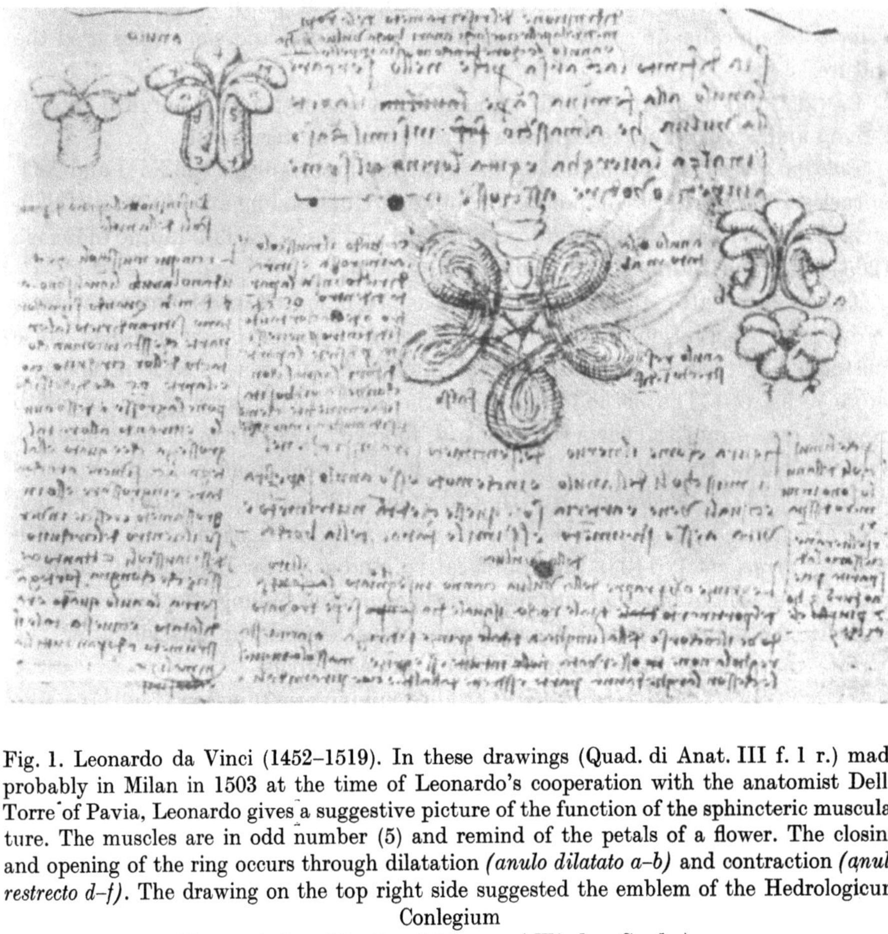

Fig. 1. Leonardo da Vinci (1452–1519). In these drawings (Quad. di Anat. III f. 1 r.) made probably in Milan in 1503 at the time of Leonardo's cooperation with the anatomist Della Torre of Pavia, Leonardo gives a suggestive picture of the function of the sphincteric musculature. The muscles are in odd number (5) and remind of the petals of a flower. The closing and opening of the ring occurs through dilatation *(anulo dilatato a–b)* and contraction *(anulo restrecto d–f)*. The drawing on the top right side suggested the emblem of the Hedrologicum Conlegium

(By permission of the Royal Library of Windsor Castle.)

J. P. DÉSAULT (c. 1885) Paris performed the ligature for a simple fistula by using a lead wire introduced through a little curved metal tube, whilst for complicated fistula he used the incision.

R. CHASSAIGNAC (c. 1770) in France used compression by means of a special instrument (écraseur).

OLINTO GRANDESSO SILVESTRI (1872) suggested the elastic ligature, of which he believes himself the discoverer, as everybody also believed. However, according to my recent investigation, this discovery was made by Ashton.

The ligature, both elastic and non-elastic – has had a revival in France recently, which may be due to the fact that the new followers of this technique had not studied the ancient authors sufficiently, who knew well the negative reasons for discouraging the use of this technique.

Modern Diathermic Syringotomy

According to my own method, the electrode is a snare of steel wire which cuts the fistula and the overlying tissues, sphincter included, by means of electrodessication, sterilizing them and fixing the wound walls in their natural place. Local anesthesia, no bleeding, no packing. Recovery is regulary achieved, no loss of control, even in the most difficult cases. Experimental studies on animals carried out in France show the perfect reestablishment of the sphincter muscles electrically incised as indicated above.

This method has been used by myself for over 30 years and made publicly known. It is now followed in many European countries and is therefore worth mentioning.

Fistula-in-Ano

H. R. Thompson, London, Great Britain

Surgeons concerned in the treatment of anorectal disease are well aware that the results of treatment of fistula-in-ano are far from satisfactory. A high proportion of patients suffering from this condition have undergone multiple operations and suffered from pain, infection and discharge from the anus for long periods.

That such a simple lesion should cause so much suffering is a reflection on the general conception and management of this disease. It is also a reflection on the inability of surgeons who have specialized in the treatment of this complaint to pass on clearly to others the knowledge they have acquired through their own experience.

It might be expected that with the possibilities of modern surgical progress, any general surgeon could treat this simple lesion without difficulty. Because this is not so, I am presenting the following general remarks:

1. *Definition.* A fistula is an abnormal communication between a hollow viscus and the surface of the body or between one hollow viscus and another. In fistula-in-ano it is a communication between the rectum or anal canal and the skin of the perianal region. This must be clearly distinguished from a sinus which is a granulating track leading from a deep-seated focus of suppuration to the surface.

2. *Pathogenesis.* A fistula-in-ano is the result of suppuration and abscess formation in the region of the anorectum. This may be caused by one of the three ways in which suppuration may occur in any other part of the body, i. e. by direct infection, by the blood stream, or by extension of infection from a local focus of disease. There is no doubt that the majority of fistulae-in-ano are due to infection of an anal intramuscular gland and it is such infections that give rise to the majority of non-specific pyogenic fistulae-in-ano. There is, however, a long list of specific diseases which are associated with fistula-in-ano and which I will enumerate later.

3. There are three ways in which a wound may heal – by first, second or third intention. First intention healing is the healing that is expected in an incised and sutured wound and I have no need to dwell on the first lesson that is taught to the surgical student. Second intention healing is the healing that occurs when there is loss of tissue and the wound surface granulates and is finally epithelialised by the squamous epithelium growing in from the periphery of the wound. Third intention healing is the healing that occurs in a granulating track where the phenomenon of wound contracture obliterates the track while the epithelium at either end grows across the internal and external opening. Very occasionally, when a fistula is short, epithelium may grow down the track and it might be said that this fistula has healed, but not become obliterated, by second intention.

4. From the patient's story, it is common knowledge that many fistulae-in-ano heal for a time, only to reappear again spontaneously and the question must be asked "Why does a fistula fail to heal?" There are three reasons:

a) The persistent passage of excretions or secretions through the fistulous track. For instance, diversion of the urine from a urinary fistula will result in immediate healing; suppression of secretion of saliva from a parotid fistula will have the same effect. The re-infection through the internal opening of a fistula-in-ano with mucus and faecal material will cause persistence or recurrence of such a fistula.

b) The lining of a part of the fistula with squamous or transitional epithelium. Under such circumstances, one of the openings of the fistula is unable to close and can become readily infected.

c) When the epithelial surfaces of two hollow viscera become united, healing is impossible without surgical intervention.

The above remarks apply to non-specific fistulae. Anorectal fistulae, however, are associated with certain specific diseases whose aetiology is directly responsible nor only for the development of fistulae but also for the delay or failure of healing of fistulous wounds. Certain constitutional states, such as malnutrition, anaemia, diabetes, syphilis and chronic cardiac failure leading to oedema of the tissues, are well-known causes of delayed healing. Other diseases which give rise to fistulae of atypical anatomy and where healing is atypical are:

i) Tuberculosis which may or may not be associated with pulmonary disease. The demonstration of the tubercle bacillus is essential before the diagnosis of tuberculous fistula-in-ano can be accepted.

ii) Ulcerative colitis.

iii) Crohn's disease associated with lesions of the small intestine, in the large intestine, or a local anal manifestation alone. In young women an ano-vaginal fistula is almost a diagnostic sign of Crohn's disease.

iv) Fungus infection, such as actinomycosis, may be the cause of a chronic anal fistula.

v) Lymphogranuloma venereum.

vi) Diverticulitis. There is no doubt that discharge of mucous from diverticular disease of the colon can cause repeated anorectal infections and resection of the diseased colon may result in the healing of a previously recalcitrant fistula.

vii) Endometriosis – sometimes endometrial implants are found in the perineum in women and when these glandular implants become infected fistulae form and their irradication may often be difficult.

viii) Malignant disease may be associated with a fistula in several ways:

a) it may develop in the fistulous track of a congenital reduplication, invariably a mucus secreting carcinoma,

b) implantation of malignant cells can take place on a chronic fistula-in-ano from a remote carcinoma of rectum or pelvic colon,

c) adenocarcinoma or squamous carcinoma may directly infiltrate the ischiorectal or perianal spaces to form a fistula,

d) where stenosis is a feature of the tumour, ulceration and perforation of the bowel above the stricture may lead to a perirectal abscess which finally discharges through the perianal skin below the tumour, thus by-passing the growth,

e) a squamous carcinoma may cause secondary infection of adjacent anal crypts and glands to form fistulae remote from the tumour site.

ix) Foreign bodies – swallowed foreign bodies may cause abscesses and fistulae by direct infection. Poultry and meat bone splinters, fish bones, pins and even pieces of cocktail sticks have been recovered from anorectal abscess cavities and fistulous tracks.

Lastly, there are three conditions, namely pilonidal disease, hydradenitis suppurativa and infected dermoid cycts, which have all the physical signs of a fistula-in-ano but which by definition are really sinuses. The failure to appreciate the possibility of these conditions may lead to disappointments in treatment.

The sending of representative pieces of tissue from a fistulous track to the pathologist for microscopic examination is an essential step in any operation for fistula-in-ano.

5. Fistulas of the anorectal region are unique as they traverse a muscular mechanism on which continence of the intestine depends. The successful treatment of a fistula-in-ano necessitates the division of a variable amount of this important muscular mechanism. It is essential, therefore, that a surgeon concerned with this work should have at least a sound clinical appreciation of such component parts of the sphincter mechanism as may be felt and seen. He should be able to demonstrate the limits of the sphincter muscles and know how much may be divided without making the patient incontinent.

6. The anatomy of non-specific fistulae. For all practical purposes there are two main fistulous types, the one a simple direct track which passes from the external opening to the internal opening in the anal canal at the dentate line. This fistula may be recognized by the fact that the track is palpable under the perianal skin and a probe passes transversely to the long axis of the rectum along the track. The internal opening is in direct line with the external opening and no induration can be palpated through the rectum. The other, the so-called horseshoe fistula, has a track which runs round the top of the ischio-rectal fossa, a probe passes vertically to the long axis of the rectum along its track, the internal opening is in the midline posteriorly and bears no direct relationship to the external opening, and considerable induration may be palpated in the rectum. The so-called pelvirectal fistula, where the internal opening is above the whole sphincter mechanism, constitutes about 0.1 per cent of fistulae and this fistula, unless it has been caused by the trauma of an inexperienced surgeon's probe, is invariably due to suppuration in the supra-levator space.

Treatment

It is not my intention to go into the details of treatment of fistulae. It is, however, interesting to note that some surgeons convert a fistulous track that fails to heal by third intention into a flat wound that will heal by second intention. Other surgeons, particularly the French school, excise the fistulous track and suture the wound, thus converting the track that fails to heal by third intention into a wound that heals by first intention. My criticism of this method is that wounds which heal by first intention should be kept cool, dry and free from infection. Wounds of the anal canal are inevitably warm, moist and the risk of infection is ever present. To counteract this, large doses of antibiotics are frequently given, which bring in their turn the complications specific to themselves.

Recent work has suggested that provided the anal intramuscular gland is excised, the fistula will heal without the creation of a classical fistula wound. Personally, I find it difficult to discipline myself or to instruct my assistants on how to excise a structure which can only exceptionally be either seen or felt.

Causes of Failure in the Treatment of Fistula-in-Ano

This is due to ignorance of the anorectal musculature, ignorance of the anatomical types of fistula, failure to identify correctly the internal fistulous opening, fear of dividing too much of the sphincter ani muscle and ignorance of the specific causes of a fistula-in-ano.

The Classification of Fistula-in-Ano

A. G. Parks, London, Great Britain

This report contains an analysis of 163 cases of fistula seen and personally treated at St. Mark's Hospital between the years 1959 and 1968. Details of the anatomy of the tracks of each fistula were carefully recorded. An attempt is made to establish a logical anatomical classification of fistula with special reference to the relationship of the tracks to the sphincter muscles.

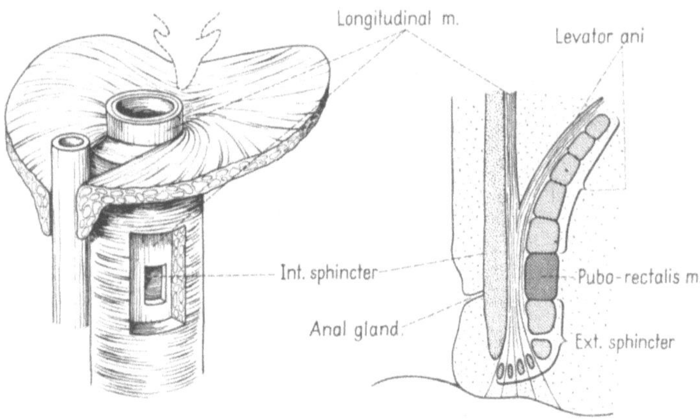

Fig. 1

It is first necessary to recapitulate briefly the anatomy of the anal sphincters (Fig. 1). The pelvic floor mechanism has two components; there is an inner tube comprised of the termination of the hindgut, surrounded by a sheath of skeletal muscle by means of which continence is maintained. The muscle of the inner component, being visceral, is composed of smooth fibres and its action is under the control of the local autonomic reflexes. The muscle of the outer component is skeletal muscle which is activated in part voluntarily, but chiefly by a spinal reflex mechanism. This component is funnel shaped (the expanded part of which is made up of the levator ani muscles); the upper expanded part divides the pelvic cavity from the perineum; above it is the para-rectal space into which infection readily spreads; below it are perineal structures, mostly ischio-rectal fat. The two components are bound together by areolar and fibrous tissue which constitutes an important plane, the intersphincteric plane. Its importance is that it is one of the major pathways of spread of fistulous infection; it has also been implicated in the pathogenesis of most fistulas (PARKS, 1960). There are three main routes in which fistulae track (Fig. 2); between the muscles (intersphincteric), outside both groups of muscles (the fat of the ischiorectal fossa), and above the levator ani muscles (the para-rectal or supra-levator space).

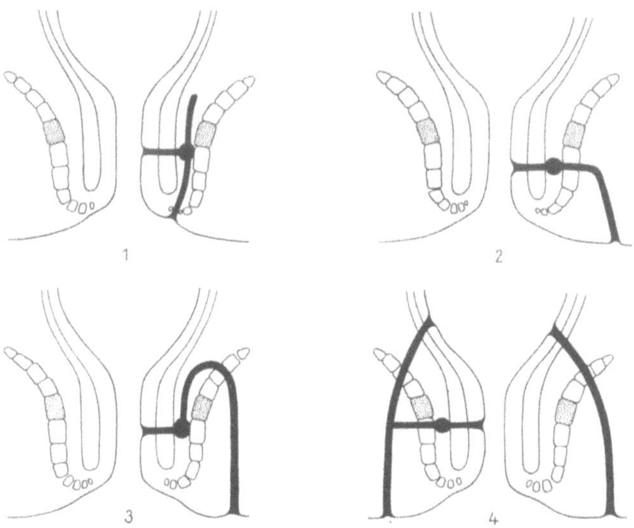

Fig. 2

In order to facilitate a more detailed discussion it can be said at once that it is possible to classify the cases into four main groups, as follows:

1. Intersphincteric Fistula (96 cases).

In this group infection spreads into and through the intersphincteric plane but not beyond it into the surrounding skeletal muscles.

2. Transphincteric Fistula (52 cases).

Here infection passes from the intersphincteric plane through the external sphincter muscle into the ischio-rectal fossa.

3. Suprasphincteric Fistula (19 cases).

Infection arises in the mid-anal canal, passes upwards in the intersphincteric plane over the top of the entire sphincter mass, including the pubo-rectalis muscle, and then dips downwards through the levator ani muscles into the ischio-rectal fossa to appear at the perineal skin.

4. Extrasphincteric Fistula (3 cases).

In these cases there is a communication between the rectum and the perineum which passes entirely outside the ring of the external sphincter muscles.

This classification has an obvious practical application. If an intersphincteric (type 1) fistula is laid open, only the internal sphincter will be divided and although this may interfere with continence slightly, it seldom does so to any great degree. In the case of the transphincteric fistula, part of both sphincters will have to be divided. Interference with continence will then depend upon the level at which the track passes through the external sphincter; fortunately this is usually at a low level. The suprasphincteric and extrasphincteric fistula present grave therapeutic problems which are out of the terms of reference of this study; it is apparent that an attempt to deal with them by section of muscle will inevitably result in incontinence.

Patients with gross ano-rectal disease due to carcinoma, ulcerative colitis or Crohn's disease have been excluded from this survey.

Detailed Analysis of Results

Type 1. Intersphincteric Fistula

There were 96 cases in this group of which 74 were of the common, simple variety.

A. Uncomplicated (74 cases). This variety passes from the primary abscess in the intersphincteric plane to the anal verge. It is easy to treat and the amount of muscle which has to be divided seldom gives rise to disturbing symptoms. It is usually referred to as the "low anal" fistula and is the commonest of all types.

B. Intersphincteric fistula with a high secondary track (7 cases). In these cases there is a high extension of the fistula between the internal sphincter and the longitudinal muscle of the upper anal canal into the rectal wall. This upper track is secondary to the primary source of the disease in the mid-anal canal and it will heal once the primary site of infection has been dealt with. However, even if the upper part of the track is also laid open, by dividing the whole of the internal sphincter, little disturbance of continence occurs because the edges of the sphincter are held together by peri-fistulous fibrosis.

C. Intersphincteric fistula with a high secondary track opening into the rectum (5 cases). This is an important variant as it is frequently misdiagnosed. A probe entering the external opening passes through the entire track into the rectum. The surgeon may be misled into believing that the track passes through the ischio-rectal fossa, that is, that the fistula is an extrasphincteric one. Indeed, in one instance in this series the patient was declared inoperable because of this misunderstanding. In fact, it is not a difficult fistula to operate as the lower half, or indeed the entire track, may be laid open without fear.

D. High intersphincteric fistula without an external opening (3 cases). Infection commences in the intersphincteric zone of the mid-anal canal and passes upwards into the wall of the rectum where it usually re-enters the gut through a secondary opening. The track lies deep to the circular muscle of the rectum but is usually, and I believe erroneously, called a submucous fistula. Treatment is simple; the track is laid open into the rectum, care being taken to open up the lowermost part which is in the upper anal canal.

E. High intersphincteric fistula with a rectal wall abscess (2 cases). This is similar to the above (type *1D*) but an abscess is present in the rectal wall instead of the high opening. It is my experience that such abscesses are always deep to the circular muscle layer of the rectum which is very thin at this level. They should be drained into the rectum.

F. High intersphincteric fistula with an extra-rectal abscess (5 cases). Here again infection commences in the intersphincteric zone of the mid-anal canal but it spreads upwards through the longitudinal layer to reach the true pelvic cavity. It lies above the levator plate and the correct treatment is drainage into the rectum. If drainage of this type of abscess is attempted through the ischio-rectal fossa (and thereby through the levator ani muscle) a suprasphincteric (type 3) fistula is created iatrogenically.

G. Intersphincteric fistula from a pelvic source (2 cases). The intersphincteric plane is natural pathway for infection from the pelvis to follow if it tracks downwards. In one case in this series this arose from infected non-absorbable suture material used to repair a femoral hernia; another case was due to diverticulitis. Treatment must, of course, be directed to the pelvic disease; once this is removed the fistula will heal.

Type 2. Transphincteric Fistula (52 cases)

A. Uncomplicated (37 cases). The common type passes from the intersphincteric plane through the external sphincter into the ischio-rectal fossa and thence to the perineal skin. Fortunately the passage across the sphincter is usually at a low level so that laying it open only results in minimal division of the lower part of the external sphincter. A few, however, pass at higher levels and obviously the higher they pass, the more difficult and hazardous the surgical treatment.

B. Transphincteric fistula with a high secondary track (15 cases). This is one of the most important of fistulae because its nature is so often misunderstood. Having crossed the external sphincter, the track divides into two, the lower half passing to the perineal skin; the higher limb goes to the apex of the ischio-rectal fossa and sometimes even passes through the levator ani muscles into the true pelvic cavity. The high limb extends above the ano-rectal ring of muscles, hence the term "ano-rectal fistula" given it by the St. Marks' surgeons. A probe passed through the external opening goes directly into the high part of the track. If the surgeon mistakes this upper part for the main primary track he may probe it with such vigour that a new opening is created into the rectum; he produces an iatrogenic fistula, a disastrous event. It is important to realize that the height and extent of the secondary track is not of paramount importance provided that it has not ruptured into the rectum. The essence of treatment is to find the primary track and to deal with that; the high secondary track will close on its own provided that it has been given adequate drainage.

C. Transphincteric fistula with a high secondary track opening into the rectum (1 case). This is, in fact, an extrasphincteric fistula and will be discussed in the next section.

Horseshoe Fistula

It is quite common for a transphincteric fistula to pass circumferentially in the ischio-rectal fossa, indeed it may pass from one ischio-rectal fossa to the other. A horseshoe fistula, which is sometimes held in great awe by surgeons, seldom creates any technical difficulty. The circumferential track must be given adequate drainage which may entail a large incision from one ischio-rectal fossa to the other. Circumferential spread can also occur in the intersphincteric and supra-levator planes. It must be emphasized that almost all difficulties in fistula surgery arise as the result of high penetration of the external sphincter, circumferential spread is not a major problem.

Type 3. Supra-sphincteric Fistula (10 cases)

The fistula usually starts in the intersphincteric plane of the mid-anal canal, then passes upwards in this plane above the level of the pubo-rectalis muscle. It passes over this muscle and then changes direction downwards to enter the ischio-rectal fossa through the levator plate; in this manner it loops over the entire sphincter mass. It is a difficult fistula to treat as any attempt to lay open the muscle below it will result in the division of all the external sphincter and must inevitably cause gross disturbance of continence. It may be subdivided into two groups according to whether there is a high track present as in *2 B*.

Type 4. Extra-sphincteric Fistula (3 cases)

In this situation a track passes from the skin of the perineum, through the fat of the ischio-rectal fossa, through the levator ani muscles and finally penetrates the rectum. It passes outside the entire ring of sphincter muscles and is therefore designated "extra-sphincteric"; any attempt to lay open the entire track of this type of fistula will result in total incontinence. A fistula opening into the rectal ampulla is subject to the high pressures which develop in it from time to time and which force mucus and faecal material into it. Attempts to close the rectal opening by suture usually fail because of the force of intra-rectal pressure; hence this must be prevented by giving the patient a temporary iliac colostomy.

A. Extra-sphincteric fistula due to specific ano-rectal disease. Fistula due to ulcerative colitis, Crohn's disease and carcinoma have been excluded from this series; treatment of the major disease is required.

B. Extra-sphincteric fistula due to pelvic inflammation (1 case). In this case infection from a segment of diverticulitis spread downwards through the levator plate, the ischio-rectal fossa and presented in the skin of the perineum. The fistula will heal once the pelvic disease has been removed.

C. Extra-sphincteric fistula due to trauma (1 case). The trauma may be external, as in my one case, or internal from a penetrating foreign body. Treatment consists in removing any remaining foreign body and then abolishing high rectal pressure by means of a temporary colostomy.

D. Extra-sphincteric fistula secondary to a transphincteric fistula (1 case). This is fortunately a rare condition; the high track from a type *2 B* fistula passes upwards through the levator ani muscle and enters the rectum. It may be caused by over-enthusiastic probing of type *2 B*. Two causes of persistent fistula are now present, the primary focus of disease in the anal canal and high pressures acting on the rectal opening. Both must be eliminated before the fistula will heal. Infection from the rectum itself is dealt with by performing a temporary colostomy. The perineal opening is then explored and the primary track through the external sphincter laid open.

There are two points of criticism which may be leveled against such a presentation. The first is that observations of anatomy made at operation are subject to error and also bias; I can only say that I have tried to be as careful and objective as possible. The second is that this series of cases is unrepresentative of the general population due to case selection. This is a valid criticism as patients who are sent to St. Mark's Hospital tend to have the more difficult type of fistula.

The Prevention of Anal Fistulas by the Correct Treatment of Anal Abscesses and Phlegmons

U. Marel, A. Davy and G. Cayron, Rouen, France

The treatment we use is only for the properly called anal region abscesses. It does not affect para-coccygeal ones, who have no connection with the anal canal, and whose treatment is quite different.

Among the properly called anal region abscesses, we must distinguish between:

the abscesses whose prime cause is about of retention of a known anal fistula;

and the primitive abscesses caused by a fistulous infection in the anal region.

Our treatment concerns only primitive, untreated abscesses that have not been lanced and who are still not fistulous.

The anatomo-pathologist provides us with some information about the way to treat them. A glandular canal originates in a Morgagni crypt, goes through the submucous membrane of the anal canal, where it sometimes stops, but most of the time, it proceeds through the internal sphincter and ends in a cyst situated in the longitudinal muscle level, close to the deep layer of the external sphincter which it usually does not go through.

The contamination of a cystic hollow by germs brought by the stool and spread by the glandular canal, creates a micro-abscess which is the source of most of the suppurations of the anal region. This abscess cannot be drained by the glandular canal, since the latter is too narrow and winding. It will try to develop a fistula to the skin.

Treatment

If the abscess is lanced, be it: a wide lancing, accompanied by a declivitous one, followed by a tent – regardless of the method, it is nearly never enough. For this form of treatment does not take the connections of the abscess with the sphincter ring into consideration. The same reproach has to be adressed to anti-inflammatory radio-therapy.

Contrary to what has been said, antibiotics are always harmful. They must never be used.

As soon as the diagnosis of an anal region abscess has been set, the patient must be operated on, regardless of the clinical form, spread and site of the abscess. For the spreading and virulent tendency of some anal suppurations is the very source of sphincter destructions. This is an argument for the early treatment of perianal abscesses.

All our patients are operated on under general anaesthesia. The operator cuts out the surface of the abscess widely. The muscle fascicle which is steeped in pus is cut out if it is only attached to the skin deep fascicle of the external sphincter.

The main part of the operation is to discover the glandular canal or path which goes through the internal sphincter to the anal canal and to cut it out. Sometimes it is easily found, but most of the time, it must be searched for with care and patience.

The operator probes the sore internal face, which is close to the muscular ring, with a blunt stylet. The path is often in the fibrous septum which separates the skin deep fascicle from the deep fascicle of the internal sphincter. Generally the path goes straight to the internal sphincter fascicle.

If the operator has discovered the path, he inserts a blunt stylet into it with care, and advances it to the anal canal mucosa, after it passes through the internal sphincter. Sometimes it is necessary to push carefully in order to get through the mucosa into a Morgagni crypt. When the path is found, the proper connections with the sphincter ring must be appreciated. If the path only gets through the skin-deep fascicle of the external sphincter, we must cut out the glandular canal right round the stylet.

To repair the sphincter, we are content with the natural retractile tendency of the wound, which closes by itself as a book and makes a solid scar on which the cut muscular fascicle will get the proper support.

If the path penetrates the deep fascicle of the external sphincter, we pass three nylon threads through a Bréger trocar to ensure proper drainage. Next we exchange the nylon threads for elastic ones, so that we bring about a gradual lowering of the fistulous path until it is deep-skin. Then we only have to lance it.

If the fistulous path proceeds through the levator muscle and gets in the upper pelvi-rectal space, we drain it in the same way.

If the abscess lies within the anal canal, close to the internal sphincter itself, that is to say an in-wall abscess or sub-mucosal abscess, it must be lanced long the anal canal to the skin, resulting in a drainage path.

The virulence of some suppurations is the source of seepages, releases, and even destruction of some muscle layers by pus.

If the operator does not know the connections of the path with the muscular ring exactly, he must always be very careful and sets threads. If the path was not found after a proper investigation, *he must not create a false path* by rude and blind handling of his stylet with which he probes the crypts of anal canal. This backward probing, which must be practised with great care, is sometimes successful, and the path is found. However, through this patient probing, the path is sometimes not found at all.

The fore-pole abscesses are more difficult to treat than the back-pole ones. The fore-pole suppurations often spread to perineum. In the male, the posterior urethra and the bulb of the penis are close by; this is the reason why a catheter must be inserted into the urethra. In the female the recto-vaginal septum is thin: in order to be sure of its integrity, a probing finger must be kept in the vagina.

After abscess and fistula have been cured, the operator must always check the rectal ampulla and search for spreading to the opposite side: this is more common when the abscess is a back-pole one. Infection may reach the opposite ischio-anal space, spreading in horseshoe formation.

Treatment Results

In twelve years, we have operated on 250 patients with anal abscesses.

We never use antibiotics, either before or after the operation. If the wound is still running after the operation it means that a part of the glandular canal is left or drainage was incomplete.

When we cut the skin-deep fascicle of the external sphincter, the direction of canal may be turned.

In the case of a muscle cut, sometimes a brief incontinence of flatus remains. This drawback will disappear quickly when the patient practices sphincter contraction excercises. *We have never had true incontinence of stool.*

In 17 patients, we did not succed in finding the path at operation. Six of these had a fistula later. In 4 patients however where we found the path and treated the abscess in the manner described above, a fistula appeared later.

Conclusion

The result of anal region abscesses which receive no treatment or are treated with antibiotics or anti-inflammatory radio-therapy or a single lancing, are anal fistulas whose cure is often quite difficult. In contrast, the correct operating technique of anal abscesses results in the prevention of anal fistulas most of the time.

Chronic Abscesses of the Ano-Rectum

N. J. Georgiadis and B. Leoutsakos, Athens, Greece

The late Lockhart-Mummery described in 1923 a chronic type of submucous abscess of the rectal wall which could simulate a malignant growth such as a sarcoma by the lack of typical symptoms and mainly by its thickened walls.

According to Gabriel, this type of formation may be due to an intermuscular abscess which discharges spontaneoulsy but incompletely into the anal canal and does not resolve.

The inflammatory elements which remain in the form of a lump or an infiltration in the anorectal wall after incomplete resolution of an ano-rectal abscess will be referred to as a "chronic abscess" in this paper; although the term abscess usually implies the collection of purulent matter within a cavity.

As mentioned by Lockhart-Mummery, a small abscess cavity may be found in the centre of such a formation and occasionally, instead of a single localized abscess, an indurated track runs up underneath the mucosa for some distance.

According to Eisenhammer's classification of ano-rectal abscesses (Fig. 1), a chronic abscess may be found at any site where a typical abscess might be formed. Nevertheless, chronic abscesses of the ano-rectum in the form of a lump with no fistulous connection to the perineal skin or the ano-rectal mucosa may be regarded as being uncommon.

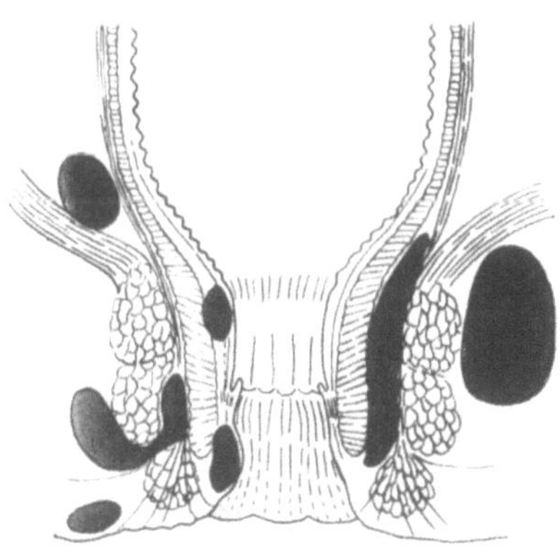

Fig. 1

During the last ten years up to 1968 we dealt with three cases of chronic abscess of this sort; in the same period we treated 217 cases of acute abscess, fistula and fissure.

Two of our patients were females, 29 and 30 years of age, and one was a 44-year-old male.

The common feature in both female cases was the lack of any history of infection, localized or diffuse, of the perineum or the pelvis. Nor did either of them mention any infectious disease in the past which could have given rise to a blood-bone invasion of the cellular tissues.

The presenting sign in our two cases was a palpable, painless lump, four centimeters in diameter, which occupied the left para-anal space. No fluctuation or signs of inflammatory lesion such as oedema or redness of the skin overlying the lump were present; the latter, ball-shaped as it was, gave the impression that it could even be enucleated at operation.

This clinical impression turned out to be erroneous at operation, as the lumps had to be dissected out by sharp dissection, because of their ill-defined limits. No fistulous track connecting the lump to the bowel or to a Bartholin gland was detected. The residual cavity was left open and healed by granulation within three weeks.

Histologically the lumps were found to consist of fibrous tissue with pronounced inflammatory infiltration (Fig. 2).

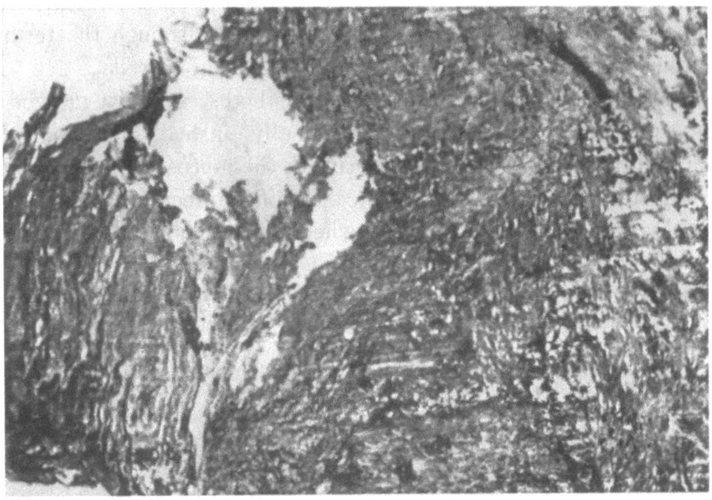

Fig. 2

As far as the third case is concerned, we believe that it can be used to support the Gabriel's previously mentioned opinion on the way a chronic abscess is produced. Indeed this male patient mentioned that thirteen years before he had had a spontaneous but otherwise asymptomatic discharge of pus per rectum; similar episodes always free of pain and temperature recurred for nearly one year. During these episodes the patient was given different kinds of antibiotics. Then he remained in excellent health for eleven years. Now he started complaining of a dull but irksome perineal pain unrelated to defecation or sitting down. No abnormality was detected on proctoscopy and sigmoidoscopy, but an irregular submucous induration was palpable just above the ano-rectal ring on the right side. The trans-rectal palpation of this induration aggravated the patient's discomfort.

We operated this patient by exposing his right ischio-rectal space widely, but we had to go even further above the levator ani in order to dissect out the entire indurated area sharply and blindly guided by a finger in the rectum. The disappearance of the patient's pain and a post-operative sinus were the initial results of the operation. After two minor operations the sinus dried up. No internal opening was ever found to explain both the chronic abscess and the post-operative sinus.

The examination of the removed induration also showed fibrous tissue with inflammatory infiltration.

We should like to make the following comments on the reported cases, knowing that we have used the term "chronic abscess" quite arbitrarily in spite of the fact that in none of them had a cavity with pus was found. We cannot imagine any other term that better describes a solid inflammatory lump in the ano-rectum, which is actually an inflammatory granuloma. We believe that the use of antibiotics as abortive treatment for an acute ano-rectal abscess may lead to the encapsulation of the latter within a thick fibrous wall and result in the appearance of what we called "chronic abscess" after a given period of time.

From our third case, we think that a high external chronic abscess of the ischio or pelvi-rectal type may simulate the picture of the proctalgia fugax condition by acting as a foreign body producing a spasm of the levator ani muscles. The surgical treatment of the chronic abscess is another noteworthy point.

For the chronic submucous abscesses, as mentioned by LOCKHART-MUMMERY, the dissection of the abscess from within the bowel, followed by washing out with an antiseptic solution must be the rule. We believe that the pre- and postoperative use of non-absorbable sulfonamides might be of great help in controlling infection. In other abscess locations as in our cases, the remaining cavity should be left open with no packing. This is easily achieved in abscesses occupying a para-anal space and could be also applied in abscesses of the ischio-rectal fossa. In case of an abscess of the pelvi-rectal space, as in our case, no widely open wound is possible and therefore it is wiser to drain the residual cavity by means of a large tube. This was the way in which we managed to dry up the sinus that resulted from the initial removal of the abscess in our case. Of course the drain should be shortened at frequent intervals and locally acting enzymes should also be used for irrigation. It is understood that a thorough search for the fistulous track must be undertaken during any operation for a chronic abscess, not only after the dissection of the abscess, but also when checking the granulating wound.

Finally, we believe that it would be advisable to renew the interest of surgeons, proctologists and pathologists in the reported condition, which seems to be almost forgotten, as there is very little reference to it in recent medical literature.

Bibliography

EISENHAMMER, S.: Surg. Gynec. Obst. **130**, 501 (1956).

GABRIEL, W. B.: The principles and practice of Rectal Surgery. Fifth Edition. H. K. Lewis and Co. Ltd. 1963.

LOCKHART-MUMMERY, J. P.: Diseases of the Rectum and Colon. London: Bailliere, Tindall and Cox 1923.

Systematic Anal Sphincter Resection and Immediate Myorrhaphy in High Anal Fistula Exeresis – Technique and Results

R. Schwartz, Paris, France

The problem of anal sphincter resection – whether partial, and even more so when complete – has given rise to much controversy at the present time but in our opinion, it is not only possible, but desirable if it is followed by an immediate muscular reconstitution at the expense of the levator ani at the same operation.

Its indication is precise in all cases when exeresis surgery obliges us to dispose of the sphincter's whole height (fistulae or tumours wedged into the muscle).

The techniques are easy but it is of the greatest importance not to neglect any detail of the principal steps:

After the course of the fistula has been flattened in successive planes: skin, cellular tissues, sphincter, ending at the anal mucous membrane, all tissues should be resected until healthy tissue is reached; it is very important for a good cicatrization that all injured tissue be removed. Temporary threads are placed in a "U" shape on each stump of the sphincter which is to be reclinated to the inside.

Each one of the anterior and posterior fascicles of the levator ani is divided in half for about 1 inch (2,5 cm); both these halves are then reclinated upon their opposites, the anterior to the back and the posterior to the front.

The halves are then crossed and the stumps of the levator ani are sutured on the stumps of the sphincter:

The split fascicles of the levator ani anterior are sutured on to the posterior stump of the sphincter;

and the split fascicles of the levator ani posterior on to the anterior stump of the sphincter.

This stitching is done with reabsorbable threads (chromatized catgut N° 1) and the stitching of the sphincter stumps with temporary threads.

This last suture has a tendency to shrink the sphincter ring which has been deprived of the resected portion; for this reason we finish the operation by a posterior sphincterectomy after exeresis of a triangular flap of skin whose superior base in bounded by the inferior edge of the anal mucous membrane; we then stitch this mucous membrane which has become free to the remaining external sphincter with two stitches right and left in a "U" shape.

Let us remind you of our dressing procedure at the end of the operation, which has become systematic for anorectal surgery, twenty years after its introduction.

Never place any kind of intra-anal drain as these always cause painful contractions; use only antiseptic and insulating pomade up to the ampulla recti in order to keep the entire surgical area free of infection of intestinal origin and to facilite the dreaded first defecation.

Gross Rectal Involvement in Crohn's Disease

T. P. Cole, S. W. B. Ewen and J. Kyle, Aberdeen, Scotland

The rectum is regularly involved at an early stage in ulcerative proctocolitis, but it has been thought that in Crohn's Disease of the colon the rectum was initially spared (Korelitz, 1967). Colonic Crohn's Disease has only been widely recognized for eight years (Lockhart-Mummery and Morson, 1960), (Lennard Jones, Lockhart-Mummery and Morson, 1968), although the frequent occurrence of fistulae-in-ano in ileal Crohn's Disease had been described earlier. The recent detection of undoubted examples of Crohn's Disease involving the rectum proper at an early stage and in gross and widespread fashion calls for a revision of the original supposition. Furthermore it raises the question whether or not such a remarkable lesion could have been missed by previous generations of surgeons and pathologists.

Present Series

During the years 1955–68, there have been 134 patients diagnosed as suffering from all forms of Crohn's Disease in North-East Scotland, which region has a population of 440,000. Twenty-four patients had colonic Crohn's Disease and of these there were five patients (Table 1) with gross rectal involvement, all occurring within the last 6 years.

Table 1. *Details of five patients with gross involvement of the rectum by Crohn's Disease*

No.	Sex	Age at onset (years)	Duration of symptoms (months)	Extent	Treatment	Result
1	F	56	18	Left colon, rectum	Steroids, Sulphasalazine	Controlled on steroids
2	M	53	12	Left colon, rectum	Left hemicolectomy	Well
3	F	19	20	Ileum, caecum, rectum	Steroids, Sulphasalazine	Controlled on steroids
4	F	78	12	Splenic flexure, rectum	Proctocolectomy	Died 1 month later
5	M	44	41	Transverse colon, rectum	Proctocolectomy	Well

The first three patients had a similar clinical course. When first seen they had short attacks of lower abdominal pain and slight diarrhoea within the preceding few weeks. Sigmoidoscopy in each case showed redness of the lower and middle rectal mucosa without ulceration. Biopsies revealed mild, non-specific inflammatory changes. Only the younger female merited treatment – with Sulphasalazine. They all re-appeared in about 18 months; all had lost weight and had troublesome diarrhoea, 4–9 times per day. The findings on rectal examination were striking. The entire rectum in each case felt as if it had been replaced by a long, tortuous malignant stricture. On attempting to perform sigmoidoscopy, distension of the rigid rectal wall was impossible and the instrument could only be introduced a few centimetres up the narrow, irregular cork-screw lumen. The oedematous, ulcerated mucosa had a cobble-stone appearance. The findings might have been interpreted as being those of rectal lymphogranuloma venereum, but Frei tests in these three patients were negative, barium enema examinations showed lesions in more proximal parts of the intestine and histological studies revealed cellular changes consistent with a diagnosis of Crohn's Disease.

The two females were treated with Sulphasalazine and with large doses of Prednisone, both systemically and by retention enemata, until they showed Cushingoid features. Thereafter the dose was gradually reduced to 10–15 mg Prednisone daily, on which dose their symptoms are minimal and their rectal walls have returned to the state they were in when first seen – reddened but distensible and with only mild inflammatory changes. Proctocolectomy was advised for Case 2, but he refused excision of his rectum. He had a colectomy, remains fairly well after 2 years, but has some rectal discharge.

The oldest female in the series, Case 4, presented with troublesome fistulae-in-ano; her other symptoms and rectal findings were similar to those in the first three patients. Although her general condition was very poor, proctocolectomy was carried out, but she died a month later of pneumonia.

Three years before the last man presented with rectal symptoms, he had had a local resection for a granulomatous lesion of the transverse colon; review of the sections showed changes consistent with a diagnosis of Crohn's Disease. His later symptomatology and rectal findings were similar to those of the other patients.

Retrospective Survey

The records of the Pathology Department for the years 1938–67 were scrutinized. During this 30 year-period approximately 144,000 specimens had been examined. Apart from the cases described above, no similar rectal lesions had been encountered.

Discussion

It seems possible that such gross rectal changes as those described could have been missed by surgeons of previous generations. The absence of any comparable histological report from the pathology records of earlier years tends to confirm the opinion that the incidence of Crohn's Disease predominantly involving the rectum must have increased during the past decade. The resolution of the marked mechanical and cellular changes in the rectal wall in response to large doses of steroids was dramatic and has not previously been described. How long the response will continue is unknown. Our experience with the management of other forms of colonic Crohn's Disease suggests that resection is preferable to medical treatment. It may therefore be advisable to recommend proctocolectomy for all patients with gross rectal involvement.

Bibliography

Korelitz, B. I.: Clinical course, late results, and pathological nature of inflammatory disease of the colon initially sparing the rectum. Gut. **8**, 281 (1967).

Lockhart-Mummery, H. E., and B. C. Morson: Crohn's Disease (regional enteritis) of the large intestine and its distinction from ulcerative colitis. Gut. **1**, 87 (1960).

Morson, B. C., and H. E. Lockhart-Mummery: Anal lesions in Crohn's Disease. Lancet **2**, 1122 (1959).

Lennard-Jones, J. E., H. E. Lockhart-Mummery, and B. C. Morson: Clinical and Pathological Differentiation of Crohn's Disease and Proctocolitis. Gastroenterology **54**, 1162 (1968).

Anal Fistulas in Regional Enteritis

J. SCHIER, Mainz, Germany

Regional enteritis (Crohn's disease) is an unspecific segmentary and granulomatous inflammation of the bowel wall. The disease shows a definite tendency to form fistulas. In the literature fistulas have been described in 60% of the cases. Of these 20 to 25% were anorectal fistulas (Table 1). Regional enteritis has also been reported to occur primarily in the rectum in a few cases.

Table 1. *Anal fistulas in regional enteritis*

Author	Number of cases	Fistulas in %
CROHN	1200	23
Collected series	1191	8
Mayo Clinic	1000	31
CATTELL	299	25
POLLOCK	108	20
DAFFNER	48	48
KÜMMERLE-SCHIER	51	20

The anal fistula is often the first symptom of regional enteritis. It may exist for many years – according to CROHN up to 14 years – before other symptoms and clinical signs reveal the true nature of the disease. Obviously the local inflammatory process of the diseased bowel wall shows a very bland reaction in these cases.

In regional enteritis, proliferative and ulcerative inflammatory processes of the bowel wall take place at the same time. Besides this concomitant inflammatory reactions in the neighbourhood and small perforations of the diseased bowel wall lead to a matted mass of several loops of bowel, usually fixed to the pelvic floor. This is the first step in the development of an anal fistula. Abscesses formed between the diseased bowel segments and the pelvic floor prepare the way for the fistulas. A diverse branched-out system of granulating ducts develops from these abscesses down between the posterior wall of the bladder and the rectosigmoid into the perirectal region. Finally they perforate the pelvic floor and appear as anal fistulas.

This mechanism of development of an anal fistula is different from the development of the common anal fistula. It therefore demands a completely different approach in operative management.

This is seen in the case of a 17-years old patient, who underwent several local surgical procedures in the anorectal area because of recurrent fistulas (Fig. 1). The anal region was completely destroyed by the surgical interventions. Fractional examination of the small intestines revealed the characteristic X-ray stenosis of the terminal ileum (Fig. 2). At operation,

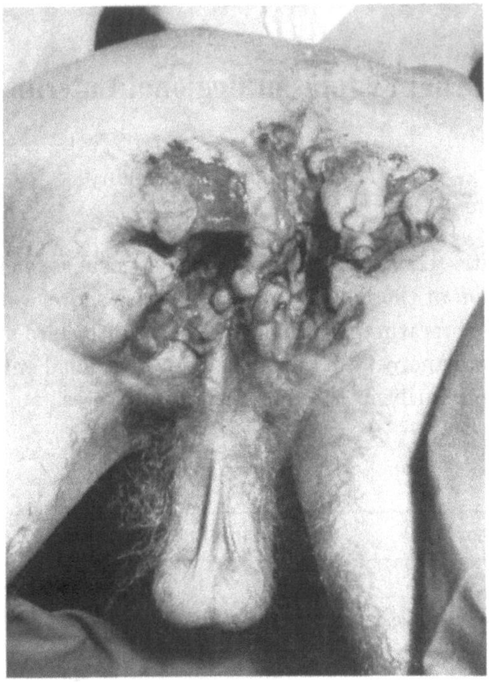

Fig. 1. Anal fistulas in regional enteritis. The perianal region is completely destroyed by local surgical interventions

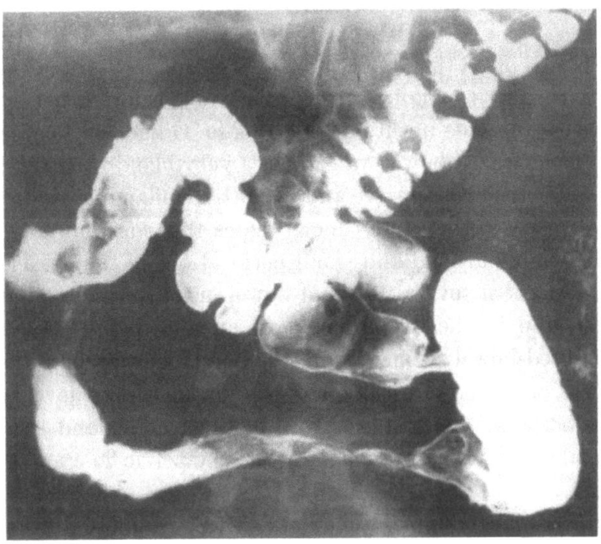

Fig. 2. Typical x-ray appearance of regional enteritis with "string sign".

a matted mass of small bowel loops was found fixed to the pelvic floor. From an intestinal fistula in the terminal ileum, a granulated duct led down into the periproctial tissues. The mass was mobilized and resected. The intestinal continuity was restored by an end-to-end ileocolostomy. At the same time a colostomy was performed in order to deviate the fecal stream. The fistulas healed, but because of the many local surgical interventions in the anal area the sphincteric apparatus was completely destroyed. The rectum had to be resected and a terminal colostomy constructed.

This case demonstrates clearly that every anal fistula should undergo fractional X-ray examination of the small intestine in order to exclude regional enteritis before deciding upon a local surgical intervention.

Of our 51 patients with regional enteritis 11 had fistulas and abscesses in the anorectal area at the same time. In 7 of these, complete healing was achieved by resection of the diseased bowel segment. In 2 patients with periproctal abscesses immediate incision and drainage was necessary. Following resection of the diseased intestinal segment, the fistulas healed without further operative treatment.

If the fistulas and abscesses are extensive and recurrent, a temporary colostomy for deviating the fecal stream is of advantage. At a second session, resection of the bowel is performed and after the anal fistulas have healed, the colostomy may be closed.

This was done in a 42-year-old woman who had had recurrent anal fistulas and abscesses for many years (Fig. 3). The fractional X-ray examination of the small intestines showed again the typical Kantor sign in the terminal ileum. At operation a mass was found in the small pelvis. From an intestinal fistula a branch system of ducts led into the perirectal region. A resection of the ileocaecal area was performed and at the same time a colostomy was performed in order to deviate the fecal stream. The anal fistulas healed completely. 8 months later the colostomy could be closed and intestinal continuity restored.

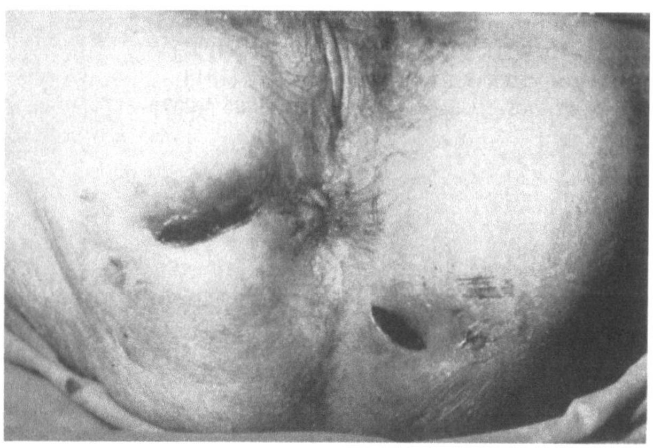

Fig. 3. Recurrent anal fistula in regional enteritis. Healed after resection of the diseased bowel and temporary colostomy.

Bibliography

Altmann, A. D., and D. Golden: Am. J. Dig. Dis. **11**, 658 (1966).

Ansell, B. M., and R. A. D. Wigley: Ann. rheum. Dis. **23**, 64 (1964).

Berning, H., W. Selberg, a. K. G. Thiele: Ileitis regionalis. Stuttgart: Ferd. Enke Verlag 1964.

COLCOCK, B. P.: Surg. Gynec. Obst. **112**, 96 (1961).
—, and C. FORTIN: Ann. Surg. **161**, 812 (1965).
CROHN, B. B.: Ref. 7. Int. Gastroenterologen-Kongreß, Brüssel, Juni 1964 **1**, 444 (1964).
—, Regional Ileitis. New York: Grune & Stratton 1958.
—, N. York Stat. J. Med. **65**, 641 (1965).
DAFFNER, J. E., and C. H. BROWN: Ann. intern. Med. **49**, 580 (1958).
FAHRLÄNDER, H., F. HUBER, u. F. DEUCHER: Ref. 7. Int. Gastroenterologen-Kongreß, Brüssel, Juni 1964 **1**, 491 (1964).
GROSS, PH.: Langenbecks Arch. klin. Chir. **303**, 547 (1963).
GRÖZINGER, K. H., W. WENZ, u. I. KRUPKA: MMW **12**, 649 (1967).
HAFTER, E.: Praktische Gastroenterologie. Stuttgart: Georg Thieme Verlag 1965.
HENNING, N.: Gastroenterology **95**, 258 (1961).
JACKSON, B. B.: Ann. Surg. **148**, 81 (1958).
KANTOR, J. L.: J. A. M. A. **103**, 2016 (1934).
KÜMMERLE, F.: Die chirurgischen Erkrankungen des Dünndarms. Stuttgart: Ferd. Enke Verlag 1963.
—, Enteritis regionalis in „Ungelöste Probleme der Chirurgie". Stuttgart: Georg Thieme Verlag 1966, 135.
LANGEN, D.: Persönliche Mitteilung.
MAINGOT, R.: Abdominal Operations. New York: Appleton-Century-Croffs 1961.
MARX, F. W.: Arch. Surg. **88**, 546 (1964).
MÖRL, F. K.: Bruns Beitr. klin. Chir. **213**, 285 (1966).
PATTER VAN, W. N., I. A. BARGEN, and M. D. DOCKERTY: Gastroenterology **26**, 347 (1954).
POLLOCK, J. H.: Brit. J. Surg. **46**, 193 (1958).
RAVDIN, I. G., and C. G. JOHNSON: Am. J. M. Sc. **198**, 269 (1939).
REIFFERSCHEID, M., u. E. WOLFRAM: Chirurg **33**, 164 (1962).
RHOADS, E.: Pennsylvania M. J. **57**, 433 (1954).
SAUTER, K. E.: Am. J. Surg. **112**, 91 (1966).
SOREN, A.: Arch. intern. Med. **117**, 78 (1966).
STELZNER, F.: Dtsch. med. Wschr. **87**, 286 (1962).
STROHMENGER, P., u. E. MÜLLER: Zbl. Chir. **48**, 1777 (1966).
VANDENBROUCKE, J. P., BODART, C. DIVE, E. CENS, u. G. VANTRAPPEN: Ref. 7. Int. Gastroenterologen-Kongreß Brüssel, Juni 1964, **1**, 451 (1964).
WALTER, L. E., and L. CHAFFIN: West J. Surg. **65**, 354 (1957).
WARREN, S., and S. C. SOMMERS: Am. J. Path. **24**, 475 (1948).
WAYE, J. D., and C. LITHGOW: Gastroenterology **53**, 625 (1967).

Anal Fistula in the Adult and Child

P. Romualdi, Rome, Italy

According to a generally held opinion, the cause of perianal abscesses and fistulas is unknown. Goligher has recently written that these affections are due to hitherto unknown factors.

Another widespread assertion is that perianal abscesses and fistulas rarely occur in children. The pediatric surgery texts agree on this point and deal with the matter along the same lines as for the pathology of the adult; some texts even fail to mention it.

I have already demonstrated in one of my previous papers, that anal fistulas in the child, besides having their own peculiar features, are anything but rare (Table 1).

Table 1. *Bambino Gesù Hospital, Rome. Anal fistulas and abscesses (1955–1967), 146 cases*

Male infant and child	antero-lateral fistulas	116
	medial fistulas	5
	total	121
Female infant and girl	ano-vulvar fistulas	20
	antero-lateral fistulas	5
	total	25

In the child, abscesses and fistulas differ, in site and clinical course from those occurring in the adult; not only that, in the child, they show a different site and behaviour depending on whether the patient is a male or female infant. In studying this affection as it occurs in children, I once again obtained clear proof that the study of pediatric surgical pathology may be useful for a better understanding of the pathology of adults. We note that in the male child, the fistula is almost always located in the anterior half of the anus, in front of the Goodsal line, and that it only rarely occurs in the posterior half. The fistula follows a radial, straigth course, moving from the primary opening to the external orifice in the skin. The primary opening is usually, at the level of the dentate margin.

In the female infant, this affection occurs less frequently, and the site is anterior. As a rule, it precedes a perineal phlegmon situated in the perineum, and extends so far as to cover one labium majus; the fistula coming from it is right in the middle, anovulvar: the primary orifice is at the level of the dentate margin, corresponding to a funnel-shaped depression, at all times well within the reach of the fingers. The orifice is always proximal to the hymen. Secondary sinuses, chiefly in the labium majus, are a frequent occurrence.

A difference between sexes is apparent also in the adult, albeit to a lesser degree. Women usually have a fistula with an anteromedian primary orifice, which very seldom bursts into the vulva; in men, the fistula usually has a posteromedian primary opening, always at the level of the dentate margin. The passage of the fistula is often twisting as Goodsal had stated. Although less frequently, an infantile-type abscess or fistula (chiefly of the male type) may be observed (Table 2).

Table 2. *Policlinico Umberto I., Rcme. 2. Surgical Service. Anal fistulas (1960–1967)*

Adult cases	192
Followed cases	109
Medial anterior fistulas	20
Medial posterior fistulas	72
Antero-lateral fistulas	17
	109

The above-mentioned typical pictures cover the large majority of cases. Atypical pictures also exist, but they are in the minority. The latter group includes fistulas with a rare pathogenesis, such as those of abdominal origin (regional enteritis, cancer of the sigmoid, diverticulitis, etc.). The origin of the horse-shoe abscess is always posteromedian, with the primary opening at the typical site, sometimes caused by a suppurating pre-coccygeal cyst.

What conclusions may be drawn from this?

It will be easy for the pediatric surgeon to draw his conclusions, accustomed as he is to observe and study all congenital malformations.

We have available some reliable basic data:

1. Fistula always have a primary orifice at the level of the dentate margin, at the margin of the crypts of Morgagni.

This statement must be chiefly credited to the English language authors (Buie, Nesselrod). It is true in regard to both adults and children.

2. In most cases, the primary orifice is postero- or antero-median.

In the child (male infant), the orifice is more frequently anterolateral; but in this case its site is also constant. This constant, or at least, preferred site can be noted in the illustrations and descriptions of cases appearing in books and papers of authors who failed to attach relevance to it. This is quite evident, for example, in Stelzner's monography, which is, on the other hand, quite a valuable book for those who devote their attention to this matter.

Bensaude writes that ,,le siège de l'orifice profond est remarquablement fixe. Il est presque toujours commissural posterieur''.

The primary orifice thus has a constant site.

Now, in my opinion, this is an extremely relevant remark, which may be the key to a satisfactory interpretation of the obscure pathogenesis of anal fistulas.

Clinical observation teaches us that when a fistula has a constant site, whether or not it is preceded by a suppurative process, it is of congenital origin. This we observe in the neck, in the head and along the spine. Many years ago, Herr Chiari, a German embryologist, gave an embryological explanation for the origin of fistulas, either congenital or developing after the birth; he affirmed that they represent suture defects and that they always occur along the suture lines. This statement goes under the name of Chiari's rule, or law, it has no exceptions and affords a satisfactory explanation of the origin, not only of fistulas, but also of those congenital cysts, whose site is constant and along the sutural lines.

I will not refrain from declaring that fistulas and congenital cysts are nothing but expressions of the same malformation process.

It is a matter of extent, not of nature.

And perhaps I am right in saying that no congenital fistulas are to be found at the level of limbs, as no suture process occurs in their growth.

If all this is true – if it is true that anal fistulas, not unlike the acknowledged congenital fistulas, have a constant site; if it is true that this site of anal fistulas corresponds to some suture lines, then I believe one cannot help thinking that anal fistulas develop as congenital malformations.

What we know about the embryological development of the anoperineal region, in no way contradicts this assumption. Of course, I refer to the classic embryology, not to that of the present-day surgeons, who often deform it to uphold their theories on the origin of anorectal malformations.

The dentate margin represents the suture line between anus and rectum; the posteromedian line of the anus represents the fusion line between the posterior extremities of the anal tubercles; the anteromedian line of the anus represents the fusion line between the anterior extremities of the same tubercles; the lateral lines along which the anal fistulas of the male infant type develop, represent the suture lines between the perineal body and the anal tubercles.

It is easy to guess that thin fistulous channels, or better "sinuses", may represent these suture defects, and become the site of a fistulous abscess. Infection occurs as a result of the usual obstruction mechanism. Sometimes, the fistulous sinus is accompanied by a cyst located either on the antero- and postero-median, or on the lateral line.

The other interpretations of the pathogenesis of anal fistula are well known.

Cryptitis may occasionally be the cause, but this is an exception, otherwise it would be difficult to explain why a normal anatomical formation so frequently becomes the site of a suppurative process; and it should also be explained why the suppuration of a cryptitis very rarely bursts into the anorectal lumen, and why the crypts on the median line are the site of choice.

Stelzner affirms that the crypts may develop abnormally, especially on the posteromedian line, i. e., where fistulas occur more frequently, thus easily becoming the site of inflammatory processes; but since this is so, some significance should be attributed to the fact that this condition may be a malformation.

The often repeated hypothesis that suppuration is the cause – that the cause of the fistula is an abscess, that the causes of the fistulous abscess (according to Eisenhammer's expression) include abrasions and lesions of the anal cutis, as well as hard stools, is naive. As Parks rightly points out, if it were really so, our operations of hemorrhoids would be frequently followed by infection and fistula.

Lastly, many authors attach paramount importance to the glands of Hermann and Desfosses, previously hinted at by Morgagni and described by Holler Luska, Sömmering and Chiari. Their significance is uncertain and controversial. The German authors call them "sinuses" rather than glands, in agreement with Luska. Since fistulas are frequently transsphincteral, and these sinuses can be found in between the bundles of the external sphincter, it is tempting to attach some importance to them at the onset of the fistulous abscess.

But in the case of the *sinus of* HERMANNI, the objection can also be raised that, since Parks found it in 100% of cases, a normal formation cannot so frequently be the site of an infective process.

This does not happen in any other gland of the digestive tract, and one should explain why the *sinuses* tend to become infected chiefly on the median line.

The intrasphinterical site of many fistulas can be easily explained by the progress of the infection between the various parts of the external sphincter, of which there are no less than three.

According to GOLIGHER, their relevance for initiating these suppurations and fistulas is periodically suggested, only to be discarded soon afterwards. By way of conclusion, I believe we can not deny the value attached to the hypothesis that the majority of abscesses and perianal fistulas originate from suture defects at the lines joining the anal tubercles to the perineal body. It may only explain the fact that most fistulas have the principal orifice at the median and anterolateral lines of the anus.

This hypothesis does not conflict with the clinical observation, with the embryology, with the anatomy or with the pathology.

It is likely, therefore, that this hypothesis is close to the truth.

Bibliography

BENSAUDE, A.: Les hemorroïdes et affections courantes de la région anale. Paris: Maloine 1967.

—, et P. L. CHIGOT: Précis de Proctologie Infantile. Paris: L'Expansion, Ed. 1960.

BUIE, L. A.: Practical Proctology. 2. Ed. Springfield, Illinois-USA 1960.

EISENHAMMER, S.: The anorectal fistulous abscess and fistula. Diseases of Colon and Rectum 7, 498 (1936).

HERRMANN, G., et L. DESFOSSES: Sur la mouqueuse Cloacale du Rectum. C. R. Acad. Sci. **90**, 1301 (1880).

GABRIEL, W. B.: The principles and practice of rectal surgery. London: H. K. Lewis and Co. 1963.

GOODSALL, D. H., and W. E. MILES: Diseases of the anus and rectum. London: Longmans, Green and Co. 1900.

GOLIGHER, T. C.: Treatment of anal abscess and fistula. Modern Trends in Surg. **1**, 39 (1962).

v. HALLER, A.: cit. by STELZNER.

MORGAGNI, G. B.: Adversaria Anatomica Omnia. Advers. III. Animadv. VI, p. II. Patavii 1719 (cit. by STELZNER).

NESSELROD, I. P.: Clinical Proctology. 3 . Ed. Phil. and London: Saunders Co 1964.

PARKS, A. G.: Pathogenesis and treatment of fistula in ano. Brit. Med. Jour. Feb. 18, 1961.

ROMUALDI, P.: Acquired recto-vaginal fistula in infancy etc. Riv. Chir. Ped. **2**, 239 (1960).

—, A new "heretical" (but not too much) approach to pathogenesis of the malformations of anus and rectum (A study on 151 cases). Riv. Chir. Ped. **4**, 113 (1962).

—, Classification of the ano-rectal abnormalities. Riv. Chir. Pod. **7**, 1 (1965).

STELZNER, F.: Die anorectalen Fisteln. Berlin-Göttingen-Heidelberg: Springer 1959

STEPHENS, F. D.: Congenital Malformations of the rectum, anus and genito-urinary tracts. Edinb. and. London: E. and S. Livingstone Ltd. 1963

III. Chronic Obstipation

Surgical Treatment of Chronic Obstipation

M. Reifferscheid, Aachen, Germany

Obstipation is a symptom of disturbed intestinal motor function. It is produced by intra- and paraintestinal as well as extraintestinal stimuli. Thus the number of possible disturbances is manifold. Hence a pathogenetic clarification is necessary before individual cases can be treated according to their cause. In practice this means that a clear line must be drawn between the intra- or para-intestinal causes of obstipation and the extraintestinal functional forms when one decides on the indication for operation (Table 1).

Table 1.

morphologically caused obstipation

- paraintestinal causes
- intraintestinal causes
  - (intramural, intraluminal)

Naturally, errors in setting the general indication can be avoided if conservative treatment is first applied so as to rule out functional influences before looking for a morphological cause. But the postulate of a timely causal treatment is not fulfilled, and can only be attained by a simultaneous diagnostic investigation which takes into account all the possible causes. The main reason for stating this precondition is experience, which has taught us that obstipation is a cardinal symptom of malignant intestinal affections.

Our present conception of the pathogenesis of obstipation is based on investigations by Chaudhary, Ritter, Connel, and in a more general sense on those by Bloom, as well as on my own observations.

In almost every form of para- or intraintestinal obstipation, the initial reaction which leads to passage obstruction is due to stenosis caused by a spasm. Chronic obstruction of the passage first sets in with the oral progression of the spastic contraction. Whether the intraintestinally produced spasm is due to local irritation or due to a morphological obstruction is of secondary importance. The obstruction may be of a paraintestinal kind – in other words brought about by external causes such as compression, pinching, folding or strangulation, – or due to intraintestinal processes proceeding from the lumen or the intestinal wall.

The first phase of obstipation, where the actual spastic cause is as yet the sole predominant feature, responds clinically to the treatment with spasmolytics. Phase two, the alternate spastic and atonic obstipation, responds only occasionally to spasmolytics. Finally, the third phase, that of atony, can be alleviated only with such tonics as Physostigmin and Hypophysin. Obstipation induced by intra- and paraintestinal causes, however, leads to an altogether different course of development of the three phases to that of the idiopathic primarily functional form, as we have learned by clinical experience, and this has dictated our policy. As a rule with very few exceptions, idiopathic primarily functional obstipation induced by extraintestinal, neural stimuli, show a more protracted course of development. Between the spasm of stage I and the complete atony of stage III there is often a period of some years. In the case of the idiopathic intestinal morphological forms, on the other hand, only a relatively short period of weeks or months lies between the same two stages. A contracted aberration of morphologically conditioned obstipation is represented by ileus. This condition can be generally regarded as exhibiting a pathophysiological course of obstipation. In the clinic, where initially effective spasmolytic treatment suddenly fails, a morphological cause of the obstipation can be assumed.

In discussing different morphological causes for obstipation, we will begin with the paraintestinal group (Table 2). Firstly, recurrent appendicitis and perityphlitis should be excluded as the most frequent cause of obstipation. Where the clinical picture is vague, a reliable basis for diagnosis is provided in younger patients if the appendix fails to appear during x-ray examination and if there are pressure-pains in this area, combined with a tympanitic caecum. A further cause is the variability in the fixation and location of the mobile ascending colon. This may by manifest either in the form of an ostensible appendicitis or in painful, chronic, intermittent obstipation. During the last years, we have operated seven such cases, mostly younger women. By affixing the mobile ascending colon, we were able to free them of their intermittent, chronic constipation. The operation of affixation is simple, and x-ray examination in combination with the clinical findings permits an easy diagnosis. Appendectomy should always be performed at the same time. Besides the mobile ascending colon, the excessively pronounced Jackson membrane should be mentioned, which constricts the ascending colon and appears on the roentgenograph picture as a pseudosphincter (Hirsch). Sometimes physiosis of the caecum and lower ascending colon accompanied by caecal rumblings dominate the clinical picture. The results achieved by this operation, due caution being exercised in setting the indication, show the significance of this malformation.

Table 2. *Paraintestinal causes*

1. Chronic relapsing appendicitis and perityphlitis.
2. Anomalies of position and fixation (Caecocolon mobile, Jacksons's membrane, malrotation, mesocolic hernia).
3. „Doppelflintenbildung" (reduplikation) of bowel flexures (Payer).
4. Adhesions.
5. Compression from the neighbourhood (pancreas, bladder, spleen).

The malformations such as malrotation and especially the mesocolic hernia can present with intermittent obstipation, even in older patients. Obstipation can present in intestinal obturation, as the small intestine is affected by malrotation. It is usually easy to diagnose these malformations with the help of a barium meal where one can see the whole of the large intestine on the left side and the whole of the small intestine on the right. Restoration in the normal anatomical position cures the patient of his complaints completly. We were able to observe this in recent years in the case of a boy aged 16 years and a female patient aged 32 years.

Till now we have discussed the paraintestinal obstruction which manifests clinically as mechanical obstipation. We shall now discuss a group of conditions which are a rather problematic chapter for the surgeon. First of all one has to mention the "Payer's double-barrel" of the left colonic flexure which one finds so often mentioned in the literature. In our experience this finding as such has no clinical significance. Only when it is the result of the linear growth due to aboral spasm or inflammation, could it cause complete obstruction with partial volvulus. And only when this is proved to be the case, do we consider the resection of the double-barrel as indicated.

The double-barrel due to the stenosis of the flexure on the other hand, is a different category. This is often seen as a result of pancreatitis with islets of necrosis in the tail of the pancreas, relaxation of the diaphragm and several other conditions in the left epigastrium. It is certainly wrong to resect the double-barrel considering it as the cause of the supposed obstipation, when one cannot demonstrate tangible morphological changes. The seriousness of operation is then in no proportion to its cause.

The abdominal adhesions which are responsible for obstipation, are even more problematic. The removal of adhesions to cure obstipation is indicated only after it is proved clinically as well as radiologically that there is a definite relation between the complaints and this cause.

In the recent years we had opportunity to observe an unusual cause of obstipation in 2 cases.

An extremely large diverticulum of the bladder caused intermittent compression of the sigmoid colon. This was diagnosed by introducing a catheter which immediately relieved the patient of his complaints.

The intramural or intraluminal causes of obstipation are characterized by the presence of the obligatory clinical phenomenon, intermittent, sometimes even colicky pain (Table 3). The resection frees the patient of the complaints.

Table 3. *Intraintestinal causes*

1. Benign and malignant tumors (sometimes with invagination).
2. Diverticulitis.
3. Inflammatory strictures (TB).
4. Mega- and dolichocolon.
5. Blind-Loop-formation.
6. Reduplication.
7. Anal findings (fissures, haemorrhoids, fistula, abscess, proctitis).

A special form of obstipation which is accompanied by intermittent colics is chronic recurrent invagination in the adult. An exophytic tumor which projects into the lumen of the bowel especially in the region of the ileocaecal valve is the usual cause. Due to the absence of a dramatic symptomatology, it often takes months or even years to find the cause.

The intermittent obstipation which sets in during the 5th decade especially in males is often the result of the stenosis which is found predominantly in the sigmoid colon. The primary cause of this stenosis is either a carcinoma or diverticulitis. Let us discuss the symptomatology of diverticulitis or sigmoiditis rather than that of the carcinoma, the latter being very well known. The inflammatory sclerosis of muscle and the connective tissue of the wall progressively constricts the lumen for the lenght of about 10 to 20 cm and this causes the typical sigmoid obstipation. Clinically localized tympanitic percussion sounds stop abruptly at this site on the left lower obdomen. This tympanitic region is often painful and disappears after defecation in contrast to the tumor palpable in front of the iliac bone. This was seen in the X-ray film as the so-called diverticulitis tumor.

But obstipation is only one of the cardinal symptoms of this progressive disease. Together with all the other symptoms and signs, clinical as well as radiological, it creates difficulties in differential diagnosis with carcinoma. This realization dictates our indication for resection. The indication is based on three considerations:

1. to get rid of the obstipation
2. as prophylaxis against the deadly complications which are certain to set in,
3. to clarify the difficult differential diagnosis between this and carcinoma.

The enlargement of the colon presents itself as a chronic obstruction occurs in many different forms. Pathogenetically we have to differentiate megacolons caused by primarily stenotic, functional or symptomatic from the primarily atonic idiopathic forms of megacolon. In the first group – megacolon due to stenosis – the disease begins with an aboral obstruction.

a) aganglionic paralytic segment (Bodian), or Hirschsprung's disease
b) in form of anal spasm, or different types of anal or sigmoid stenosis.

The obstruction blocks the lumen and initially gives rise to increased spastic activity of the colon which attempts to overcome the obstruction with the following results:

a) the wall of the bowel hyperthrophies
b) the bowel increases in width and length.

Aboral stenosis, spasm, hypertrophy, increase in width and length are the hallmarks of this process. The bowel thus deformed is no longer able to transport its contents and slowly becomes itself an obstructive element. This form of obstipation could be cured by removal of the cause of the megacolon i. e. stenosis, anal spasm and the paralytic segment. But with that alone we cannot relieve the patient of his obstipation, we also have to resect the elongated and widened colon which has become an obstruction. The removal of the original obstruction alone is sufficient only at an early stage, i. e. before the oral end of the colon starts increasing in size.

Simple dilatation of the anal canal is sufficient to remove the main obstruction, not only in cases of advanced stenosis with secondary megacolon of the pediatric patients. With this therapy we can see immediate good results in cases of painful anal conditions such as fistula, haemorrhoids and fissures which are usually accompanied by spasm. Good results are also obtained in cases of obstipation personality who are psychologically cramped. Anal spasm has more than one way of influencing the motor activity of the entire colon i. e. in its role as an obstructive agent, it also affects the activity of colon through the retrocolic inhibitory reflex.

With that we approach the form of obstipation, running over the reflex arches (extraintestinal obstipation), idiopathic megacolon being the first and the foremost type. It has no spastic or mechanical basis for the obstipation, which is typical for the morphological forms. The resection of the colon in this case only has a symptomatic effect as the increase in the width and length of the bowel are only secondary phenomena. Even then, the subtotal resection of the colon with subsequent treatment with ergot-alcaloids can be regarded as a successful form of treatment.

Other types of obstipation are the result of the viscero-visceral reflex caused by foci of diseases other than those of the bowel, for example diseases of the gall bladder and bile ducts, of the pancreas, of the urogenital system and portal hypertension due to liver cirrhosis. Finally pheochromocytoma and parathyroid adenoma may cause chronic obstipation (Table 4). The operative removal of the tumor is indicated in every case.

Table 4. *Extraintestinal causes*

Viscero-visceral reflexes	Neurogenic	
gallstone	idiopathic megacolon	pheochromocytoma
gastric- and duodenal ulcers	diseases of central	adenoma of the parathy-
pancreatitis	nervous sytem	roid glands
stone of ureter	diseasis of peripheral	
prostatitis	nervous system	
gynecological findings	psychogenesis pathological	
liver cirrhosis with portal	behaviour	
hypertension		

We follow the following scheme for diagnosis, indication and therapy:

The diagnosis is based on:

1. case-history with special reference to the earlier obstipations and the possible causes of the obstipation.

2. digital examination per rectum, gynecological examination, percussion, auscultation and palpation of the abdomen. The visual examination of the feces is as important as the laboratory results of blood sedimentation rate, blood cell count, serum proteins, electrolytes, haemoglobin and haematocrit. With the help of barium-meal and barium-enema, we can exclude the malignant tumor. Function is tested with diagnostic doses of spasmolytics and tonics. Only after the morphological causes are diagnostically excluded can one be content with the diagnosis "functional obstipation".

The following requirements must be satisfied for setting the indication for the operation in cases of obstipation:

1. extreme and chronic obstipation with detrimental effects on the general condition of the patient.

2. rapid transition of the spastic phase into the atonic phase.

3. the congruent localization of the clinical and radiological examinations.

4. the identical localization according to the palpatory, auscultatory and percutory examination of the colon.

5. constancy of the pathological findings in the X-ray of the colon such as an anomaly of the position, changes of the width of the lumen and increase in the length.

At operation, the following technical points have proved to be helpful:

1. preoperative sterilisation of the bowel with energetic purgation and antibiotic medication.

2. the resection of the obstructive agent, i. e. spastic bowel, the segment that has undergone inflammatory alteration and the hypertrophied, dilated and elongated oral part with end to end anastamosis in two layers.

3. postoperative dilatation of the spincter.

4. early laxation of the operated patient with measures ensuring the stimulation of the peristaltic movements:

I. castor oil in case of colon to colon anastamosis

II. paraffin medication in case of anastamosis between large and small bowel

III. ergot-alcaloids for increasing the tone in cases of the primarily atonic form.

Bibliography

BLOOM, A., PH. LO PRESTI, and J. T. FARRAR: Motility of the intact human colon. Gastroenterology **54**, 232 (1968).

CHAUDHARY, N. A., and S. C. TRUELOVE: Colonic Motility. Amer. J. Med. **31**, 86 (1961).

CONNELL, A. M.: The Motility of the pelvic colon. Gut **2**, 175 (1961); **3**, 342 (1962).

DEMLING, L., u. R. OTTENJANN: Motilitäts- und Sekretionsstörungen des Darms. In Klinik der Frauenheilkunde und Geburtshilfe, SCHWALM-DÖDERLEIN, München, Berlin: Urban u. Schwarzenberg 1965.

FINSTERER, H.: Resultate der operativen Behandlung der chronischen Obstipation. Arch. klin. Chir. **268**, 174 (1951).

—, Colonresektion bei chronischer Obstipation. Arch. klin. Chir. **138**, 449 (1925).

ORESTANO, F.: Zur Pathohistologie des Auerbach-Plexus beim sogen. sekundären Megacolon. Brun's Beitr. klin. Chir. **216**, 233 (1968).

RITTER, N.: Untersuchungen über die Motorik des Darmtraktes. Gastroenterologie (Basel) **86**, 80 (1956).

NIEBERREITHER, H.: Die Hemicolectomie zur Behandlung der chron. Obstipation. Brun's Beitr. klin. Chir. **183**, 166 (1951).

Current Problems in Constipation[1]

R. OTTENJANN, Erlangen, Germany

When BAYLISS and STARLING stated that "in no other sector of physiology do opinion and fact differ so widely as in the physiology of intestinal motility" in 1899, they could have had no idea that, more than half a century later, the situation would hardly have changed. The physiology and pathophysiology of intestinal motility and of the passage of ingesta through the intestine, have become interesting again in the last decade. Results of animal experiments and clinical findings have often been at odds with the generally accepted teachings. Even today, for example, the opinion is widespread that intestinal hypermotility leads to accelerated passage and thus to diarrhoea, while the intestinal movements in constipation are characterized predominantly by hypomotility and "atony".

The information on the pathophysiology of intestinal movements is based almost exclusively on results produced by cineradiography and intraluminal manometry. The results can in as much as a definitive judgement is possible at this stage – be summarized by saying that the intestinal transport of ingested material is subject to similar laws as those pertaining to the blood circulation. The dominating factors are the pressure gradients between the proximal and distal parts of the intestine, and the peripheral resistance, which inhibits the transport and which is chiefly based on the segmental contraction of the intestinal wall [16]. Segmental intestinal contractions such as are also manifested in the formation of haustra, are the chief intestinal activity reponsible for increasing the intraluminal pressure and can thus be recorded manometrically [15]. Propulsive intestinal movements usually lead to no, or only insignificant, manometric waves. Pressure measurements in the small and large intestines provided apparently paradox results. They showed that in constipation, the intestinal activity tending to promote an increase in pressure, is often increased or normal, while in diarrhoea, a striking manometric "calm" is usually recorded in the intestine. Segmental intestinal activity, which inhibits the passage of ingesta, is thus less often recorded than in healthy persons [2, 5, 7]. Diarrhoea means accelerated passage as a result of reduced local intestinal contractions, while constipation is, in the main, the expression of an obstruction of the passage of ingesta resulting from increased segmental activity. Thus the constipative effect of codein and opium is not – as is generally believed – due to the lowering of the intestinal tone, but results from an increase in the intensity of segmental intestinal contractions [14]. For this reason, anticholinergic drugs can, in cases of constipation not only act "spasmolytically", but can also accelerate the transit of ingesta so that they usually remain without effect in cases of diarrhoea.

[1] With the support of the Deutsche Forschungsgemeinschaft.

Personal Investigations

The influence of sympathetic and parasympathetic nerves on the activity of the intestine in vertebrates becomes progressively less, from the amphibian onwards. In higher vertebrates, when both the sympathetic and parasympathetic nerves supplying the intestine are severed, intestinal activity still continues apparently normally [8]. Sympathectomy has no effect, and vagotomy no clinically recognizable effect on intestinal motility [3] in most cases. In addition to this nervous regulation, the intestinal activitiy is also influenced by humeral and hormonal factors. Constipation is a symptom of *primary hyperparathyroidism* and of other *hypercalcemia syndromes*. A direct effect of the parathormone on the intestinal musculature was not proved. Both *acute* and *chronic hypercalcemia* stimulate the gastric secretion of acid and the functional activity of endocrine cells [1, 12]. An increase in the extracellular calcium concentration promotes the inter- and intracellular spread of excitation. In many functions, magnesium acts as an antagonist to calcium. In three separate series of investigations, we examined the influence of acute *hypercalcemia* and *hypermagnesemia* on the activity of the intestinal musculature tending to promote an increase in pressure. During intravenous infusion of calcium with subsequent hypercalcemia, a significant increase in intestinal motility (wave frequency, length of activity and motility index) compared with the resting motility and with placebo infusion (fructose) was demonstrated. In the second and third experimental series, hypermagnesemia was induced. The result was a statistically significant inhibition of the resting motility and of the colon motility associated with pressure activity and induced by hypercalcemia (wave frequency, length of activity, motility index and wave amplitude). All in all, these experimental results allow us to draw the conclusion that hypercalcemia stimulates the smooth muscles of the intestine to pressure-active segmental activity, and in this way delays the intestinal passage of ingesta. Hypermagnesemia inhibits both this influence of hypercalcemia and the pressure-active resting motility, and thus produces intraluminal pressure curves such as are often recorded in cases of diarrhoea. Our results are, to some extent, at odds with clinical observations in patients with hypomagnesemia and diarrhea which could only be influenced by the administration of high doses of magnesium [9].

The peptide hormones which influence intestinal motility, include bradykinin, vasopressin and others, as well as *gastrin*, which has been analysed and synthesized in the meantime. In experiments, both with animals and human subjects, a motility-enhancing effect has been demonstrated in both small and large intestine [10, 11]. As a result of his investigations, LOGAN [10] has spoken of a physiological mediator role played by gastrin in the gastrocolic "reflex". Our information on the hormonal physiological regulation of intestinal motility is still completely inadequate. Above all, we know too little about these hormones in the pathophysiology of intestinal movement. The same is true for *serotonin*, which acts not only as a direct stimulant of the intestinal musculature, but which also works as a carrier substance of the newly discovered nonadrenergic neurons in the myenteric plexus, and thus indirectly inhibits the intestinal musculature. A third point of attack for serotonin is provided by the afferent nerve fibres in the intestinal mucosa, which are stimulated [6, 7]. Scientific interest is at present concerned with the potential significance of serotonin in the pathogenesis paralytic ileus and of diverticulosis coli.

Until recently the diagnostic methods used to differentiate between functional constipation and organic constipation were limited to X-ray examination and sigmoidoscopy. A new technique, *transintestinal intubation*, appears suited to extend our diagnostic facilities [4, 13]. The oral-anal, end to end, tube technique allows biopsy tubes, catheters and fully flexible glass fiberscopes to be introduced retrograde into the intestine as far as BAUHIN'S valve and into the caecum. To date, we have been able to carry out transintestinal intubation in twenty-three patients, and have introduced various probes and instruments as far as the ascending colon. This possibility opens new avenues for scientific investigation. For example, solid state detectors can be introduced as far as BAUHIN'S valve and, by means of radioactive substances, the passage of ingesta through the small and large intestines can be distinguished exactly.

Bibliography

1. BARRERAS, R. F., and R. M. DONALDSON: Effects of induced hypercalcemia on human gastric secretion. Gastroenterology **52**, 670 (1967).
2. BLOOM, A. A., P. LO PRESTI, and J. T. FARRAR: Motility of the intact human colon. Gastroenterology **54**, 232 (1968).
3. CHRISTENSEN, J.: The adrenergic nerves and gastrointestinal smooth muscle function. Gastroenterology **55**, 135 (1968).
4. COLAGRANDE, C., P. ARULLANI, and C. CASALE: A suction-biopsy procedure for obtaining specimens of mucosa from the right and left colon. Amer. J. dig. Dis. **11**, 389 (1966).
5. CONNELL, A. M.: Recording of intestinal motility: routine or research? Gut **8**, 527 (1967).
6. FARRAR, J. T., and A. M. ZFASS: Small intestinal motility. Gastroenterology **52**, 1019 (1967).
7. GERSHON, M. D.: Serotonin and the motility of the gastrointestinal tract. Gastroenterology **54**, 453 (1968).
8. HIATT, R. B., I. GOODMAN, and A. ALAVI: Hormonal control of intestinal motility. Ann. Surg. **166**, 704 (1967).
9. HOLTMEIER, H. J., u. P. RIECHERT: Magnesiummangel bei Krankheiten des Magen-Darmtraktes. In: Aktuelle Gastroenterologie, hrsg. von H. BARTELHEIMER, N. HEISIG, S. 369. Stuttgart: Thieme 1968.
10. LOGAN, C. J. H.: Gastrin as an intestinal activator. Brit. J. Surg. **54**, 297 (1967).
11. MIKOS, E., and J. R. VANE: Effects of gastrin and its analogues on isolated smooth muscles. Nature **214**, 105 (1967).
12. OTTENJANN, R., F. WIDMAIER, u. L. DEMLING: Magensekretion bei akuter Hyperkalzämie und Hypermagnesiämie. Verh. Dtsch. Ges. inn. Med. **69**, 160 (1963).
13. OTTENJANN, R.: Endoskopie und Biopsie des Colon. Dtsch. med. Wschr. **93**, 1372 (1968).
14. PAINTER, N. S., and S. C. TRUELOVE: The intraluminal pressure patterns in diverticulosis of the colon. Part I: Resting patterns of pressure. Gut **5**, 201 (1964).
15. PAINTER, N. S., and D. OBST: The correlation of the pressures in the human colon with the shape of the colonic lumen as shown by cineradiography combined with simultafeous pressure recording. Amer. J. dig. Dis. **13**, 468 (1968).
16. TEXTER, E. C.: Pressure and transit in the small intestine. Amer. J. dig. Dis. **13**, 443 (1968).

Psychosomatic Aspects in Chronic Constipation

J. M. GARRIGUES and C. A. BRUERE-DAWSON, Montpellier, France

ERIK BRIKSON, the American psychoanalyst, sees the excessive tendencies of Martin Luther toward constipation as the underlying cause of the reformation. Without wanting to make his statement ours, we recognize as he does the importance of the psychological factor in chronic constipation.

This widespread affection has many causes – some functional, other psychogenic. In reality, these factors are almost always both involved.

Our purpose is to show the existence of these interactions and the importance of knowing about them, not only to establish an effective treatment but to see through the constipation and find an underlying personality problem.

In the first chapter we will summarize the psycho-physio-pathological bases of the syndrome according to the emotional concept which PIERON defined psychologically as "An intensive affective reaction of diencephalic origin and involving vegetative manifestations".

In the second chapter we consider the clinical manifestations by showing that a purely psychic disorder can change functional disorders into organic troubles, and conversely that an organic ailment can result from psychic or neurovegetative troubles which evolve on their own when the somatic lesion is gone.

"The abdomen is the echo chamber of the emotions" according to WEISS and ENGLEISH. In fact, certain popular expressions recognize the soundness of this conception ("to feel fear in the stomach . . .") and in the same light, experimentally one can create digestive troubles by means of emotional stress.

The psycho-physio-pathological bases of these manifestations are well known. Actually, the entire neuroendocrine system participates here, but to simplify matters we will say that the hypothalamus plays the main role as the central integrator of the emotions and as a relay zone between the neighboring centers above and below: fronto-orbital pole of the cortex, rhinencephalus, hypophysis and the ortho- and para-sympathetic autonomic nervous systems.

The hypothalamus modulates the humor, the affective and emotional expressions, the springing up of needs . . .

Experimentally, stimulation of the posterior and lateral nuclei causes a hypokinesis and a fall in intestinal secretion, while stimulation of the anterior nucleus gives the opposite results.

The fronto-orbital anterior pole of the cortex and the rhinencephalus also play an important role in the integration of emotions.

Their stimulation almost always affects the vegetative function and above all the digestive motility.

The hypothalamo-pituitary interaction explains the importance of the endocrine factors on the behavior of the digestive tract.

In the case of the hypothyroid, the endocrine aspect is pure and results in a true and persistent constipation – it can also come from the neuro-psychic domain of the subject. Among these "hypersympathicotonics", women known as "orthosympathicotonics" are witness to the fact that their constipation is aggravated during the premenstrual period. The association of constipation and sclero-cystic ovaritis is rather frequently the organic expression of emotional troubles and sexual irritation.

The ortho- and parasympathetic autonomic nervous systems represent the somatic expression of the emotions. Under the predominant influence of the parasympathetic system the individual abandons his external problems and retires into the depth of his vegetative existence. Conversely, by stimulating of the orthosympathetic system, this same individual neglects or even inhibits the functions of reconstruction and growth and directs his attention towards solving these external problems (ALEXANDER).

The function of colonic motility for example, is the result of an antagonism or symbiosis of the two autonomic nervous systems: "The orthosympathetic makes the colon longer, wider, drier, and sluggish while the parasympathetic makes the colon shorter, narrower, increases both the secretion and the motility, in short, more active" (B. HENRY).

These facts allow us to understand the slim margin of dependance which exists between defecation, a banal act in itself, and the cultural and psycho-affective tonus of the individual. DAVÈNPORT was able to show the variations of peristalsis and the color of the secretions according to the change of moods in a patient with a colostomy.

C. QUARTI, J. RENAUD and CH. DEBRAY were able to record variations in the tone of the colon in a patient subjected to stress by means of a balloon catheter. This brings us to the discussion of the pyschological and clinical expression of chronic constipation.

The clinical manifestations of chronic constipation are not singular. They are sometimes permanent and well tolerated, entailing only some functional neurovegetative troubles. Sometimes, however, they are transitory, poorly tolerated, and end up by causing organic troubles. Occasionally they even come about, after a lesion has long been cured. This is what we call "after effect constipation".

The most simple and most common form is that which is imposed by the trepidant rhythm of our daily lives. It is particularly frequent among women whose activities consist of both domestic and professional duties. They are mostly hypersympatheticotoniques with a touch of hyperthyroidism with shiny, animated eyes, they are slim, eat very little, constantly on the go and refuse to relax long enough to allow physiological conditioning for defecation. Usually their constipation is well tolerated. It is among such patients as these that splanchnic infiltration gives such beneficial results.

In this category falls the "bad habit constipation". It is by far the most frequent. It is an ailment of our times. The rhythm of our lives, the expediency permits neither child nor adult to satisfy at any desired moment, the need to defecate. It is thus that the physiological reflexes gradually fade and disappear.

Another type of simple constipation is that encountered during voyages where rhythm and habits are interrupted thus reducing rectal sensitivity. This condition could be the beginning of a chronic constipation initiated by poor habits.

A form slightly more complex is the constipation which comes about after a serious or radical change of living habits. An example is the young girl who enters a boarding school and having lost the rhythm and family framework, becomes des-orientated and anxious. A temporary amenorrhea is often associated which is proof of a deep commotion resulting in diencephalo-pituitary trouble. This can be compared to the cases of temporary amenorrhea (6 months), sometimes permanent, which are often observed among young girls dedicating themselves to religion.

Another type of psychogenic constipation raises a new factor: inhibition. This is seen in patients, who pay too much attention to defection; this can modify and even inhibit colo-rectal motility. The most effective treatment here is psychotherapy plus tranquilizers, a treatment which is also applied in cases of impotence of non hormonal origin. But constipation can also be an expression of more serious personality troubles.

ALEXANDER estimates that the chronically constipated patient has a particular attitude; he is a pessimist, a defeatist, lacking confidence in himself, and having the feeling of not being liked and being rebuffed. And pushing it to the extreme, he might be a paranoid or a melancholic. It is this which makes him say "the chronic constipated patient has the suspicions of a paranoid and the pessimism of a melancholic". For these patients, constipation is an attitude. Being anxious, inhibited, and not having confidence in others, they hold on to their fecal matter as well as everything else vital to them.

The psychoanalysts hold to the idea that the origin of these psychogenic troubles of intestinal function stem from childhood and the manner in which the problem was resolved: should he give or should he keep that which is his, concerning the fecal matter. This conflict can be seen in all levels of life. The response to this problem depends to a great extent to the experiences in training and to the attitude of an overprotective mother or on the other hand, one without affection.

The encopresia of childhood and chronic constipation represent the somatic component of a hostile refusal to give, to waste, or of a reaction of protest which might be directed against an obsessional conformite or an excessive maternal solicitude. It must be said that encopresia can be a means of attracting attention for the child. It can also cover up a sexual component; in the act of refusing the urge to defecate, a certain joy is realized.

We can see then that these psychic disturbances can cause purely functional troubles. However, it is not always this way. The states of emotional tension produced by situations of conflict, (even though they may not result in spectacular effects of violent emotion) will produce all sorts of endocrino-vegetative functional disturbances which became important in the long run. The transformation of emotion to lesion is one particular case of a general law which states: a neuro-vegetative disorder entails functional manifestations which produce organic disturbances by their intensity and repetition (CLAUDE BERNARD, RAYNAUD, REILLY). Two examples can be cited: a resistant constipation which accompanies a sclero-cystic ovaritis and an irritable and spastic colon.

It is well known that, sclero-cystic ovaritis is frequently seen together with important emotional problems and irritative sexual factors such as dyspareunia. QUARTI, who studied these problems in regard to biliary dyskinesis, noted that these patients showed disturbances of mood and affectivity with significant emotional reactivity and almost uncontrollable neuro-vegetative reactions. He also noted that they have a tendency to direct emotional forces against themselves. In all these cases, the functional and organic disorders become established after the patient has suffered from psychosymatic disturbances, particularly from chronic constipation for a long time.

We may find the explanation for an irritable and spastic colon in the studies by REILLY. They show that non-specific irritation of the vegetative system can cause intestinal lesions which range from stasis to edema, and from leucodiapedesis and erythrodiapedesis to infarction with its consequences – ulcerations and necroses. One can easily understand why, in a predisposed individual, a colon which reacts to emotional solicitations as violently as DAVENPORT witnessed in his patient with a colostomy, presents organic disorders after a time. Patients with irritable colon syndrome are above all depressive hypochondriacs and hysterical women with considerable neuro-vegetative lability. Constipation alternates with diarrhea and is accompanied by many other symptoms such as insomnia, asthenia, headaches, vertigo, nausea, flatulence . . .

Laxophilia often creates or at least complicates functional troubles. It is common among patients who have a normal daily defecation and who imagine the volume to be insufficient; because they are afraid of getting dirty or because they worry about a pseudo-intestinal comfort which they should have felt after an evacuating enema, they use and abuse a large number of laxatives, thereby creating a laxophilia. In other cases, the patients are really constipated. They are usually women, who are anxious and emotional, having a mental comportment similar to that seen in mental anorexia. They cannot tolerate their constipation whether real or relative either because it provokes the symptoms already described or because consciously or not they fear stercoral intoxication through their dislike for getting dirty and their need for cleanliness. The only solution seems to lie in the taking of laxatives which irritate, thereby creating a true colitis and often serious hydro-electrolytic disturbances which can only aggravate their problems. The result is that they have the laxative disease. The third part of our triptych is the one we call "after effect constipation". It is a psychogenic constipation secondary to an already present organic lesion.

It can be a neurovegetative souvenir. It is the case with post-amibian constipation which is part of the post-amibian syndrome occurring during metamibien enteritis or tropical neurasthenia of MANSON-BAHR and CRAIG. This colitis acts above all by a neuro vegetative mechanism giving a psychic impression of insecurity, anxiety, asthenia and fatigue. It is in such a manner that the intestinal dyskineses which have become resistant to treatment, bring about nervous and psychic troubles. All this is embraced by the somato-psychic domain.

It can also be the conscious and obsessive remembrance of an intolerable pain during defecation. JEAN DUHAMEL studied this syndrome in the child and thinks it occurs in the particular case where it is associated with an encopresia. It is usually seen among anxious children who are sometimes even phobic, often overprotected by their mothers. We have also seen this syndrome in a 40-year-old man operated on for a very painful anal fissure who would not defecate after the operation, so great was his obsession. After the twelfth day, he had to be anesthetized so that the fecal matter could be removed. The anesthesia was performed as psychotherapy. Afterwards the patient went to the toilet normally, having been persuaded that now that the fecaloma had been removed, he would have no more pain.

Sigmoid Fixation Syndrome

T. WILENSKY, Lansing, Michigan, U. S. A.

Chronic non-tumorous incompletely obstructing colopathy deserves much more frequent and earlier clinical recognition.

Characteristically following abdominopelvic surgery, this somewhat obscure syndrome is marked by poorly localized, deeply-seated left-sided pain frequently associated with the sensations of weight and pressure and ungratified bowel evacuations.

Extensions of pain into the left sacroiliac region is common. The urge to defecate and repeated unsuccessful efforts to secure relief by this means has very often resulted in the use of frequent enemas and/or laxatives which at best have provided temporary and unsatisfactory symptomatic improvement.

Most often patients with this syndrome have been referred by gynecologists although a few have had orthopedic and neurosurgical consultations. A positive diagnosis had not been made in any instance although a number had been submitted to barium enema examinations. Strangely enough, the one woman referred from a neurosurgeon with the probable diagnosis of dysfunctional pelvic colon disease was after investigation referred elsewhere for reconsideration of intervertebral disc disease since it had not been possible to incriminate her pelvic colon. This diagnosis was confirmed and laminectomy was performed with excellent effect.

Many have been obsessed with the frequently given opinion that this is a neurosis or the irritable bowel syndrome. Exploratory operations that have failed to recognize the anatomical deviations are, I suspect, rather common. Such surgical interventions are of no value and will more than likely complicate the problem further. This introduction will suggest that the sigmoid fixation syndrome is not usually established with the first consultation. Obviously the possibility must be considered if it is to be recognized at all.

A detailed and searching history is absolutely essential. The painstaking physical examination including abdominopelvirectal palpation and proctosigmoidoscopy is followed by roentgenography. The roentgenologist is best treated as a consultant and his informed cooperation will be rewarded with observations especially during fluoroscopy that are indispensable.

Unfortunately the barium enema examination may seriously mislead in this syndrome by failing to reveal the character and degree of deformity present.

Diagnostic failure with roentgenography in the small bowel matting syndrome has similarly contributed to serious delay in management. Many such afflicted patients have been dismissed as confirmed neurotics and not rarely have resorted to alcohol or habituating drugs for pain relief. These facts have been attested to in numerous publications.

In this presentation all conditions marked by low abdominal pain and the passage of mucus and blood rectally must be considered. Pathologic states involving the genitourinary and neuroskeletal systems must be ruled out, of course. Irradiation injury to the small and/or large bowel is frequently overlooked and the essential surgical correction consequently withheld.

Roentgenographically observed colonic abnormalities of the so-called prediverticular state received considerable attention in the recent literature. Prediverticular disease of the colon or unmistakable active diverticulitis of any grade can be the sole cause of the sigmoid fixation syndrome or a contributing factor. On the other hand, it can be an incidental discovery which may seriously delay the recognition of the adhesive deformities and fixations, internal herniations or volvulus which so seriously incapacitate this patient.

Here again it is pertinent to observe that the X-ray evidence can mislead and must be incorporated into the total picture with care.

When the diagnosis of obstruction in the iliac colon is supported by clinical and roentgenographic observations, the surgical implications are clear. Not rarely, a searching investigation will fail to establish a firm diagnosis. When an uneasy suspicion persists that organic disease or mechanical factors may be present and when symptoms fail respond to well-directed treatment and when familiarity with the patient discloses no contraindications, an exploratory laparotomy may be the only answer.

Occasionally, deforming and immobilizing adhesive formations have been observed in the iliac colon during operations carried out to relieve obstruction of the small intestine. When such procedures demand time-consuming dissection, the sigmoid colon has frequently been left untouched for fear of extending the procedure beyond reasonable bounds.

When such a patient fails to reach a comfortable postsurgical status and when his or her complaints suggest strongly the sigmoid-fixation syndrome reoperation for correction will be mandatory. More commonly patients submitted to surgery for small intestinal mechanical obstruction are not explored fully and the anatomical state of the colon remains unknown. Such patients who continue to complain bitterly and in whom the X-ray examination is less than diagnostic are readily labelled with the irritable bowel syndrome and followed, if at all, with mounting reluctance.

Numerous patients suggesting this diagnosis in varying degrees of severity have been seen. Many have secured acceptable symptomatic relief without surgery by dietary control, weight reduction, improved bowel habits and even reconstructive anorectal surgery when significant local disease, particularly iatrogenic anal stenosis and rigidity was found.

Within the past five years abdominopelvic surgery has been performed specifically for the sigmoid fixation syndrome in twelve women and two men. In all cases without exception deformities and fixations were encountered that far exceeded the roentgenographic statements.

Most frequently the sigmoid colon has been redundant and has been fixed into every conceivable distortion and location. Not rarely its apex has become fixed deeply into the right iliac fossa in which situation the right-sided pain provided additional diagnostic confusion. A most frequent deformity consisted of the accordion-pleated rectosigmoid and distal sigmoid colon packed vertically and deeply into the sacral hollow from which it had to be elevated by sharp dissection. This condition was encountered in its most marked form in women who had been submitted to abdominal hysterectomy and in whom the pelvic cul-de-sac had deepened grossly because of a supported vaginal vault.

How does one deal with the redundant iliac and rectosigmoid segments once the dissection has been completed?

Noble's method of plication has been used by me several times with good to indifferent results. It has been particularly useful when the sigmoid colon was of average length and the plicated single wing had been prepared with care to direct its apex toward the liver. More often and with distinctly better results, I have elected to excise the redundant colon which has been anastomosed end-to-end in two layers over a sterile rubber tube introduced through the anastomosis into the rectum just before the suture line is completed.

This tube is recovered from below by the circulating nurse and is later pushed up from below and guided to the descending splenic flexure. It serves less as a drain than as an internal stent and is withdrawn after about five to seven days. In addition and when the anastomosis is quite low in the pelvis, further protection is secured by adding a tube caecostomy.

The results in this small group of patients have been extremely gratifying from the surgical standpoint and perhaps even more so for the sociological and personal benefits extended to a number of men and women who felt to some degree abandoned to their nondiagnosable pain and misery.

Bibliography

Abrams, B. L.: Sigmoid Volvulus. Arch. Surg. **87**, 1033, Dec. 1963.

Bocca, C. R.: Dolichocolon and Painful Abdominal Crises. J. méd. Lyon **19**, 507 (1938).

Dhallium, A., and M. Verhaeghe: Pericoloc Pelvic Stenosis of Adnexal Origin. Mem. Acad. Par., **76**, 291 (1950).

Levene, G., and E. A. Bragg: Mobility of the Rectosigmoid. A New Diagnostic Sign.: Radiology **54**, 717 (1950).

Ligat, D., and T. D. Overend: Recurrent Volvulus of Pelvic Colon. Brit. med. J. **2**, 42 (1933).

Noble, T. B.: Sigmoid Fixation. Amer. J. Surg. **88**, 282 (1954).

Spackman, J. G.: Obstructive Lesions of the Small Intestine and Sigmoid due to Irradiation. Ann. Surg. **127**, 121 (Jan. 1948).

The Pathology of Megacolon

W. MEIER-RUGE, Basel, Switzerland

Four types of megacolon are recognized at present. They are:

1. Hirschsprung's disease,
2. secondary megacolon,
3. acquired megacolon and
4. functional megacolon.

Until just recently, it has been difficult to differentiate these 4 types with certainty by the convential histological techniques. Now however this is possible, using some simple histochemical reactions [26, 27, 28] such as those demonstrating the activity of acetylcholinesterase [1, 9, 20], catecholamines [7,35] and dehydrogenases [10, 11].

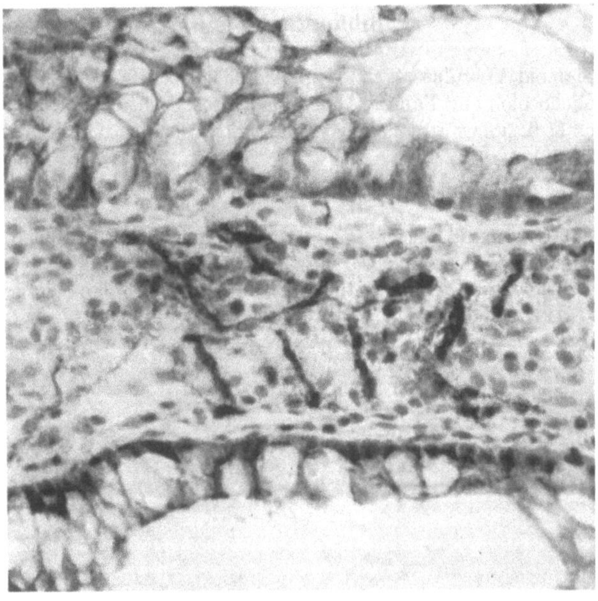

Fig. 1. Intestinal biopsy of the mucous membrane of a segment of spastic colon in Hirschsprung's disease showing the characteristically increased activity of acetylcholinesterase in parasympathetic nerve fibers. (Acetylcholinesterase shown with hematoxylin as counterstain. Enlargement 320 times.)

Hirschsprung's disease – all too often wrongly called Megacolon congenitum, it is typified by aplasia of the intramural ganglion cells [4, 5] in spastic intestinal segments. In addition, there is an extremely high activity of acetylcholinesterase (Fig. 1) in the extramural parasympathetic nervous system [15, 19, 26, 27]. Normally, this cannot be shown by conventional enzymatic histochemical methods.

This increased cholinesterase activity can be shown even in tiny pieces of mucosal biopsies and provides a positive diagnosis of Hirschsprung's disease [26, 27, 28]. Thus more dangerous deep biopsies of the mucosa and intestinal wall are unnecessary. The nerve fibers of the sympathetic system as well as those of the parasympathetic system are increased [2, 27].

Spasticity of the aganglionic intestinal segment is caused by the constant secretion of acetylcholine by the extramural parasympathetic fibers [27, 28] whereas active intestinal dilation is brought about by pressure stimuli on the myenteric plexus and the submucosal plexus [21, 23]. During this active dilatation, the extramural parasympathetic system is blocked to a great degree and comes into action only after the removal of pressure stimuli which are needed for peristaltic contractions of the ring musculature [19, 25] (Fig. 2). This also explains, why the nor-

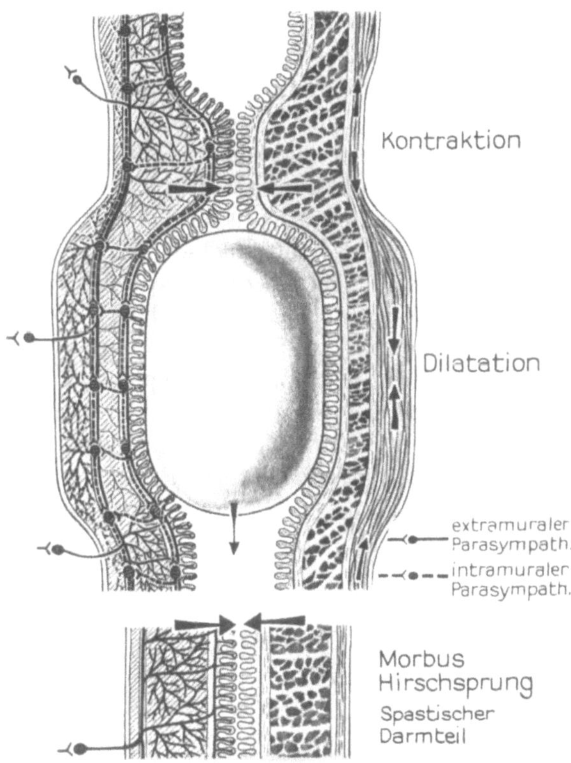

Fig. 2. Schematic presentation of neural structures stimulated by contraction and dilation of the colon. In the lower part the relationship in Hirschsprung's disease are shown. (W. MEIER-RUGE, Virch. arch. path. anat. **344**, p. 67 (1968).

mal peristaltic contractions of the spastic intestinal segment are supressed [12, 16].

The fact that only the distal segment of the colon is affected in Hirschsprung's disease is the result of the special innervation found throughout the distal colon [27]. This innervation is requisite since a greater amount of pressure must be exerted [34] by the ring musculature in the distal colon because of the consistency of the fecal matter here.

Secondary megacolon is found proximal to the narrow segment of Hirschsprung's disease and is similar to other peripheral stenosing processes. In secondary megacolon, the intestine has a normal innervation and merely displays some hypertrophy of the intestinal wall musculature after prolonged stenosis. Our experience has shown that a positive diagnosis on the basis of intestinal wall hypertrophy [27] is possible only after intestinal resection or at autopsy.

Acquired megacolon is easier to diagnose. There is more or less pronounced atrophy of the intramural ganglionic cell plexuses *and* the extramural parasympathetic nerve fibers. In contrast to Hirschsprung's disease, the area between the longitudinal and ring muscular layers is occupied by connective tissue. Besides numerically ascertainable ganglionic cell atrophy, sometimes degeneration of ganglion cells can be seen – especially in Chagas' disease and ulcerative colitis.

Signs of atrophy in the intestinal wall musculature in accordance with the degree of damage found to the intestinal innervation may occasionally be seen. The most important causal factors of acquired megacolon are ulcerative colitis [23, 26], Chagas' disease [8, 17, 18] and virus or toxin-induced ganglionic cell disease; the latter has connection to hypoganglionosis in elderly persons.

According to experimental evidence, it seems unlikely that acquired megacolon is caused by ischemia following surgical intervention [13, 14, 31, 32].

The chief characteristic of acquired megacolon is subtotal atrophy of the neural structures leading to an insufficiency of intestinal motility.

Lastly it should be pointed out that *functional megacolon* induced psychogenically [3] or by anticholinergic substances and ganglionic blockade [27, 29, 33] cannot be diagnosed by biopsy.

In Pseudo-Hirschsprung's disease or congenital hypoganglionosis [30] however, a hypoplasia of both intramural and extramural parasympathetic nerve fibers can be seen. According to our present knowledge, hypoganglionosis is etiologically a "forme fruste" of Hirschsprung's disease. However, there are no pathogenetic relationships between the two conditions since Pseudo-Hirschsprung's disease displays neither hyperplasia of the extramural parasympathetic nerve fibres nor aplasia of the ganglionic cell plexuses.

Rather Pseudo-Hirschsprung's disease is characterized by the hypoplasia of neuronal and ganglion cells of the parasympathetic system (Fig. 3). It can be seen that normal acetylcholinesterase activity is present in the parasympathic nerve fibers of the intestinal wall. As a rule, there is a sharp transition from the poorly innervated intestinal segments to the normally stimulated intestine [27, 30] (Fig. 3).

An important observation is that often a more or less lengthy strip of hypoganglionic intestinal segment is joined to an aganglionic segment of Hirschsprung's disease. This led us to the assumption that Pseudo-Hirschsprung's disease could be a "forme fruste" of Hirschsprung's itself. In this sense it would seem that the "acquired megacolon" – described by Ehrenpreis in 1965 – following resection of an aganglionic segment [6] would best correspond to a segment with congenital hypoganglionosis.

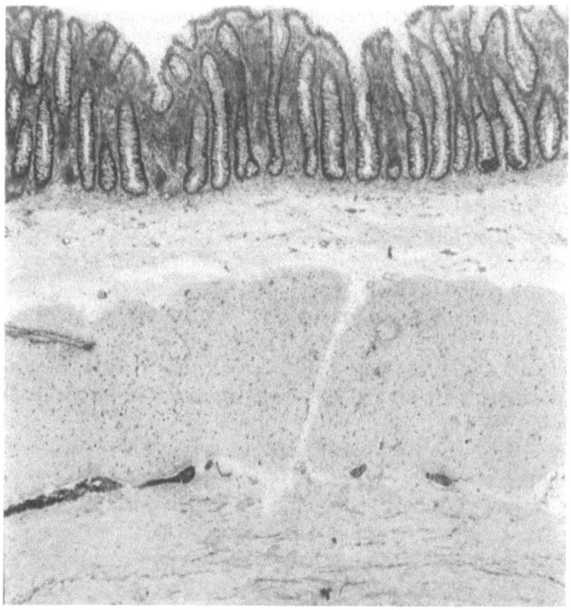

Fig. 3. Intestine showing congenital hypoganglionosis. Note relative short transition from normally innervated intestinal segment (left) to hypoplastic parasympathetic fibers in intestinal wall (right), which is typical for congenital hypoganglionosis (Pseudo-Hirschsprung's disease). (Acetylcholinesterase, with hematoxylin as counterstain. Enlargement 30 times.)

The fact that an aganglionic segment of intestine can adjoin a segment with a hypoplastic nervous system emphasize the importance of the enzymatic histochemical diagnosis of megacolon. With the help of such histochemistry we are able to set a more accurate diagnosis than has been the case up now with conventional means [26, 28, 30]. At the same time we can acquire more profound knowledge concerning the pathophysiology of megacolon – knowledge which lends greater security to surgical procedures and therapeutic measures.

Bibliography

1. El-Badawi, A., and E. A. Schenk: Histochemical methods for separate, consecutive and simultaneous demonstration of acetylcholinesterase and norepinephrine in cryostat sections. J. Hictochem. Cytochem. **15**, 580–588 (1967).
2. Bennett, A., J. R. Garrett, and E. R. Howard: Adrenergic myenteric nerves in Hirschsprung's disease. Brit. med. J. **1**, 487–489 (1968).
3. Berger, H.: Das große atonische Colon bei gewissen Obstipationsformen der Kinder und seine Behandlung mit Sympathicolytica. Ann. paediat. (Basel) **178**, 187–206 (1952).
4. Dalla-Valle, A.: Contributo alla conoscenza della forma famigliare del megacolon congenito. Pediatria (Barcelona) **32**, 569–599 (1924).

5. Ehrenpreis, T.: Megacolon in the newborn. A clinical and roentgenological study with special regard to the phathogenesis. Acta chir. Scand. **94**, Suppl. 112 (1946).
6. — Acquired megacolon as a complication of recto-sigmoidectomy for Hirschsprung's disease. Arch. Dis. Childh. **40**, 180—182 (1965).
7. Falck, B., and C. Owman: A detailed methological description of the fluorescence method for the cellular demonstration of biogenic monoamines. Acta Univ. Lundensis, Sectio II, No 7 (1965).
8. Ferreira-Santos, R.: Megacolon and megarectum in Chagas' disease. Proc. roy. Soc. Med. **54**, 1047—1053 (1961).
9. Gomori, G.: Histochemical demonstration of sites of choline esterase activity. Proc. Soc. exp. Biol. **68**, 354—358 (1948).
10. Hess, R., D. G. Scarpelli, and A. G. E. Pearse: The cytochemical localization of oxidative enzymes. II. Pyridine nucleotide-linked dehydrogenases. J. biophys. biochem. Cytol. **4**, 753—760 (1958).
11. — — — Cytochemical localization of pyridine nucleotide-linked dehydrogenases. Nature (Lond.) **181**, 1531—1532 (1958).
12. Hiatt, R. B.: The pathologic physiology of congenital megacolon. Ann. Surg. **133**, 313—320 (1951).
13. Hukuhara, T., S. Nakayama, and T. Sumi: The role of the intrinsic mucosal reflex in the fluid transport through the denervated intestinal loop. Jap. J. Physiol. **9**, 406—418 (1959).
14. —, T. Sumi, and S. Kotani: The role of ganglion cells in the small intestine, taken in the intrinsic reflex. Jap. J. Physiol. **11**, 281—288 (1961).
15. Kamijo, K., R. B. Hiatt, and G. B. Koelle: Congenital megacolon. A comparison of the spastic and hypertrophied segments with respect to cholinesterase activities and sensitivities to acetylcholine, DFP and the barium ion. Gastroenterology **24**, 173—185 (1953).
16. Keefer, G. P., and J. F. Mokrohisky: Congenital megacolon (Hirschsprung's disease). Radiology **63**, 157—175 (1954).
17. Köberle, F.: Die Chagaskrankheit. Eine Erkrankung der neurovegetativen Peripherie. Wien. klin. Wschr. **68**, 333—339 (1956).
18. — Die Chagaskrankheit - ihre Pathogenese und ihre Bedeutung als Volksseuche. Z. Tropenmed. Parasit. **10**, 236—268 (1959).
19. Koelle, G. B.: Autonomie und pharmacologic control of colonic activity. Ann. N. Y. Acad. Sci. **58**, 307—315 (1954).
20. —, and J. S. Friedenwald: The histochemical method for localizing cholinesterase activity. Proc. Soc. exp. Biol. (N. Y.) **70**, 617—622 (1949).
21. Lenz, H.: Zur Physiologie der Peristaltik des Dünndarms. Dtsch. med. Wschr. **90**, 1657—1663 (1965).
22. Lewitan, A., L. Nathanson, and W. R. Slade, Jr.: Megacolon and dilatation of the small bowel in Parkinsonism. Gastroenterology **17**, 367—374 (1951).
23. Marshak, R. H., L. J. Lester, and A. J. Friedman: Megacolon, a complication of ulcerative colitis. Gastroenterology **16**, 768—772 (1950).
24. Mc Inernney, G. R., W. G. Sauer, A. H. Baggenstoss, and J. R. Hodgson: Fulminating ulcerative colitis with marked colonic dilation: A clinicopathologic study. Gastroenterology **42**, 244—257 (1962).
25. Mei, N.: Nouvelles données sur la décharge des mécanorécepteurs vagaux de l'intestin. C. R. Soc. Biol. **160**, 2382—2387 (1966).
26. Meier-Ruge, W.: Zur Pathologie und bioptischen Diagnostik des Morbus Hirschsprung in Relation zum Megacolon acquisitum und functionale. Verh. dtsch. Ges. Path. **51**, 323—328 (1967).
27. — Das Megacolon, seine Diagnose und Pathophysiologie. Virchows Arch. path. Anat. **344**, 67—85 (1968).
28. —, and R. Morger: Neue Gesichtspunkte zur Pathogenese und Klinik des Morbus Hirschsprung. Schweiz. med. Wschr. **98**, 209—214 (1968).
29. McLamed, M., and E. Kubian: Relationship of the autonomic nervous system to "functional" obstruction of the intestinal tract: report of four cases, one with perforation. Radiology **80**, 22—29 (1963).

30. MORGER, R., u. W. MEIER-RUGE: Pseudo-Hirschsprung. Mschr. Kinderheilk. **114**, 579 bis 581 (1966).
31. OKAMOTO, E., and T. UEDA: Embryogenesis of intramural ganglia of the gut and its relation to Hirschsprung's disease. J. Ped. Surg. **2**, 437—443 (1967).
32. —, T. IWASAKI, T. KAKUTANI, and T. UEDA: Selective destruction of the myenteric plexus: Its relation to Hirschsprung's disease, achalasia of the esophagus and hypertrophic pyloric stenosis. J. Ped. Surg. **2**, 444—455 (1967).
33. SCHARAR, L. L., and H. J. BURHENNE: Megacolon associated with administration of an anticholinergic drug in a patient with ulcerative colitis. Amer. J. dig. Dis. **9**, 268—274 (1946).
34. SMITH, A. N., and M. RIDGEWAY: Use of telemetering capsules in disorders of alimentary tract. II. Application to study of human gastrointestinal motility. Gut **3**, 371—376 (1962).
35. SPRIGGS, T. L. B., J. D. LEVER, P. M. REES, and J. D. P. GRAHAM: Controlled formaldehyde-catecholamine condensation in cryostat section to show andrenergetic nerves by fluorescence. Stain Technol. **41**, 323—327 (1966).
36. ZYPEN, E., VAN DER: Licht- und elektronenmikroskopische Befunde am vegetativen Nervensystem des Colon bei Colitis ulcerosa des Menschen. Dtsch. Z. Nervenheilk. **187**, 787—836 (1965).

Surgery of Megacolon

R. Morger, St. Gallen, Switzerland

1. Introduction

By the term "Hirschsprung's disease" we understand an aplasia of the intramural parasympathetic cells in conjuction with hyperplasia of the extramural parasympathetic and sympathetic cells, resulting in a narrow, spastic segment of bowel (Meier-Ruge). As a consequence a megacolon develops above this narrow segment and the sphincter is affected by achalasia. Operation is the only remedy in the vast majority of cases. The aims of surgical treatment are as follows:

1. Regular, spontaneous defaecation and elimination of meteorism;
2. Complete continence;
3. No loss of potency in male patients.

2. Surgical Methods

The aganglionosis of the narrow segment and of the rectum induced Swenson in 1948 to elaborate his rectosigmoidectomy technique (Fig. 1).

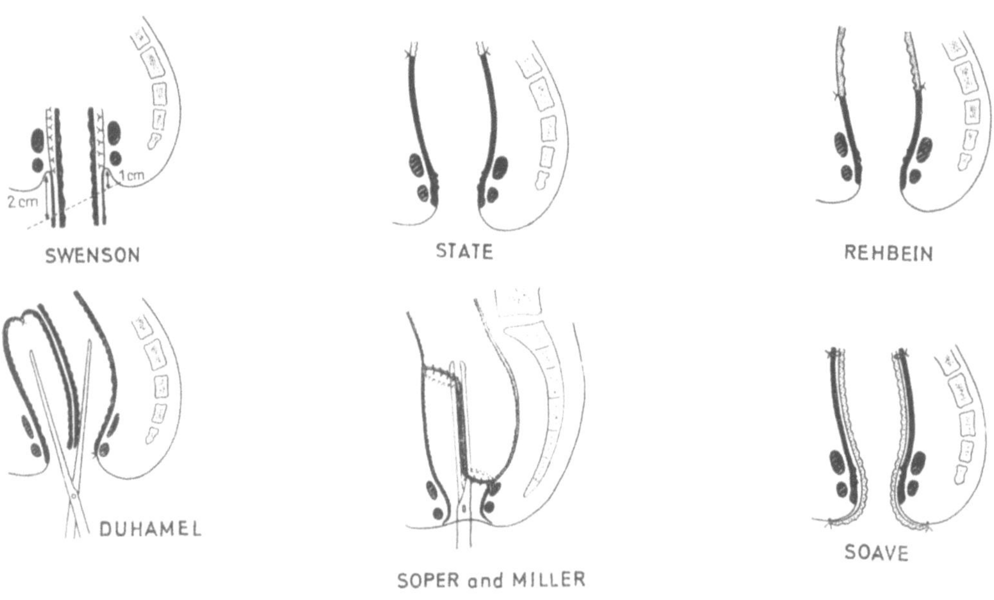

Fig. 1. Different methods of operation in Hirschsprung's disease

Gaining access through an abdominal incision, he mobilised the lower sigmoid and the rectum, immediately along the intestinal wall, and divided them at two places: in the sigmoid about 12 cm proximal to the narrowing, which is clearly visible, and aborally just above the internal sphincter, i. e. about 2–3 cm above the anus. The external sphincter is distended and the peripheral segment of the rectum intussuscepted. The rectum is now incised outside the sphincter. Dressing forceps are introduced from below and the residual sigmoid or colon is pulled through the pelvis and the distal segment of the rectum. Anastomosis between the residual rectal segment and the proximal colon is thus effected extraperitoneally in front of the sphincter. The reunited bowel is then allowed to slip back through the spincter. More recently SWENSON prefers to leave somewhat more of the anterior wall of the rectum intact and thus carry out an oblique anastomosis. The introduction of an intussusception tube by GROB simplified the method to some extent.

In 1952 STATE published his anterior resection method, in which he resected the colon as far as the left flexure, saving the rectum (Fig. 1).

Since 1953 REHBEIN has employed a method in which, after resection of the rectosigmoid and sigmoid, anastomosis is performed intraabdominally between the peripheral segment of the rectum and the colon (Fig. 1).

The anastomosis is however extraperitoneal. It lies 3–7 cm above the anus, according to the age of the child, and not (as in SWENSON's method) 2.5 cm. One never ceases to be amazed how far down it is possible to penetrate into the pelvis minor from the abdomen when the patient is in the correct position. For this, he needs a cushion under his buttocks and the operative field should be well exposed by means of a retractor especially designed by REHBEIN.

The posterior wall of the bladder and the peritoneum of the pouch of Douglas are anchored canopy-like to the abdominal tensor by a line of stay sutures. The pelvic floor is thereby raised and the rectum rendered accessible. Moreover as a result of this exposition, the operative field remains unchanged throughout the procedure. A very important point to note is that the sphincter must be well distended at the end of the operation.

In 1956 DUHAMEL made known his retrorectal pull-through operation (Fig. 1).

From a lower median incision, the peritoneum in the pouch of DOUGLAS is opened above the rectum and the two ureters located. The rectum is transected and closed by means of an inverting suture. The sigmoid is freed upwards and the distended, hypertrophic portion resected. The retrorectal space is then freed with the finger as far as the pelvic floor. A semicircular retroanal skin incision is now made with a thermocauter and the wall of the anal canal exposed with a pair of blunt scissors. The colon is then delivered and sewn to the skin of the anus. Two Kocher's clamps forming a V grip the posterior rectal and the anterior colonic wall, which converge at the orifice, so that a wide rectocolic anastomosis forms within a few days.

In 1959 GROB proposed a modification of the method to protect the internal sphincter, and more recently SOPER and MILLER described a valuable improvement. (Fig. 1).

A further method of operating was described by SOAVE in 1963: he leaves the rectum intact and, like REHBEIN and ROMUALDI in the operation for anal atresia or von EKESPARRE in that for ulcerative colitis, removes the mucosal cylinder of the rectum and draws the sigmoid or the descending colon through (Fig. 1).

3. Time of Operation and Preoperative Measures

In the neonatal period both the diagnosis and the therapy can be difficult. In the event of severe ileus as a result of intestinal perforation with peritonitis, the most minor intervention, i. e. laparotomy, provision of a colostomy and suturing of the perforation, promises the most success. In all other cases conservative treatment with an intestinal tube and enemas, which is not entirely without danger on account of possible perforation, however, should be undertaken.

If the general condition of a patient with Hirschsprung's disease can be rendered satisfactory with conservative measures, the present-day anaesthetic techniques are such that the operation discussed above can be carried out at any time. I am of the opinion that an artificial anus should be avoided as far as possible and that, circumstances permitting, everything should be definitively corrected at one session. Needless to say, if conservative measures prove problematical, the opportunity should not be missed to fashion a colostomy at the right site, i. e. according to REHBEIN just above the narrow segment, at the right time. But a new-born infant with an artificial anus requires an experienced team of doctors and nurses. In the other cases, once the infant is out of the neonatal period, he can be prepared for the operation by regular intestinal flushing with physiological saline, possibly supplemented by a little liquid paraffin.

4. Results

A critical comparison of the figures given in the communications of DUHAMEL, REHBEIN and SWENSON shows that with equivalent experience the same results can be achieved with any of the three methods. The figures for STATE's method and SOAVE's pull-through operation are too small to allow comparison with the other three.

Discussion

From the point of view of the results obtained, there is little to choose between the methods of SWENSON, DUHAMEL and REHBEIN. All three take account of the pathophysiological situation. While extension of the sphincter is explicitly advocated only in REHBEIN's method, it follows automatically in those of SWENSON and DUHAMEL. SOAVE's pull-through technique involves the risk of rectal incontinence, since we now know that the short mucosal stump in the anal canal does not contain sufficient nerve endings to ensure complet control. STATE's method is doubtless not radical enough, and takes no account whatsoever of the sphincter problem.

If we now consider the three methods, with the improvements mentioned, from the point of view of their technical difficulty, I should say that of SWENSON is the most difficult to execute. Next comes DUHAMEL's operation with GROB's and SOPER's modifications. The method of REHBEIN is doubtless the simplest, and can thus be employed by a surgeon with little experience in this operation. Furthermore the duration of the intervention is very short. REHBEIN's fifteen years of experience have shown that the operation is well tolerated at all ages. It is rendered particularly simple in infants and small children by the fact that the rectum is readily accessible via the abdomen at this age. The anastomosis is generally situated 3 cm from the anus in infants and up to 7 cm in older children. It thus lies very low and can always be reached and examined with the finger from below. The larger rectal segment, which in contrast to SWENSON's method is retained, i. e. remains as part of the tract, and which is very often at the centre of discussion, is in reality only a few centimetres long.

I have attempted to make a comparison of the different methods of operating Hirschsprung's disease. It is not my intention to reject the other methods, and we are well aware of the fact that they can bring good success. I only wanted to counter unjustified arguments which have on occasion in the past led to a rejection of the method of intraabdominal resection.

Bibliography

DUHAMEL, B.: Technique Chirurgicale Infantile. Paris: Masson, 1957. Rectorectal and Transanal Pull-Through Procedure for Treatment of Hischsprung's Disease. Dis. Colon. Rect. **7**, 455 (1964).

v. EKESPARRE, W.: Radikale, kontinenzerhaltende Operationsmethode bei Colitis ulcerosa. Z. Kinderchir. **1**, 156 (1964).

GROB, M.: Lehrbuch der Kinderchirurgie. Stuttgart: Thieme 1957. Intestinal Obstruction in the Newborn Infant. Arch. Dis. Childh. **35**, 40 (1960).

MEIER-RUGE, W., u. R. MORGER: Neue Gesichtspunkte zur Pathogenese und Klinik des Morbus Hirschsprung. Schweiz. med. Wschr. **98**, 209 (1968).

MEIER-RUGE, W.: Die Pathologie des Megacolon. Hedrologicum Conlegium 3rd International Congress, 11.–12. Oktober 1968 Erlangen-Nürnberg.

MORGER, R., u. W. MEIER-RUGE: Pseudo-Hirschsprung. Mschr. Kinderheilk. **114**, 579 (1966).

REHBEIN, F.: Angeborene Verschlüsse des Anus und Rectums. Kinderärztl. Prax. 26. Echter Hirschsprung. Mschr. Kinderhk. **114**, 581 (1966)

—, R. MORGER, J. G. KUNDERT, and W. MEIER-RUGE: Surgical Problems in Congenital Megacolon. J. Pediat. Surg. **1**, 526 (1966).

—, u. J. NICOLAI: Operation der Hirschsprung'schen Krankheit. Dtsch. med. Wschr. **88**, 1595 (1963).

—, u. H. WUERTENBERGER: Die intraabdominelle Resektion bei der Hirschsprung'schen Krankheit. Langenbecks Arch. klin. Chir. **308**, 322 (1964).

—, u. H. V. ZIMMERMANN: Ergebnisse der intraabdominellen Resektion bei der Hirschsprung'schen Krankheit. Zbl. Chir. **84**, 1744 (1959).

ROMUALDI, P.: Eine neue Operationstechnik für die Behandlung einiger Rectalmißbildungen. Langenbecks Arch. klin. Chir. **296**, 371 (1960).

SOAVE, F.: Hirschsprung's Disease: A New Surgical Technique. Arch. Dis. Childh. **39**, 116 (1964).

SOPER, R. T., a. F. E. MILLER: Modifications of Duhamel Procedure: Elimination of Rectal Pouch and Colorectal Septum. J. Ped. Surg. **3**, 376 (1968).

STATE, D.: Surgical Treatment for Idiopathic Congenital Megacolon (Hirschsprung's Disease). Surg. Gynec. Obstet. **95**, 201 (1952).

—, Segmental Colon Resection in the Treatment of Congenital Megacolon (Hirschsprung's Disease). Amer. J. Surg. **105**, 93 (1963).

SWENSON, O., et al.: Hirschsprung's Disease: A New Concept of the Etiology: Operative Results in 34 Patients. New Engl. J. Med. **241**, 551 (1949).

—, A New Surgical Treatment for Hirschsprung's Disease. Surgery **28**, 371 (1950).

—, Follow-up on 200 Patients Treated for Hirschsprung's Disease during 10-year Period. Ann. Surg. **146**, 706 (1957).

—, Partial Internal Sphincterectomy in the Treatment of Hirschsprung's Disease. Ann. Surg. **160**, 540 (1964).

The Surgical Treatment of Megacolon

K. Schwemmle, Erlangen, Germany

Chronic obstipation in infancy and childhood is frequently caused by one of the various forms of megacolon.

Unless they are given enemas, these children fail to have a bowel movement for days or even weeks. The course is interspersed with bouts of diarrhoea which may contain blood. Diarrhoea in infants rapidly leads to anemia, electrolyte imbalance and exsiccosis. After the introduction of a rectal tube or during the rectal examination, large quantities of foul-smelling gases and stool escape. In cases of symptomatic megacolon the stenosis can easily be palpated at rectal examination. In Hirschsprung's disease, the ampulla contains no stool and the terminal bowel is narrow, whereas idiopathic megacolon is characterized by a dilatation of the colon just beyond the anus. Stool incontinence automatically excludes the presence of Hirschsprung's disease. Agangliosis of the bowel is a congenital defect which appears in infants and young children, while functional megacolon develops gradually and therefore presents in older children. The extent and degree of megacolon and often even the form can be detected on a barium enema. In symptomatic and idiopathic megacolon, the dilatation extends as far as the anus or the mechanical block, while a narrow segment appears in Hirschsprung's disease. The dilatation of the intestine in idiopathic megacolon remains unchanged even after the bowel is emptied (Meier-Ruge, Morger). The diagnosis is particularly difficult in new-borns where a megacolon has not developed yet. If meconium fails to appear on the first day after birth, then agangliosis must enter the differential diagnosis. At an early stage, sometimes even on the second day already, the abdomen becomes distended and dilated loops of bowel can frequently be seen. Bilious vomiting indicates an increasing degree of ileus; the X-ray of the abdomen reveals numerous fluid levels as a sign of ileus of the terminal ileum. The mortality in the first month of life is 28–80% (Hofmann and Rehbein, Fraser, Dormann); this is very high in contrast to the mortality of congenital megacolon which is 5–10%. Occasionally the distension of the colon leads to perforation (Atrell). Perforation of the appendix in agangliosis has also been described (Martin and Perrin). We ourselves have seen 2 perforations of the ascending and transverse colon in a 6-day-old boy.

Of special significance appears to us to be the fact that the first symptom of congenital megacolon in infants can be dyspepsia and not stool retention (Schäfer).

Swenson has recommended the biopsy of the rectal musculature in order to confirm the diagnosis of agangliosis. However, this procedure is not without danger. Cases of death have been described (Fraser). Furthermore the extent of the agangliotic zone cannot be determined. Therefore we share Soave's opinion that muscle biopsy can be avoided if the X-ray examination unequivocally reveals a narrow segment. In new-borns and infants, however, the biopsy is a valuable aid since the X-ray signs are not characteristic here yet. Recently MEIER-RUGE has shown that the muscle excision can be avoided even in these small patients. A biopsy of rectal mucosa removed without an anesthetic is enough to demonstrate or ecxlude the presence of acetylcholinesterase and thus to diagnose Hirschsprung's disease. Nevertheless, a muscle biopsy is still necessary if an infant or child has to undergo laparotomy for an ileus and the exact cause fails to be found. Even if there is no stenotic segment, agangliosis may still be present. The proximal edge of the segment can be determined by means of frozen section examinations.

Treatment

If conservative measures do not achieve a cure in idiopathic and symptomatic megacolon, surgical treatment should not be delayed too long.

Operation must be performed in cases of congenital megacolon because this is the only method of curing these children. The mortality of the conservative treatment of Hirschsprung's disease is 50% (DORMANN).

In 1948 SWENSON took the decisive step in the surgical treatment of megacolon by performing a rectosigmoidectomy. The other techniques of resection have been described by MORGER. As a rule, we prefer the pull-through method of SOAVE where the rectal mucosa is removed while the musculature of the rectum is spared. In order to preserve sensation in the anal region which is important for continence, we leave a 2–3 cm long border of rectal mucosa above the anus. The advantages of this technique are its simplicity, the avoidance of an anastomosis (and thus the danger of insufficiency of the anastomosis) as well as the preservation of vegetative nerve fibres to the pelvic organs.

REHBEIN has repeatedly pointed out the importance of sphincter dilation. He believes that the success of all the operations described depends on the elimination of sphincter achalasia.

We do not regard a colostomy as a prerequisite in every case. However, in cases of ileus or severe dyspepsia in new-borns and infants, the anus praeter is the only life-saving treatment and it is important not to hesitate in carrying out this procedure. The function of the artifical bowel outlet depends on the fact that it is made above the stenotic segment. At the same time the length of the aganglionic segment should be determined by means of frozen sections of muscle biopsies. Final surgery is carried out at the age of one year (SWENSON, LEE). REHBEIN operates at the age of 6 months already (REHBEIN and ZIMMERMAN). In infants with a completely aganglionic colon, ileostomy must be performed immediately. This is the only way of lowering the high mortality (73% EDELMANN).

While idiopathic and symptomatic megacolon do not pose any special diagnostic problems, the high mortality of Hirschsprung's disease in new-borns and infants must be lowered by early diagnosis and timely surgical treatment.

IV. Incontinentia Alvi

Problems of Continence in Atresia Ani and Congenital Megacolon

F. Rehbein, Bremen, Germany

Problems of continence and incontinence play an important role in the treatment of megacolon congenitum and atresia ani.

In the case of Hirschsprung's operation, incontinence, when it appears, is not a problem inherent in the disease but one of operation method and technique. This applies particularly in Swenson's operation. Only when it is skillfully carried out, as by Swenson himself, can the danger of incontinence be disregarded.

With Duhamel's operation, too, it has been proved that a loss of continence threatens only when the "pull-through" is effected below the internal sphincter, i. e. when the internal sphincter is by-passed. For this reason, Grob has recommended effecting the pull-through at a higher point. In this way, the indispensible sphincter segment remains functional and the danger of incontinence is banned.

In the correctly executed operation after Soave a loss of continence need not be feared either.

If we now confine ourselves to the intra-abdominal resection, which we have been doing since 1953, the anastomosis is situated at some distance from the sphincter, approx. 4–8 cm above the anus. There is no involvement of the sphincter apparatus during the operation. A specific problem does, however, arise. It has been shown that in every case of congenital megacolon, continence is enhanced, or, as Stelzner expressed it, a hypercontinence occurs which belongs to the clinical picture. This behaviour of the sphincter can be termed an achalasia, when compared with the conditions prevailing at the cardiac portion of the stomach. The significant point about this defect is, that the sphincter does not relax during defaecation. The reason for this behaviour of the sphincter is still completely unknown. Indeed, the fact first became clear through the use of the intra-abdominal resection technique. As long as the operation itself contains a manipulation to weaken the sphincter, the condition of achalasia associated with every megacolon does not become manifest. If the sphincter remains untouched during the operation, the condition manifests itself in all its severity.

I do not wish to repeat here what Morger has already said. I should like to say only this: In every Hirschsprung operation, in addition to the resection of the aganglionic segment of the bowel, continence must be reduced, i. e., the sphincter must be weakened not merely slightly but permanently and sufficiently if success is to be achieved. If the weakening of the sphincter is performed as an integral part of the operation, nothing additional needs to be done. If this is not the case, something must subsequently be done to reduce continence. I should like to go even further and maintain that, the actual problem of the Hirschsprung operation is to be found in the reduction of continence and in the removal of the achalasia. From this point of view, the argument as to the method of operation is basically without foundation. A reduction of continence is generally possible by performing one or two vigorous dilations of the sphincter.

We performed follow-up examinations on 200 children or received information from the parents; we lost 19 and were unable to contact 12 further children. In a group of 158 children the results were very good – the children passing unassisted movements 1–3 times daily. The second group contains the difficult cases. Some of these children are mentally retarded or live in poor social circumstances. Others are cases in which no aganglionic segments were obtained, so-called low cases, in which the disease was, as it were, concentrated in the sphincter apparatus.

We are convinced that a portion of these cases can yet be regraded into group one, with appropriate post-operative treatment. This postoperative treatment consists of a repetition of the sphincter dilation. In particularly stubborn cases a sphincterotomy, the simple division of the sphincter or, what we have lately been doing, a myectomy, the excision of a muscular strip from the whole sphincter, can be carried out. These procedures are possible without loss of continence.

With the 158 children manifesting "very good" results, 1–3 dilations were generally sufficient. The condition of achalasia returned only in a few cases and made repeated dilation or sphincterotomy necessary. Here it must be mentioned that a child can be considered as cured when the good results have remained constant over a period of 3–4 years.

The conclusions may be drawn from these observations:

1. During the operation for congenital megacolon, the operative method is of secondary importance. Of primary importance is that weakening of the sphincter must be achieved. If constipation again occurs this does not indicate that the operation method is poor but that achalasia of the sphincter has returned.
2. The condition of hypercontinence, or achalasia of the sphincter, is always present but is varyingly severe. It can be remedied either
   primarily during the operation or
   by means of a sphincter dilation.
   In special cases a
   sphinctcrotomy or
   a myectomy
   is required.

In anal and rectum atresia, subsequent continence or incontinence is dependent not only on the deformity itself but also on the operative procedure. The cases with a vestibular fistula, simple membranous occlusion and the so-called covered anus with a subcutaneous fistula, usually become continent. With these malformations the sphincter apparatus, particularly the puborectalis muscle is properly developed and there are no defects in respect to sensitivity either.

If the occlusion is situated at a higher point, continence problems occur. This applies particularly in males with urethral fistulas. In such a case the operative method is decisive. A muscular apparatus that is just sufficient, may be damaged during the operation; this must be avoided at all costs. We believe that, with the procedure we have been using for the last 10 years, the least damage is caused.

The rectum is divided transversely and the mucosa removed from the blind pouch. A canal is prepared for the perineum, and the colon, which is situated higher, is pulled through. There is no doubt that a disadvantage of this method is the loss of mucosa and thus of sensitivity especially in view of the fact that the sensitivity of the proctodaeal skin and the sensation of contact in the normal anal canal are lacking. Despite this fact, the continence results are good and even very good in a considerable number of cases. This can only be explained by assuming that there are further receptors outside the rectal mucosa in the remaining wall of the rectum or in the pelvic fibrous tissue, which provide information as to the state of filling. These receptors would be lost and damaged if, the entire blind pouch were to be mobilized and pulled through as was done earlier.

With the predominantly occurring low forms with a fistula to the urethra, the distance between the blind pouch and the perineum is small. It is our experience that, as is the case with the vestibular fistula in the female, the muscle groups of the sphincter organ, in particular the puborectalis, are present. These cases deserve our particular attention for it should, as in the female comparison group, with careful work, be possible to achieve satisfactory continence. This procedure is, admittedly complicated and, as we have already said, not without its faults. It is, however, virtually dictated by the presence of the recto-urethral fistula, which must be eliminated at all costs.

A mistake which can easily be made is to effect the "pull-through" too far to the rear and not through the sling of the puborectalis. If this occurs, continence can, of course, not be achieved. Kiesewetter and Turner have both drawn attention to this mistake and its consequences.

We do not know exactly whether, in all low cases, the blind pouch, in its development, pushes the levator ani together with the puborectalis muscle in front of it or whether the pouch has already pushed through the muscles towards the perineum. It is certain that in medium-high and high forms this is not the case so that the danger of missing the sling when preparing the canal is particularly great. This is especially so as in these cases the puborectalis muscle forms a close ring around the urethra or the vagina.

In these cases, which can in part be described as anorectal agenesis, it is necessary to use the sacral approach suggested by Stephens in addition in order to be able to localize the sling exactly. Unfortunately, in these high forms, which are often associated with sacral deformities, the sphincter musculature and its innovation are only slightly developed. Despite this, the attempt must be made to achieve the best possible results.

In the last few months we have examined all those cases of anal atresia operated on in the period from 1959–1967 in accordance with the procedure described. During this examination special attention was paid to the question of continence. 81 cases were operated on in the abdominoperineal approach. 13 cases were exclusively of the high form. The good and very good results account for approximately $^1/_3$ of the total number. This picture will improved as, in our experience, some of the children with very poor function in the 3rd and 5th groups will later move up into group 2.

In general, one might say that in the operation for anal atresia, the method has now reached a final stage of development. A number of valuable suggestions, e. g. by Kottmeier, Nixon and Stephens, might produce still further improvements.

There will, however, always be a not inconsiderable number of children remaining, in whom the achievement of a satisfactory condition will not be possible.

The gracilis plastic operation after PICKRELL can bring improvements in continence in some of these cases. This is confirmed by the results of GELBKE, HECKER and KÖLLERMANN in the clinic of Erlangen. To date we have performed 10 such operations and have achieved significant improvement in at least 4 cases. The possibilities of this operation must not be overestimated however. Perhaps, in a number of these cases, the transplanted muscle merely acts as a support for the pelvic floor and thus provides better conditions for the function of the remaining sphincter musculature. Perhaps it sometimes functions as nothing more than an elastic pad.

A wide field of application will, in future, probably open up for the electronic pacemaker in conjunction with the Pickrell plastic operation. At any rate, the ini tial results obtained by NIXON seem very promising.

Electrical Treatment of Anal Incontinence and Rectal Prolapse Using an External Stimulator with Intra Anal Electrodes

B. R. Hopkinson and R. Lightwood, Birmingham, Great Britain

Introduction

Parkes [1] showed that the normal pelvic floor is always in a state of electrical activity and tone. Phillips and Edwards [2] suggested that the activity of the pelvic floor is more important than anal sphincter tone in the mechanism of continence. Incontinent patients generally have very poor pelvic floor and sphincter tone, but Caldwell [3, 4, 5] Hopkinson [6, 7] and Lightwood [8] have described patients who have been made continent by electrical stimulation of the muscles involved. Caldwell implanted electrodes directly into the sphincter muscles and Hopkinson used an intra anal plug bearing two electrodes to stimulate the anal muscles. Some patients are made continent of urine as well as faeces by this treatment, presumably because of increased pelvic floor tone as demonstrated experimentally by Alexander and Rowan [9]. This paper describes further experience with the use of intra anal electrodes to treat patients with anal incontinence and rectal prolapse.

Methods

Most of the 45 patients in this report had symptoms for at least 2 years before treatment using the commercially available stimulator and plug described previously [7] and illustrated in Fig. 1. Some of the children required smaller plugs which were handmade from cold curing

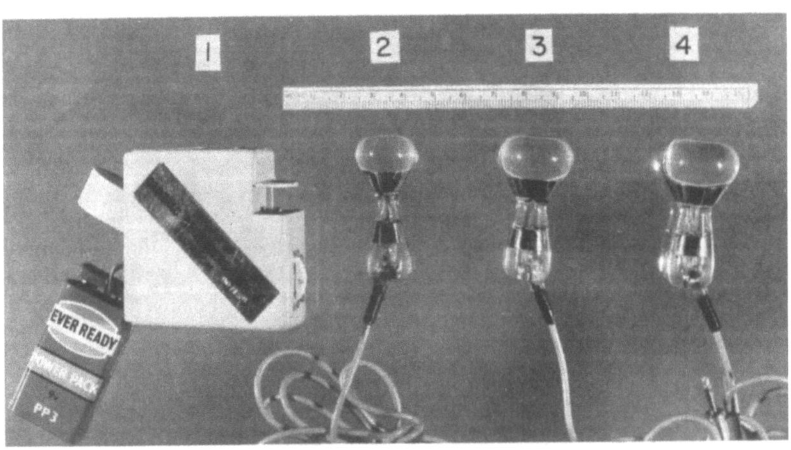

Fig. 1 (1) Electrical stimulator, (2, 3, and 4) three standard intra anal plugs each bearing two electrodes. Note the 15 cm rule above the plugs

acrylic with dental gold electrodes connected to the standard stimulator. The entire apparatus was easily secreted beneath the patient's clothes. The appropriate plug size was selected at an out-patient visit as the smallest one to be easily retained on walking. Before the current was turned on, the plug position was checked to ensure that both electrodes were inside the anal canal and making a good contact. The current was slowly increased until the patient was just aware of the stimulation; gentle traction on the wire lead confirmed that the plug was being held in place. The patient was now encouraged to walk around. Most could do this easily. The duration and frequency of treatment was largely determined by the patients themselves. Some used the apparatus continuously day and night, only removing it to defaecate or urinate; some used it at night only, and some for as little as 30 minutes daily. The plug and electrodes had to be kept clean by washing with soap and water at each removal. The batteries lasted from one to three weeks or more according to the amount of time they were used.

Table 1. *Summary of 45 patients treated up to August, 1968*

	Cured	Good Control	Partial Control	Day Trial only	Failed
Anal incontinence without prolapse	1	5	—	2	2
Massive rectal prolapse with incontinence	—	2	3	3	5
Massive rectal prolapse without incontinence	—	3	3	—	2
Children with anal incontinence	2	3	5	4	—
Total	3	13	11	9	9

i. e. 27 of the 45 patients have benefited.

Results (Table I)

1. Adults with Anal Incontinence Without Rectal Prolapse

All 10 patients tolerated the plug well at the first session. Only one refused further treatment and another who suffered from encopresis through a normal sphincter, abandoned it after six weeks; he was continent during the day but unhelped by the plug at night. The remaining 8 patients were enthusiastic about their treatment. After two months daily treatment for periods of one hour, one male patient was quite continent and only used his stimulator for 20 min once a week. He was regarded as a cure. Five other patients were dry while using the plug for 2–4 hours daily but occasionally soiled themselves without it. Several of them were able to attend normal social activities while using the plug.

2. Adults with Massive Rectal Prolapse and Faecal Incontinence

At first only two of the 13 patients in this group were able to retain the plug while walking. These two patients, after five months and two years respectively were achieving good control of their prolapse and incontinence by using the plug for 2–6 hours daily. Their prolapses only came occasionally with attacks of diarrhoea. Three were achieving some measure of control by using the stimulator for 2–4 hours daily but without the plug in place the prolapse usually came down. Five patients abandoned treatment, being unable to retain the plug satisfactorily. These failures were usually associated with diarrhoea, loss of awareness of rectal fullness and impaired awareness of the stimulating current.

3. Massive Rectal Prolapse Associated with Faecal Continence

Initially all but two of the eight patients in this group were able to retain the plug while walking. These two patients turned out to be the two failures and they were still unable to retain the plug after some weeks practise despite good visible contractions of their anal sphincter muscles. After 2–6 months daily treatment, 3 patients were well-controlled and found that their prolapses only occasionally recurred at times of stress or with diarrhoea. Three other patients achieved partial control of their prolapses after less than three months of daily treatment.

4. Children with Anal Incontinence

Two of the fourteen children treated had neurological defects associated with spina-bifida. All of the others had various forms of congenital anal deformities corrected surgically soon after birth. The youngest child treated was 4 years of age. The majority were first seen between 8 and 10 years. The two children with neurogenic defects also had urinary incontinence and after 2–3 months both were showing signs of improvement with partial faecal and urinary control. The two cures have occurred in a boy of 9, left incontinent after a "pull-through" for Hirschsprung's disease, and a girl of 12, left incontinent of urine and faeces after a "cut-back" procedure for imperforate anus with a recto-vaginal fistula. After six months of daily treatments lasting from 30 min to 2 hours, both had achieved a marked hypertrophy of the pubo-rectalis muscle and became continent without further use of the stimulator. After six months, two other children had develop marked hypertrophy of the anal sphincter but were unable to achieve complete continence from lack of awareness of rectal fullness. The other children have generally not been treated fo so long a time.

Discussion

PHILLIPS and EDWARDS [2] showed that the resting and maximum voluntary pressures in the anal canal are only small compared with the large intra abdominal pressures encountered during coughing and exercise, suggesting that the anal sphincter alone is not responsible for the maintenance of normal continence. They advanced the "Flutter Valve" theory, illustrated in Fig. 2 to show the place of the pelvic floor in maintaining continence. As the intra-abdominal pressure is raised, the pelvic floor contracts and draws up the anal canal, kinking it and holding it firmly by a narrowed slit in its diaphragm. The small additional pressure of the anal muscle supported above this slit is enough to maintain continence. Voluntary contraction of the sphincter can usually hold up intra rectal faeces until the urge to defaecate has passed. Defaecation is achieved when faeces are in the rectum, by relaxing the pelvic floor, while raising the intra-abdominal pressure to push down and straighten out the anal canal. A similar mechanism of continence is thought to apply to the other exits from the abdomen, the urethra and the oesophageal hiatus, where floppy tubes pass through slits in a muscular diaphragm. Weakness of the sphincter muscles and pelvic floor can lead to incontinence of faeces and urine. CALDWELL [3, 4, 5] showed that continuous electrical stimulation of the appropriate sphincter muscle could achieve continence and subsequent hypertrophy of the muscles could in some cases lead to recovery of continence without electrical stimulation. Case reports are given here showing that electrical stimulation via electrodes on an intra anal plug can also achieve continence of faeces and urine; in some cases tone has recovered sufficiently for patients to be continent without stimulation. The control of urinary continence is thought to be due to pelvic floor contraction as demonstrated experimentally by ALEXANDER and ROWAN [9] in dogs.

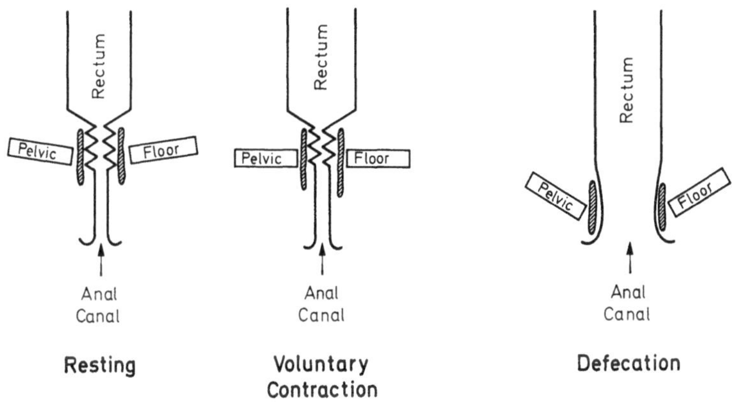

Fig. 2. Diagrammatic representation of the movements of the pelvic floor from the resting to the voluntary contraction and defaecation position (After Phillips and Edwards [2])

The results from treating patients with rectal prolapse are poor in patients who have difficulty retaining the plug on walking. They often find themselves pushing down their prolapses mistaking them for faeces. Prolapse is not always associated with a weak sphincter or pelvic floor; one of the patients in this series had a 2″ prolapse, through a good continent sphincter. She was unable to retain a plug after a few minutes walking despite a good visible contraction of the sphincter when the stimulator was turned on. CALDWELL's method of surgically implanting the electrodes into the muscle does not introduce a foreign body into the lumen of the anal canal and seems to give good results for the treatment of prolapse [5].

The non-operative method of stimulating the anal muscle and pelvic floor via an intra-anal plug has the advantages of immediate application in the out-patient clinic and the ready availability of the electrical apparatus for maintenance or repair. It is giving satisfactory results for the treatment of anal and urinary incontinence and for some patients with rectal prolapse.

The electrical stimulator and a range of plug sizes are available from: Cardiac Recorders Ltd., 375–7 City Road, London, E. C. 1., England.

Bibliography

1. Parkes, A. G., N. H. Porter, and J. Melzak: Experimental study of the Reflex Mechanism Controlling the Muscles of the Pelvic Floor. Dis. Colon Rect. **5**, 407—414 (1962).
2. Phillips, S. F., and D. A. W. Edwards: Some Aspects of Anal Continence and Defaecation. Gut **6**, 396—406 (1965).
3. Caldwell, K. P. S.: The Electrical Control of Spincter Incompetence. Lancet **2**, 174—175 (1963).
4. —, et al.: Urinary Incontinence following Spinal Injury Treated by Electronic Implant. Lancet **1**, 846—847 (1965).
5. — The Treatment of Incontinence by Electronic Implants. Ann. Roy. Coll. Surg., Engl. **41**, 447—459 (1967).
6. Hopkinson, B. R., and R. Lightwood: Electrical Treatment of Anal Incontinence. Lancet **1**, 297—298 (1966).
7. — — Electrical Treatment of Incontinence. Brit. J. Surg. **59**, 802—805 (1967).
8. Ligthwood, R.: A shaped Electrode for the treatment of incontinence. Proc. R. Soc. Med. (in press).
9. Alexander, S., and D. Rowan: Closure of the Urinary Spincter Mechanism in Anesthetized Dogs by means of Electrical Stimulation of the Perineal Muscles. Brit. J. Surg. **53**, 1053—1056 (1966).

Surgical Tactics in the Treatment of Rectal Sphincter Insufficiency

J. M. MATYASHIN and V. V. BUKHTEYEV, Donetsk, UdSSR

Rectal sphincter insufficiency is a severe affliction which deprives the patient of his ability to work and makes him a burden to society. Numerous operative methods of treatment are not devoid of essential defects, so that relapses are frequent.

In our series there were 52 cases with different degrees of rectal sphincter insufficiency. Women predominated (34 cases). They are classified according to etiology.

The cause of sphincter insufficiency was postpartum rupture of the sphincter in 26 cases, sequelae of rectal and perineal operations in 18 patients and perineal injuries in 8 cases.

Some patients had already been operated on more than once in other hospitals (12 cases) before being admitted to our clinic. The duration of illness varied from six months to eight years.

All patients admitted to the clinic were operated. The character of the restorative operation depended on the degree of sphincter lesion and on the state of adjacent tissues which are used as plastic material. Besides the physical examination (inspection, rectal examination), great importance was attached to junctional tests; of these, special mention should be made of sphincterometry with A. M. AMINEV's method and electrophysiological methods to study muscular excitability.

To restore the anal sphincter, we used various operative methods: sphincteroplasty with the gracilis muscles and gluteal muscle segments; use was also made of alloplasty of the sphincter with various synthetic materials. These procedures are too bulky and do not always prove effective. Operations to strengthen the sphincter with the gracilis muscle and gluteal muscles are frequently fraught with danger of the graft necrosing as a result of excessive mobilization and overextention of the muscular grafts. In three out of twelve operations made by us, the transplants necrosed and relapse of disease occured.

Experience with restorative operations using various femoral and gluteal muscles have shown that these interventions demand the surgeon's skill and caution.

Nonetheless, the special features of the vasculature in this area are such that the success of the operation cannot be ensured by surgeon's high skill and carefulness alone. In a number of cases, it was impossible to mobilize transplants with the necessary dimensions. In this connection we succeeded in elaborating this operation by experiments on cadavers and animals (dogs) – graft lengthening was ensured by stitching the lavsan tapes up to their distal parts.

Counterstitching of these tapes around the anus is conducive to its active obturation when muscles used for the plastic begin to make contact.

Technically, the operation is simple and results obtained were quite satisfactory. Complexity and reliability of the above mentioned operative methods made us start surgical management with a more simple operation, namely sphincteroplasty. This operation limits itself to the excision of the cicatricial tissues of the defect followed by suturing the muscles with two or three layers of stitches. To close the defect the final suture is placed on the skin and mucous membrane. Occasionally our operation is successful in cases of postpartum sphincter rupture. All 25 patients recovered. The good functional results persisted subsequently.

The success of restorative operations on the rectal sphincter depends on efficient preoperative preparation and good anesthesia. Before the operation, the intestine must be emptied. This was achieved with the help of oil enemas. Such measures allowed us to rest the affected sphincter during the 5–7 days of the postoperative period. Absence of the stool in this period was also ensured by a limited diet and the administration Tinctura Opii. Asepsis at operation was achieved by the administration of antibiotics (colimycin, neomycin).

Of all existing methods of anaesthesia, we prefer spinal anesthesia with 1% solution of novocaine. From our point of view, this form of anesthesia is the most harmless and at the same time is able to ensure prolonged (2–3 hours) anesthesia and muscle relaxation in the operative area.

The solution of novocaine was administered in the space between the second and third lumbar vertebrae.

Conclusion

1. Of all the existing methods of restoration of the anal sphincter the most simple and reliable is sphincteroplasty which consists of suturing the ruptured muscle fibres.

2. Restoration of the sphincter using gluteal muscles and gracilis muscles are complicated and less reliable in view of the possible necrosis of the mobilized muscular segments. Results of this operation may be improved by stitching lavsan tapes to the distal parts of the graft.

3. The success of restorative operations on the anal sphincter is ensured by the effective preoperative preparation and reliable anesthesia.

We consider spinal anesthesia with 1% solution of novocaine to be the method of choice.

Myokinetic Sphincterplasty with Incontinentia Alvi after Anal and Rectal Atresia

R. Daum and W. Ch. Hecker, Heidelberg, Germany

It is of utmost importance to take optimal care of muscles and nerves when a correction of anal and rectal atresia is performed in order to avoid an incontinentia alvi. Rehbein has described very clearly the problems that result and operating techniques necessary to achieve continence.

In spite of this, incontinence may result after abdomino-perineal pullthrough. The rate of failures in the literature is between 20 and 40%. In our patients, 74 children, who were examined very carefully after the operation, a bad result, i. e. an incontinentia alvi, was found in about 9% of the cases (Tab. 1).

Table 1. *Functional results of operation for Anal and Rectal Atresia*

Author/Hospital	Excellent or good	Fair	Poor
Robert Gross	60%	20%	20%
Scott	55%	7%	37%
Kiesewetter	55%	14%	30%
Swenson	55%	8%	37%
Children's Memorial Hospital Chicago	43%	14%	43%
Babis Hospital New York	54%	20%	26%
H. B. Lynn	77%		23%
Rehbein, Hagen	55%	18%	27%
W. Schmitt	60%	20%	20%
Breyton	52%	6%	42%
Own Results	62%	29%	9%

The following three methods can be applied to achieve better closing function of the anus and rectum after an abdomino-perineal pullthrough operation:

The fascial sling plastic according to Wreden-Stone and the myokinetic substitution operations as described by Shoemaker and Pickrell. The disadvantages of the first method is that secondary megacolon can result due to the lack of elasticity of the fascia wheras the myokinetic operations are to be recommended as very valuable methods under certain conditions. We must emphasize, however, that a sphincteroplasty can never be as good as normal sphincter function.

The principle of the myokinetic substitution operations is utilization of a neighbouring muscle which undergoes a partial change in function after the transfer under the active cooperation of the patient.

According to SHOEMAKER's method, a muscle segment about 4 cm in width is dissected out under conservation of the nerve-blood-vessel-bundle from the gluteus maximus muscle. To get a possibly longer segment, an adequate incision up to the trochanter major must be made to get the tendon part of the muscle. The plastic can be one- or doublesided. We prefer the preparation of both sides in order to get a completely circular sling, which is not possible if only one muscle is used. After building a perineal tunnel, both muscle segments are slung around the anus, one from the perineal side and the other from the coccygeal side. Both muscle segments are fixed together and then attached to the ischial tuberosity. The tension of the muscle segments is controlled by the forefinger in the rectum.

The disadvantages of SHOEMAKER's method are: firstly, the operation is very bloody, secondly, the muscle segment is not large enough and thirdly an adequate blood supply must be maintained. The gracilis plastic, due to the topographical and anatomical location of the muscle (m. gracilis) takes less time and operating field, the muscle is, furthermore, long enough so that only one muscle is needed for the entire anal sling. The danger of an infection is also reduced because the skin incisions are not near the anus.

To expose the tendon of the gracilis muscle, an arched incision, somewhat dorsal, on the internal surface of the knee-joint is laid. The search for the tendon which is the middle one of the pes anserinus is made easier by locating the sartorius muscle which is the most distal. The gracilis should be detached as much as possible at the distal end, i. e. in the region of the head of the tibia. The muscle can be traced and pulled through another incision which is proximally laid. The small blood vessel can be detached without any damage. Care should be taken to avoid injury to the nerve-blood vessel bundle of the muscle. Our further application of this method varies somewhat from the original method as stated by PICKRELL. In accordance to the modification by GELBKE we refrain from four perineal incisions after the tunnel has been laid. In our experience, two incisions at 6 and 12 o'clock are fully sufficient. Constructing the tunnels in boys poses no problems. In girls, especially when an anal and rectal atresia with an ectopic perineal anus is present, great care should be taken to avoid a perforation of the vagina. Like GELBKE, we reject patching of the gracilis with the levator ani muscle because we presume that some nutritional disturbances may occur. After having constructed the perineal tunnel, we sling the gracilis muscle which is always taken from the right side, twice around the anus, always in a clockwise direction, and fix it to the left ischial tuberosity. The tension of the muscle must be regulated by the finger in the anus.

The success of the operation can be nullified by too great or too little tension. At this moment in the operation the surgeon's skill is put to a hard test. After the wound has healed tension-exercises and later on muscle exercises (of contraction) are carried out in order to achieve a controlled anal closure. Electrical therapy is not necessary in all cases.

Apart from the exact technical procedure of the operation the success of the myokinetic substitution plastic of the sphincter depends mainly on the cooperation of the patient. A prerequisite is a sufficiently high intelligence quotient of the patient which guarentees the adaptation to the altered function of the muscle. The optimal age for the operation is between 8 and 10 years but operations between 7 and 8 are often successful.

The social and home background are just as important for the success of the operation as the factors mentioned above.

The muscle substitution plastic cannot be an equivalent of the normal muscle, because the tension of a voluntarily innervated muscle lasts only for 2–3 min. The purpose of the operation is to give the patient the possibility of sufficient continence,

i. e., to bring the urge to relieve the bowels under control for a short while. The urge to relieve the bowels is generally unaltered in cases of anal and rectal atresia. Thin stools and gases cannot be held back hence dietary precautions are indicated.

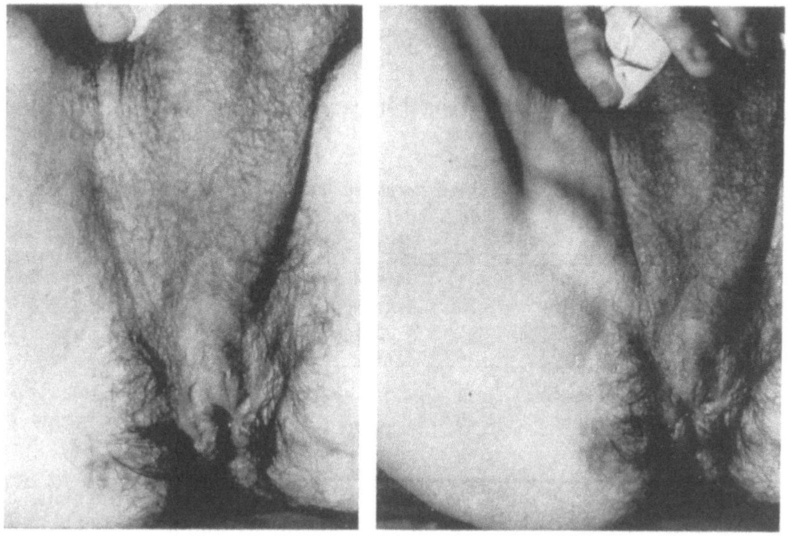

Fig. 1

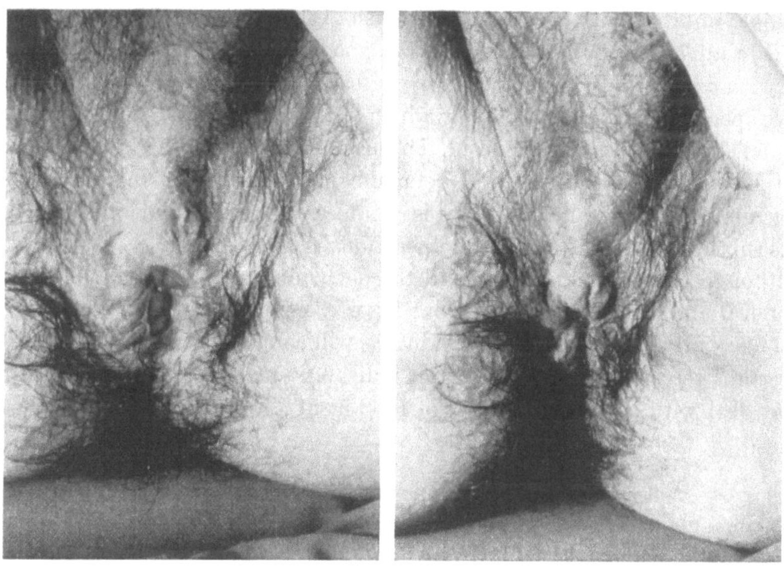

Fig. 2

18 year old (Fig. 1) patient with gracilis plastic on the gaping anus and on the right, the closed anus following the contraction of the gracilis muscle with its muscle-roll on the inner side of the thig. (Fig. 2) Showing the gaping anus on the left and closed anus after the contraction of gracilis muscle on the right.

In the last 6 years (Tab. 2) we operated 10 patients between the age of 4 and 18 years, who had an incontinentia alvi as a result of anal and rectal atresia. The first 4 patients were operated according to Shoemaker's method and the rest according to the Pickrell gracilis plastic because of the simplicity of this method. The results of the Shoemaker's plastic were: two cases were good, one satisfactory and one, although it showed an improvement, failed to achieve an adequate functional result. Re-examination of the 6 cases of gracilis-plastic operation showed three very good results. One case was satisfactory and two cases were as incontinent as before.

Table 2. *Results of myokinetic sphincterplasty with incontinentia alvi after anal and rectal atresia*

Method	No.	Result Excellent or good	Fair	Poor
Shoemaker	4	2	1	1
Pickrell	6	3	1	2
	10	5	2	3

We interprete the two failures mentioned above as follows: the first child, six years old, lives in a social home where the supervision and care which are needed are not present. The second child is only 4 years old. One can feel a good muscle bulge in this child which, however, cannot be innervated. We hope that this condition would improve with age and if not, we shall then transfer the left gracilis muscle. All in all 7 out of 10 children showed good results hence the problem which arises with a colostomy is avoided. Two cases, one 14 and the other 18 years old, deserve special mention. A colostomy which both patients had, could be closed and a normal intestinal outlet achieved. Through an abdomino-perineal pullthrough operation with breakthrough and detaching of the mucous membrane of the rectum, an outlet at the normal place is obtained. The social and emotional disturbances subsided after the successful operations (Fig. 1 and 2).

Although the latest knowhow and the deepening of the understanding of the anatomical and physiological functions have brought a certain success, the cases with unfavourable pre-operative conditions will continue to have incontentia alvi in a certain percentage. An operation is indicated in all cases and one can achieve a great deal with a certain amount of intelligent cooperation on the part of the patient.

Bibliography

Gelbke, H.: Wiederherstellende und plastische Chirurgie. Bd. 2. Stuttgart: Thieme 1963.
Pickrell, K., N. Georgiades, E. F. Richard, and F. Morris: Gracilis muscle transplantation for the correction of neurogenic rectal incontinence. Surg. Clin. N. Amer. **39**, 1405 (1959).
Shoemaker, J.: Un nouveau procédé opératoire pour la reconstitution du sphinkter anal. Sem. Méd. **29**, 160 (1909).
Stone, H. B.: Plastic operation for anal incontinence. Arch. Surg. **18**, 845 (1929).
— Imperforate anus with recto-vaginal cloaca. Ann. Surg. **104**, 651 (1936).
Wreden, R.: A method of reconstruction a voluntary sphincter ani. Arch. Surg. **18**, 841 (1929).

V. Colon Polyps and Cancer Relationship

Colonic Polyps and Carcinoma Risk

F. DEUCHER, F. NÖTHIGER, and A. WIDMER, Aarau, Switzerland

Carcinoma of the colon constitutes a great challenge to all physicians, for it is not only common, but – unlike many other tumors – also curable. The five-year survival rate varies between 30 and 66%, depending upon the initial extent of the lesions [3, 16, 17, 18, 22]. Early diagnosis of recto-colonic tumors should therefore be particularly rewarding, and in this connection it is naturally very important to elucidate the relation between the occurrence of polyps in the large bowel and the risk of carcinoma development.

The polyp, however, remains first and foremost a clinical entity, for every growth that projects above the level of the mucous membrane into the lumen of the intestine is a polyp. The pathologist whose task it is to examine biopsy material therefore has to rely on the clinical findings, because the microscope often reveals only hyperplastic or inflamed, infiltrated colonic mucosa.

Hence, by definition, there is really no such thing as a pseudopolyp. It would be more correct to speak of *inflammatory polyps* when the elevation consists of oedematous or shrunken mucosal islands, such as those typical of acute or chronic ulcerative colitis; these are not neoplasms and are consequently not precancerous. Post-colitic carcinoma develops after many years and has no connection at all with these inflammatory polyps. Obviously, a patient with genuine neoplastic polyps can also have ulcerative colitis. In one 59-year-old male who was referred for recto-colectomy because of his severe chronic ulcerative colitis, we discovered a sessile, benign papilloma of the rectum, which is probably a rare chance finding. The papilloma grows autonomously, of course, and malignant degeneration can take place; the presence of the two diseases at the same time doubles the risk of malignant neoplasia.

Enlarged anal papillae are also not neoplasms, but reactive, inflammatory, hyperplastic processes displaying no real tumorous growth. The transient polyps of adolescence show mucus retention in the goblet cells and are also known as retention polyps. ACKERMAN [1, 2] regards these as inflammatory processes, whereas MORSON [29] believes they are *hamartomata*. The hamartoma is a malformation of normal tissue and not a genuine tumour, and there is no danger at all of malignant degeneration. The same applies to fibromata and lipomata as well as to the polyps of the Peutz-Jegher syndrome [1, 2, 29, 36, 37].

The genuine, initially benign, epithelial neoplasms – the *adenomatous polyp and the villous papilloma* – are entirely different. For purposes of macroscopic differentiation, DUKES' hypothesis [10, 11, 12] that the adenomatous polyp originates in the crypts, where it develops to a stalked tumour owing to lack of space, may be helpful. The villous papilloma is said to arise from superficial epithelial cells, where it has room to proliferate unimpeded. Others assume that it is a special form developing from an adenomatous polyp [13, 14, 38].

Pathologists stress the fact that it is not always easy to differentiate histologically between adenomatous polypi and villous papillomata [19]. Frequently, villous elements can be found in an adenomatous polyp [15, 42]. MORSON [29] even describes a papillary adenoma. *The villous papilloma* is relatively rare: GRINNELL [17, 18] quotes an incidence of 7.9% of all epithelial tumours of the colon, and HELLWIG [20] found that this type accounts for 10.5% of all polyps. The lesions are usually but not necessarily single and are invariably located in the rectum and rectosigmoid and occasionally also in the caecum. Now and again, a villous papilloma is found adjacent to a carcinoma. In several specimens we even discovered one between a pedunculated adenomatous polyp and a dish-shaped invasive carcinoma. The villous papilloma is typically sessile and flat and remains soft as long as it is benign. Generally, however, an enormous cauliflower-like tumour develops gradually. In the light of our own clinical experience, we tend to share the opinion of GRINNELL [17, 18] and ACKERMAN and SPRATT [2] that this is a particular type of tumour with intrinsic biological potency. Of 29 papillomata, 14 displayed atypical cell structures or a carcinoma-in-situ; one even contained an invasive carcinoma, which had, however, just broken through the basal membrane [7]. SUNDERLAND and BINKLEY [38] first drew attention to the relative malignancy of these tumours, which has since been confirmed by most authors [5,7,13,26,29,36,41]. In our comparatively small series of patients we found carcinomata in situ in 50% of papillomata; other authors [17, 18, 20] reckon with an incidence of 33%. TURRELL [39], however, classes the villous papilloma as a benign tumour, no more prone to carcinomatous degeneration than normal colonic mucosa. He maintains that it is only dangerous because its folds may always conceal a carcinoma that might escape endoscopic inspection and biopsy. This controversy has not yet been resolved, but from the clinical point of view it is mainly of theoretical interest, for the papilloma must be removed in any case.

Carcinoma should always be suspected in the event of a relapse following complete surgical extirpation of a papilloma. In one of our patients, a papilloma without any cell anomalies had been removed sigmoidoscopically one year before he was referred to us for treatment. At the same site, we found a small, fresh growth, which we removed by segmental resection; upon microscopic examination this was found to be a clear-cut invasive adenocarcinoma.

The main topic of the discussion is the potential malignancy of *adenomatous polyps*. Whereas only a few years ago, scarcely anyone doubted that the adenomatous polyp degenerated via the carcinoma in situ to an adenocarcinoma [3, 8, 10, 11, 12, 34], many recent reports stress the innocence of the adenomatous polyp [1, 2, 5, 37, 39]. The risk of carcinoma development in patients with polypi is said to be no greater than in the remaining population. So far, neither of these views has been proved conclusively. SCARBOROUGH [33] nevertheless observed the development of a carcinoma after two to eighteen years in ten patients with polyps that had not been removed. BUIE [4] describes the development of carcinomata from polyps after eight years. The argument that carcinomata must already have been present at the first examination, at which, of course, no histological study was undertaken, does not appear to us to be very convincing, but it cannot be refuted. In this connection, it should be borne in mind that KOPPEL [24] followed up one group of patients with polyps and a comparable group without polyps and found that the incidence of adenocarcinomata in both groups was the same.

The fact that both polyps and carcinomata occur predominantly in elderly patients, with the highest incidence in the sixth decade of life [35], that they show the same regional distribution, primarily involving the rectosigmoid and caecum, and that they are more frequent in males (1.6:1) no doubt indicates that there is a close relation between the two.

Moreover, ACKERMAN [1, 2] was able to produce polyps and adenocarcinomata in the mouse with 3:2 dimethyl – 4 aminophenyl, although no transition from polyps to carcinomata could be detected. The demonstration of an elevated deoxyribonucleic acid content in carcinoma cells and in the atypical epithelia of polyps [6, 25, 40] marked a significant step forward in the elucidation of the relation between the two lesions; nevertheless, despite the most intensive research, in view of the great differences in the latency period it will remain largely a matter of chance whether any direct link between malignant tumours and precancerosis can be established.

In two large-scale studies, one involving 200 and the other 1,000 polyps, various degrees of hyperplasia and atypia and all the transitional stages were carefully recorded. WYCHULIS et al. [42] found a large number of mixed forms with adenomatous and villous structures. Moreover, they observed five times as many instances of atypical cell structure and carcinomata in situ among their 200 polyps of 0.5–1 cm diameter as PAGTALUNAN [30] and his group, who examined 1,000 small polyps of less than 0.5 cm diameter and discovered a direct correlation between the incidence of malignant degeneration and the number of polyps.

The adenomatous polyp originates from a minute, pale nodule that scarcely rises above the level of the mucous membrane. When it grows and becomes darker in colour than the mucosa, it is no longer inactive. When the polyp increases in size, it is often attached by a pedicle, which may be long and thin or may remain short and thick. Now and again, the various stages are visible side by side, e. g. next to a carcinoma or regularly dispersed over the entire large bowel. In 39% of the specimens from rectal carcinomata the Veterans Administration Study Group on Adjuvant Cancer Chemotherapy also found benign polyps. In the resection specimen from a 58-year-old patient, we discovered a whole carpet of adenomatous polyps in the rectosigmoid, surrounding two invasive carcinomata. According to our pathologist's report, one of the tumours appeared to have developed from a polyp [7]. *Multiple polyps* are always suspect and should never simply be removed locally, rather they should be treated by resection of the affected portion of the colon. RIDER et al. [32] found carcinomata twice as frequently in patients with multiple polyps as in those with a solitary adenomatous polyp.

In the case of one 66-year-old man, radiography revealed four tumours; in the colectomy specimen, our pathologist subsequently discovered three adenocarcinomata and multiple benign epithelial polyps, three of wich contained a carcinoma in situ. In another specimen, with four colonic carcinomata, there was also a small benign polyp, which could be regarded as the precursor of a fifth carcinoma with reasonable certainty. PORTNOW [31], one of our students, has summarized the relationship between primary multiple colon carcinomata and polyps in tabular form (Table 1): the solitary carcinoma is isolated in 80% of cases and accompanied by polyps in 20%. Where primary multiple carcinomata of the colon are involved, however, only 55% of cases are free of polyps, carcinomata occurring in conjunction with polyps in 45%.

Table 1. *Presence of polyps and relation to age in cases of single and multiple carcinomata of the colon*

	Single carcinoma			Multiple carcinomata								
				concomitant			non-concomitant**			total		
	N°.	%	Agc**	N°.	%	Age**	N°.	%	Age**	N°.	%	Age**
With polyps	92	19.5	57.4	38	41.8	56.2	19	51.4	51.9	57	44.5	54.8
Without polyps	381	80.5	55.6	53	58.2	53.8	18	48.6	57.0	71	55.5	54.6
Total	473	100	56.0	91	100	55.2	37	100	54.4	128	100	54.7

* Age at time of diagnosis of second lesion.
** Average age.

Familial carcinoma of the colon also appears to develop from polyps: the colectomy specimen of one 27-year-old man revealed three invasive carcinomata and two polyps, one of which contained a carcinoma in situ. The genealogical table, which was drawn up and published by Mathis [27], another of our students, caused a sensation among geneticists (Table 2). Out of 24 siblings and descendants, no fewer than 11 had single or multiple colonic carcinomata. The condition is passed on from one generation to the next by dominant and non-sexlinked transmission. McConnell [28] comments that it is difficult to deny the inference that this high familial incidence could only be ascribed to a combination of genetic factors or a rare mutation of a single gene. Our conclusion is that the progression from polyp via carcinoma in situ to invasive carcinoma can either be the result of extraneous noxious substances or an inherited characteristic [7].

Table 2. *Family tree of a Swiss family with 11 confirmed cases of rectal or colonic carcinoma (simplified after* Mathis).

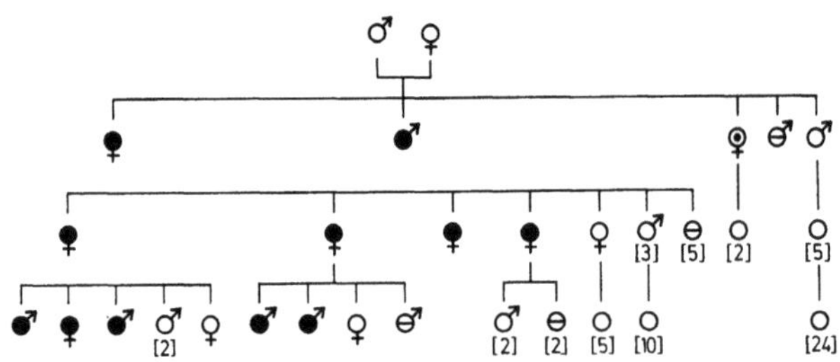

○ cancer-free, ⊖ early death, ● carcinoma of rectum or colon, ⊙ hepatic carcinoma

Nevertheless, we do not believe that this progression is inevitable in every case, as DOCKERTY [8] postulates. Like SPRATT and ACKERMAN [37] with their 20 small carcinomata, in two cases of tumour scarcely the size of cherry stones we found no indication of previous polyps but simply an adenocarcinoma, which was presumably a primary malignant growth.

The only context in which there is any real unanimity about the danger of malignant degeneration is *familial polyposis* of the colon, which is generally accepted as the most clearly defined precancerous condition known to medicine. Opinions differ only as to whether the individual polyps have a greater potential malignancy than ordinary adenomatous polypi, or whether the increased risk is attributable to the large number of polyps involved [33]. According to DOCKERTY and DUNPHY [8, 9], 50% of polyposis patients show evidence of malignant degeneration before their 30th year already. Among our six cases, one 35-year-old man and one 30-year-old woman had carcinomata. Even in Gardner's syndrome, which is characterized by polyposis, desmoid tumours and osteomata, the polyps must be classified as genuine epithelial neoplasms and hence precancerous.

The potential malignancy of colonic polyposis thus being proved, that of villous papillomata scarcely doubted, and only that of quiescent adenomatous polyps still debatable, the *therapeutic implications* are clear-cut. Even the confirmed opponents of the theory of progression from polypus via carcinoma in situ to carcinoma, such as ACKERMAN [1, 2], SPRATT [36, 37], and CASTLEMAN and KRICKSTEIN [5], concede that the malignancy of a polyp cannot be assessed clinically or radiologically. If the lesions exceed 1–1.2 cm in diameter, they recommend polypectomy and subsequent histological examination, even if this involves laparotomy, colotomy or colectomy. Their finding that all radiographically visualized polyps of more than 3 cm diameter and two thirds of those between 2 and 3 cm in diameter are malignant does not alter the fact that the entire question of the potential malignancy of polyps is largely an academic one, for the plan of treatment remains the same for advocates and opponents of the progression theory alike.

1. Familial polyposis necessitates proctocolectomy at an early stage. If the rectum only contains isolated polyps, it is sufficient if colectomy is performed and the rectal polyps excised locally or fulgurated, with subsequent ileoproctostomy. HUBBARD [21] and also COLE [6] and DUNPHY [9] have described spontaneous apocatastasis of the polyps in the rectal stump after this operation, and maintain that the shorter the stump is, the more certain it is that this will take place.

2. In the rectum only, villous papillomata may be removed locally through the proctoscope, if their size permits this in otherwise healthy patients and if regular check-ups can be made. All other papillomata must be removed by segmental resection or total proctectomy.

3. Adenomatous polyps of the rectosigmoid that can be reached endoscopically must always be removed and subjected to histological examination. Those in the lower portion can be removed through the anus and the mucous coat closed with a continuous suture. Polyps in higher portions of the colon that can only be reached by laparotomy should be removed if they are more than 1 cm in diameter, whether they are pedunculated or not. The solitary stalked type is removed by colotomy at the base of the stalk. Multiple polyps and pedunculated or unpedunculated polyps, in which the frozen section performed during operation reveals a carcinoma in the

pedicle, should be removed by segmental resection. The mortality following this operation – 0.7–2% after polypectomy and 3.2–4% after segmental resection – is lower than the incidence of threatened or actual malignant degeneration, which lies between 2.1 and 6% (Table 3).

Table 3.

Size of polypus in cm		Risk: Threatened or actual malignant degeneration	Risk: Mortality of segmental resection	Risk: Mortality of Colotomy and Polypectomy	Risk: Five-year survival
Smith	1.0–1.4	2.1%	4.0%	0.9%	
	1.5–1.9	5.6%			
Behringer and Welch	1.5	6.0%		2.0%	
Bacon			3.2%	0.7%	97%

Finally it must be stressed that all patients in whom colonic polyps are diagnosed must report for check-ups at regular intervals. Five-years follow-up in 246 patients at the Mayo Clinic [23] have revealed that the relapse rate after conservative polypectomy of multiple polyps amounts to 50%, and that, in addition, 60% of the patients later develop carcinoma of the colon. Every relapse is suspect of carcinoma and should, whenever possible, be treated by radical resection.

Bibliography

1. Ackerman, L. V.: Trans. Stud. Coll. Physns Phil. **32**, 1, 5 (1964).
2. —, and J. S. Spratt: Gastroenterology **44**, 905 (1963).
3. Bacon, H. E.: Cancer of the colon, rectum and anal canal. Philadelphia: J. B. Lippincott 1964.
4. Buie, L. A.: Practical proctology, 2nd edn. Springfield, Ill.: C. Thomas 1960.
5. Castleman, B., and H. J. Krickstein: Surg. Gynec. Obstet. **116**, 752 (1963).
6. Cole, J. W., A. McKalen, and J. Powell: Dis. Colon Rectum **4**, 413 (1961).
7. Deucher, F., and Z. Cotar: Schweiz. med. Wschr. **97**, 501 (1967).
8. Dockerty, M. B.: Proc. Staff Meet. Mayo Clin. **33**, 157 (1958).
9. Dunphy, J. E., W. B. Patterson, and M. A. Legg: Ann. Surg. **150**, 488 (1959).
10. Dukes, C.: Proc. roy. Soc. Med. **40**, 829 (1947).
11. — Ann. R. Coll. Surg. **10**, 293 (1952).
12. — Dis. Colon Rectum **1**, 413 (1955).
13. Enterline, H. T., G. W. Evans, R. Mucado-Lugo, L. Miller, and T. W. Fitts: J.A.M.A. **179**, 322 (1962).
14. Ewing, M. R.: Ann. R. Coll. Surg. **6**, 413 (1950).
15. Ferraro, L. R., and T. R. Stuart: Dis. Colon Rectum **8**, 144 (1965).
16. Fletcher, W. S., W. W. Crippaehne, C. E. Hardwick, and J. E. Dunphy: Am. J. Surg. **105**, 117 (1963).
17. Grinnell, R. S., and R. B. Hiatt: Surg. Gynec. Obstet. **94**, 526 (1952).
18. — Surg. Gynec. Obstet. **96**, 31 (1953).
19. Hedinger, C.: Schweiz. med. Wschr. **97**, 508 (1967).

20. HELLWIG, F. C.: Dis. Colon Rectum **3**, 343 (1960).
21. HUBBARD, T. B., jr.: Am. Surg. **23**, 6 (1957).
22. HUGHES, E. S. R.: Brit. med. J. 1963/II, 9.
23. JUDD, E. S., and J. C. CARLISLE: Archs Surg., Chicago **67**, 353 (1953).
24. KOPPEL, M., J. C. BAILOR, F. L. WEAKLEY, and M. B. SHIMKIN: Dis. Colon Rectum **5**, 349 (1962).
25. LEUCHTENBERGER, C.: Lab. Invest. **3**, 132 (1954).
26. MACKIE, J. A., L. D. MILLER, and W. T. FITTS: Surg. Clins N. Amer. **42**, 1451 (1962).
27. MATHIS, M.: Schweiz. med. Wschr. **92**, 1673 (1962).
28. McCONNELL, R. B.: In: Recent Adv. Gastroenterology. Ed. J. BADENOCH and B. N. BROOKE. London: Churchill 1965, p. 2.
29. MORSON, B. C.: J.A.M.A. **179**, 316 (1962).
30. PAGTALUNAN, R. J. G., M. B. DOCKERTY, and R. J. LACKMAN: Surg. Gynec. Obstet. **120**, 1259 (1965).
31. PORTNOW, S. L.: Thesis, University of Zurich, 1956.
32. RIDER, J. A., J. B. KIRSNER, H. C. MOELLER, and W. L. PALMER: Am. J. Med. **16**, 555 (1954).
33. SCARBOROUGH, R. A.: Dis. Colon Rectum **3/4**, 336 (1960).
34. SCHMIEDEN, V., and H. WERTHUES: Dtsch. Z. Chir. **202**, 1 (1927).
35. SMITH, R. A.: Am. J. Gastroenterology **47**, 485 (1967).
36. SPRATT, J. S., jr., L. V. ACKERMAN, and C. A. MOYER: Ann. Surg. **148**, 682 (1958).
37. —, — Dis. Colon Rectum **3**, 330 (1960).
38. SUNDERLAND, D. A., and G. E. BINKLEY: Cancer **1**, 184 (1948).
39. TURRELL, R.: Am. J. Surg. **112**, 805 (1966).
40. WATTENBERG, L. W.: Am. J. Path. **35**, 113 (1959).
41. WELCH, C. E.: Polypoid lesions of the gastrointestinal tract. Philadelphia: W. B. Saunders 1964.
42. WYCHULIS, A. R., M. B. DOCKERTY, R. J. LACKMAN, and O. H. BEAHRS: Surg. Gynec. Obstet. **124/1**, 87 (1967).

Incidence of Polyps and Carcinomas in the Colon and Rectum in Current Autopsy Material

K. Arakawa, Tokyo, Japan

According to vital statistics in Japan, mortality rates for malignant neoplasms have been increasing gradually for the past 15 years. In cancer of the colon, the incidence of cancer death has increased 170 per cent in men and 150 per cent in women, and in cancer of the rectum 141 per cent in men and 144 per cent in women. The incidence of malignant neoplasms of the intestine (except the rectum) and of the rectum in Japan, Germany and United States in both sexes were compared to each other as shown in Table 1. In the case of the rectum, the differences between the incidences in the three countries were not so remarkable, but for the intestine, there were wide differences between them in both sexes. Many investigators emphasized that a polyp or an adenomatous polyp is the main precancerous factor in the gastro-intestinal tract. If this theory is true, the incidence of polyp in the large bowel, especially in the colon, should be low in Japan.

Table 1. *Incidence* (%) *of intestinal and rectal cancer among malignant neoplasms* (WHO Statistics Annual, 1963)

	Male		Female	
	Intestine*	Rectum	Intestine*	Rectum
Japan	2.1	3.2	3.1	3.6
Germany	5.7	4.8	7.0	4.1
U.S.A.	9.3	3.8	13.0	3.5

* Except Rectum.

The material was selected from 4,000 cases autopsied at the Keio University Hospital in Tokyo from September 5th, 1954 to October 22nd, 1967. Distribution of the sample by age and sex is shown in Table 2. Autopsy records of each case were examined carefully, and cases giving a macroscopic description of polypous and/or cancerous lesions in the large bowel were brought to subsequent histological examination.

In the series of 4.000 autopsies, there were 44 cases of carcinoma of the colon making an incidence of 1.1 per cent (Table 3). 6 out of 44 cases had another primary carcinoma in addition to that in the colon and rectum. In 18 instances, there was a clinical history of radical operation. The number of cases of carcinoma in the rectum was 46, an incidence of 1.15 per cent. 2 of these had 2 forms of cancer. 26 out of 46 cases had undergone radical operation previously. In the case of anal carcinoma, large excavating lesions were observed in the lower rectum and in the anal canal. The histology was squamous cell carcinoma. The case of a malignant carcinoid had the primary lesion in the rectum and metastases in the lung, liver and other sites.

Table 2. *Distribution of sample by age and sex*

Age (yr.)	Male	Female	Totals	(%)
0~ 9	436	30	756	(18.9)
10~19	108	627	175	(4.4)
20~29	164	112	276	(6.9)
30~39	229	167	396	(9.9)
40~49	321	242	563	(14.1)
50~59	446	262	708	(17.7)
60~69	508	222	730	(18.2)
70~79	230	111	341	(8.5)
80~89	29	19	48	(1.2)
90~	4	3	7	(0.2)
Totals	2465	1535	4000	(100.0)

Table 3. *Malignant neoplasms of the colon, rectum and anus in 4000 autopsy cases*

	Colon	Rectum	Anus
Carcinomas	44	46	1
Sarcomas	3	0	0
Malig. Carcinoid	0	1	0

In the 4,000 autopsies there were 50 cases of polypoid lesion of the colon and rectum making an incidence of 1.25 per cent (Table 4). The size of these polypoid lesions ranged from 0,2 cm to 3 cm. They were classified by means of histological examination as shown in Table 4. In 4 instances, a polypoid carcinoma of small

Table 4. *Polypoid lesions of the colon and rectum in 4000 autopsy cases (4000 = 100%)*

	No. of cases	%
Adenomas	39	0.95
Adenomatous Polyps	33	0.83
Villous Tumors	4	0.10
Juvenile Polyps	2	0.05
Small Polypoid Carcinomas	4	0.10
Carcinoid Tumors	2	0.05
Polypoid Lymphangiectasis	1	0.03
Granuloma in Submucosa	2	0.05
Cavernous Hemangioma	1	0.03
Hyperplasia of Mucous Memb.	1	0.03
Totals	50	1.25

size was recognized to be a polyp on gross examination. In 2 cases, submucosal granulomas in the rectum were recorded as polyps, and further histological examination revealed the presence of eggs of Schistosoma japonicum in the granulomas. There was not a single case of diffuse familial adenomatosis in this series.

In the series of 4,000 autopsies, there were 39 cases of adenoma making an incidence of 0.95 per cent. This incidence is quite low when compared with the figures in western countries such as 2.7 per cent reported by LAWRENCE in the United States and 4.2 per cent by STEWART in England. A classification of these adenomas has been based upon the character of the morphological and histological structure of the tumors. There were 33 cases of adenomatous polyp, 4 cases of villous tumor and 2 cases of juvenile polyp. Incidences of these subtypes of adenoma are shown in Table 4. 3 out of 4 villous tumors showed atypical proliferation of tumor cells. No malignant change was obeserved in 2 cases of juvenile polyp.

19 out of 33 cases of adenomatous polyp had single lesions and the remaining 14 cases had multiple lesions. The incidence of multiplicity was 42 per cent. There were 72 adenomatous polyps in 33 cases; with the exception of 2 all polyps were pedunculated. Table 5 shows the relationship between the size of an adenomatous polyp and malignancy. Most of them were smaller than 1 cm in diameter. The incidence of atypical proliferation of the tumor cells was 6 per cent in this group. In polyps over 1 cm and more, the incidence increased as shown in this table. In one case of over 2 cm, invasive proliferation of carcinomatous tissue was observed next to adenomatous tissue.

Table 5. *Relation of size of adenomatous polyps to malignancy*

Size in cm.	No. of Polyps	Atypism No.	Atypism %	Carcinomatous Change
~1	76	4	6	0
1~2	3	1	33	0
2~	2	2	100	1
Totals	72	7	9.7	1

The fact that polyps may become malignant brings up the question whether or not there is any correlation between the distribution of carcinomas and that of adenomatous polyps. Anatomic distribution of 72 adenomatous polyps and 90 carcinomas in the colon and rectum is shown in Table 6. It is clear that about half of the carcinomas are located in the rectum while polyps are distributed rather irregularly. This result alone suggests that polyps are by no means the only precancerous factor in the large bowel in my series. Table 7 shows the anatomic distribution of adenomatous polyps in the large bowel reported by 3 authors. Although the incidences are different, the polyps are distributed with surprising similarity in the 3 series of autopsy material. Fig. 1 illustrates the age incidence of adenomatous polyps and that of carcinoma in both sexes. After the third or fourth decade, the incidence increased progressively, but carcinomas have another peak of incidence in both sexes, namely in the second decade. This result suggests that another precancerous factor should be considered in the cases of carcinoma in the young generation.

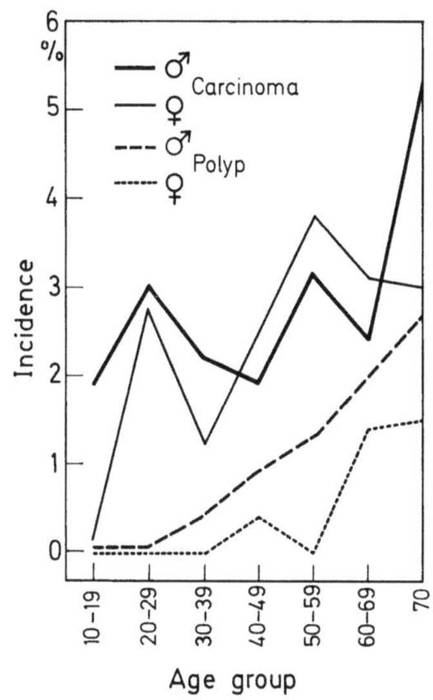

Fig. 1

Table 6. *Anatomic distribution of adenomatous polyps and carcinomas in 4000 autopsy cases*

	Polyps No.	Polyps %	Carcinomas No.	Carcinomas %
Cecum } Ascend. Colon	20	27.7	8	8.9
Ascend. Colon			8	8.9
Hepatic Flexure	3	4.2	3	3.3
Transv. Colon	11	15.5	3	3.3
Splenic Flexure	2	2.8	3	3.3
Descend. Colon	10	13.8	7	7.8
Sigmoid Colon	19	26.3	12	13.4
Rectum	7	9.7	46	51.1
Totals	72	100.0	90	100.0

Table 7. *Anatomic distribution of adenomatous dolyps in 3 reports*

		Arakawa	Helwig	Lawrence
Size of Sample		4000	1460	7000
Incidence of Polyps		0.83%	9.5%	2.7%
Distribution in %	Cecum } Ascend. Colon	27.7	11.8	14.5
	Ascend. Colon		15.4	15.1
	Hepatic Flexure	4.2	4.4	5.7
	Transv. Colon	15.5	11.8	15.1
	Splenic Flexure	2.8	4.8	7.3
	Descend. Colon	13.8	8.1	15.1
	Sigmoid Colon	26.3	27.9	17.7
	Rectum	9.7	15.8	9.5

Statistical Analysis of Polyps of the Colon and Rectum in Japan with Consideration of their Malignant Degeneration

S. Yamagata, H. Watanabe, T. Takebe and T. Narasaka, Sendai, Japan

We report here the results of statistical observation of polyps of the colon and rectum basing both on the annual report of autopsies in Japan during the last 5 years and on the clinical material obtained in our department in the last 10 years with special reference to the probable etiological correlation between polyps and cancer. Polyps in this report do not include histologically confirmed malignant tumors, benign nonepithelial tumors and ulcerative colitis. Multiple polyps i. e. more than two in one patient, is also treated as polyposis in this report occasionally.

Table 1. *Distribution of polyps in the intestinal tract according to the annual report of autopsy in Japan (1962–66)*

		polyp no. of cases	%	polyposis no. of cases	%
small intestine	duodenum	28	0.03	2	0.002
	jejunum	13	0.02	0	0
	ileum	23	0.03	13	0.02
	recorded as small intestine	8	0.01	4	0.005
	total	72	0.09	19	0.02
large intestine	appendix	0	0	0	0
	ileocecum	2	0.002	8	0.01
	cecum	17	0.02	1	0.001
	ascending colon	14	0.02	0	0
	hepatic flexure	0	0	0	0
	transverse colon	5	0.006	0	0
	splenic flexure	1	0.001	0	0
	descending colon	9	0.01	0	0
	sigmoid colon	23	0.03	3	0.004
	rectum	68	0.08	3	0.004
	anus	1	0.001	0	0
	recorded as large intestine	67	0.08	60	0.07
	total	207	0.26	75	0.09
small and large intestine				12	0.02
	total	271	0.33	106	0.13
		total of autopsied cases 81,229			

We found 294 cases of polyps of the colon and rectum among 81,229 cases autopsied in the last 5 years in Japan, which is a frequency of only 0.36%. Table 1 shows that the site where polyps are seen most frequently is the rectum, then follows the sigmoid, the cecum and the ascending colon. Table 2 deals with the distribution of cancer of the colon and rectum detected at autopsy during the same period; it shows the same tendency as in polyps.

Table 2. *Distribution of cancer in the intestinal tract according to the annual report of autopsy in Japan (1962–66)*

		No. of cases	% of all intestinal cancer cases	% of all autopsied cases
small intestine	duodenum	42	3.1	0.05
	papilla of Vater	82	6.0	0.10
	jejunum	6	0.4	0.007
	ileum	4	0.3	0.005
	recorded as small intestine	4	0.3	0.005
	total	138	10.0	0.17
large intestine	appendix	11	0.8	0.01
	ileocecum	48	3.1	0.05
	cecum	53	3.9	0.07
	ascending colon	69	5.0	0.08
	hepatic flexure	15	1.1	0.02
	transverse colon	58	4.2	0.07
	splenic flexure	12	0.9	0.01
	descending colon	24	1.7	0.03
	sigmoid colon	166	12.1	0.20
	rectum	638	46.4	0.79
	anus	12	0.9	0.01
	recorded as large intestine	139	10.1	0.17
	total	1237	90.0	1.52
	total	1475	100.0	1.82
		total of autopsied cases 81,229		

In 286 autopsied cases there were 203 males and 83 females, giving a sex ratio of 1:0.41 in favour of males. Age also affects the incidence of both polyps and cancer in almost the same manner showing the gradual increase of incidence with age as seen in Fig. 1. The same tendency is found in the frequency, calculated on the basis of the population autopsied in each group, as shown in Fig. 2.

Meanwhile, we found 167 cases of polyps clinically by means of x-ray and romanoscopic examination during the last 6 years including 2 cases of Peutz-Jegher syndrome and 2 cases of familial polyposis. Table 3 shows that 164 cases of polyps were detected by the romanoscope in the same period; this corresponds to 7.8% of 2,103 cases examined by romanoscope. In these cases, 108 are male and 56 cases female, giving the sex ratio of 1:0.52. The distribution of polyps according to age shows the peak incidence during the fifth decade followed by the sixth, seventh and fourth decade as seen in Fig. 3. The same tendency is noticed in 120 cases of cancer diagnosed clinically in the last 10 years (Fig. 3). However, the frequency in each age group is highest in the seventh decade followed by the eight, sixth and fifth decade. This coincides with the results obtained in autopsy cases.

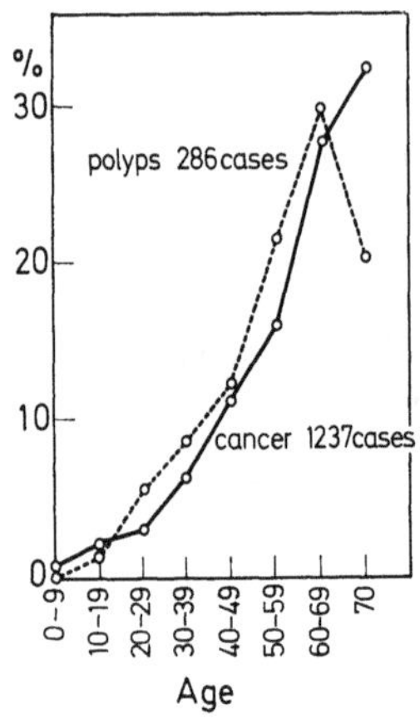

Fig. 1

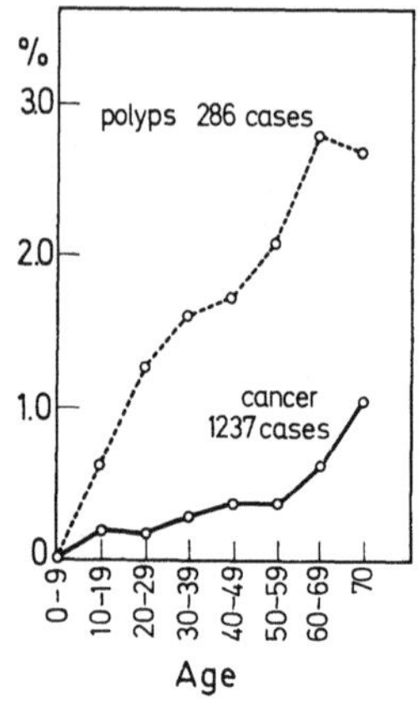

Fig. 2

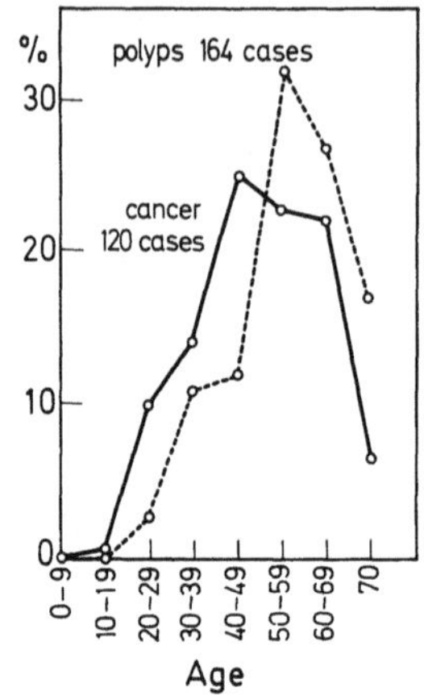

Fig. 3

Table 3. *Diseases of the large intestine detected by romanoscopic examination (1962–67)*

	no. of cases	%
polyps	164	7.8
cancer	49	2.3
ulcerative colitis	46	2.2
melanosis coli	9	0.4
amebic colitis	5	0.2
tuberculosis	2	0.09
sarcoma	1	0.04
total	2103	100.0

Table 4. *Size of polyps detected by the romanoscope (1962–67)*

size	male no. of cases	%	female no. of cases	%	total no. of cases	%
smaller than rice	55	50.9	30	53.6	85	51.8
red bean	32	29.6	22	39.3	54	32.9
bean	10	9.3	1	1.8	11	6.7
little finger tip	5	4.6	1	1.8	6	3.7
thumb tip	3	2.8	0	0	3	1.8
bigger than walnut	3	2.8	2	3.6	5	3.0
total	108	100.0	56	100.0	164	100.0

As to the size of polyps in these 164 cases, one can easily see that almost half of all cases have tumors of rice size or smaller and one third of red bean size, and tumors bigger than the tip of the small finger are seen in only 8.5% as shown in Table 4. Table 5 shows the number of polyps found clinically in each case. In two-thirds the single polyps and two or three polyps were seen in 13.8% and 11.4% respectively, while innumerable polyps of familial polyposis were encountered in only two cases. One also sees that four-fifths of our cases were found in the rectum and then relatively often in the sigmoid, but only 4.2% in the portion higher than the sigmoid where the romanoscope cannot be used.

Table 5. *Number and site of polyps detected clinically (1962–67)*

		no. of cases	%
number	1	109	65.3
	2	23	13.8
	3	19	11.4
	4 ~ 10	11	6.6
	11 ~ 20	2	1.2
	21 ~	1	0.6
	innumerable	2	1.2
site	rectum	135	80.8
	sigmoid colon	53	31.7
	descending colon	6	3.6
	transverse colon	3	1.8
	ascending colon	3	1.8
	cecum	3	1.8
	total	167	100.0

Biopsies of 119 polyps from 117 cases revealed that more than half of the cases are adenomatous polyps, then comes the so-called hyperplastic polyp (Lane et al.) seen in Table 6.

Table 6. *Histologic findings of polyps biopsied at romanoscopic examination (1958–67)*

histologic findings	no. of cases	%
adenomatous polyp (including villous adenoma)	65	55.5
so-called hyperplastic polyp (Lane et al.)	18	15.4
juvenile polyp	5	4.3
inflammatory polyp (excluding ulcerative colitis)	6	5.1
lymph follicle hyperplasia	4	3.4
normal mucosa	21	17.9
total	117	100.0

To see the possible etiologic link between polyps and cancer, the combined occurrence was surveyed using both autopsy and clinical cases.

Table 7 shows that the rate of cancer found in 207 cases of polyp autopsied during the last 5 years is 6.3%, while that in 87 cases of polyposis is 29.9%. On the contrary, the rate of polyps found in 1,227 cases of cancer autopsied during the same period is 2.9% and that in 10 cases of so-called polyp cancer is 40% as shown in Table 8. The same survey done using 174 cases of clinically detected polyps during the last 6 years is summarized in Table 9. In these cases, cancer is seen in 9.2% and so-called polyp cancer in 1.7%. In some cases, both cancer and so-called polyp cancer were observed together, leaving the final frequency at 9.8%.

Table 7. *Incidence of combined occurrence of cancer found in cases of polyps of the large intestine according to the annual report of autopsy in Japan (1962–66)*

	no. of cases	cancer no. of cases	%	so-called polyp cancer no. of cases	%	total no. of cases	%
polyp	207	13	6.3	0		13	6.3
polyposis	87	22	25.3	4	4.6	26	29.9
Peutz-Jeghers syndrome	2	0	0	0	0	0	0

Table 8. *Incidence of combined occurrence of polyps found in cases of cancer of the large intestine according to the annual report of autopsy in Japan (1962–66)*

	no. of cases	polyp no. of cases	%	polyposis no. of cases	%	total no. of cases	%
cancer	1227	13	1.1	22	1.8	35	2.9
so-called polyp cancer	10	0	0	4	40.0	4	40.0

Table 9. *Incidence of combined occurrence of cancer found in clinically detected cases of polyps of the large intestine (1962–62)*

	no. of cases	cancer no. of cases	%	so called polyp cancer no. of cases	%	total no. of cases	%
polyp	110	7	6.4	0	0	7	6.4
polyposis	60	8	13.3	2	3.3	9	15.0
Peutz-Jeghers syndrome	2	0	0	0	0	0	0
familial polyposis of the colon	2	1	50.0	1	50.0	1	50.0
total	174	16	9.2	3	1.7	17	9.8

The existence of cancer among polyps is also studied according to the histological findings of polyps. It is seen in Table 10 that 69 cases of adenomatous polyp contain 12 cases of cancer, that is 17.4% and 3 cases of so-called polyp cancer, that is

4.3%, while 18 cases of so-called hyperplastic polyp contain 4 cases of cancer that is 22.2%. Cancer of the colon and rectum resected in the last 10 years combines polyps of various histologic findings as shown in Table 11. It is seen that 88 cases of cancer include 10 cases having adenomatous polyps somewhere in the large intestine (11.4%) and 4 cases of so-called hyperplastic polyp (4.5%). 3 cases of cancer and so-called polyp cancer occurring together include 2 cases of adenomatous polyp and one of the 2 so-called polyp cancers also had an adenomatous polyp.

Because of the similar tendency seen in the distribution of both polyps and cancer concerning the site and age, because of a significantly high incidence of cancer in polyps especially in adenomatous polyps or so called hyperplastic polyps, it is suggested that an etiological correlation exists between polyps especially of the adenomatous or hyperplastic type and cancer of the colon and rectum.

Table 10. *Combined occurrence of cancer in cases of polyps of the large intestine examined clinically and histological findings of polyps*

	no. of cases	cancer no. of cases	cancer %	so called polyp cancer no. of cases	so called polyp cancer %	total no. of cases	total %
adenomatous polyp (including villous adenoma)	69	12	17.4	3	4.3	13	18.8
adenomatous polyp + so called hyperplastic polyp	2	0	0	0	0	0	0
so called hyperplastic polyp (LANE et al.)	18	4	22.2	0	0	4	22.2
juvenile polyp	8	0	0	0	0	0	0
inflammatory polyp (excluding ulcerative colitis)	6	0	0	0	0	0	0
lymph follicle hyperplasia	4	0	0	0	0	0	0
normal mucosa	21	0	0	0	0	0	0

Table 11. *Histological findings of polyps found in resected cases of cancer of the large intestine (1958–67)*

	no. of cases	adenomatous polyp no. of cases	adenomatous polyp %	so called hyperplastic polyp no. of cases	so called hyperplastic polyp %	histology unknown no. of cases	histology unknown %	total no. of cases	total %
cancer	88	10	11.4	4	4.5	5	5.7	19	21.6
cancer + so called polyp cancer	3	2	66.7	0	0	0	0	2	66.7
so called polyp cancer	2	1	50.0	0	0	0	0	1	50.0
total	93	13	14.0	4	4.3	5	5.4	22	23.7

Adenomatous Polyps of the Rectum and Recto-Sigmoid – Benign and Malignant – Surgical Management

H. BERNHOFT, Buffalo, N. Y., U. S. A.

The incidences in which adenomatous polyps, solitary or multiple, are found in the rectum or recto-sigmoid range from 7–10%. That many of these may undergo malignant transformation if not removed is the consensus of clinicians and pathologists. These may or may not become metastasizing, "killing cancers". This is not possible to prognosticate with accuracy. Therefore, surgical removal and histologic study of all adenomatous polyps found at the time of sigmoidoscopy is most essential.

In a review of 6335 patients routinely examined sigmoidoscopically to the 26 cm level, we found 439 to have one or more visible adenomatous polyps. 17 or 3.9% were of the villous type. This review was conducted since 1956 thus giving a 12-year-period for follow-up examinations every six months for five years, then yearly.

I wish to emphasize that none of these were biopsied. The polyp was removed in its entirety and sent for histologic study. When it was necessary because of size, it was removed in several pieces. Care was taken to send the stalk or base separately on these occasions.

The electro-surgical snare is most satisfactory for use in polypectomies. If used, it is essential that the operator be skilled technically and aware of the complications that may occur, such as explosions or over-coagulation of the tissue with subsequent hemorrhage or perforation when the coagulum sloughs.

In this series of polyps, all were removed as office procedures. There were no perforations and only 2 hemorrhages. Both developed 10–12 days after the polypectomy. One required hospitalization for blood replacement – the other did not. Neither required more than clearing the site of old clot and coagulation of a bleeding site without further complication.

Whether or not one elects to perform laparotomy, when the polyp is above the peritoneal reflection, depends on his own judgement. If the risk of anesthesia, operative and post-operative mortality and morbidity is considered less than that of sigmoidoscopic polypectomy, then the surgeon may elect the abdominal approach.

In 26.6% of our patients, the polyps were considered to be above or at the peritoneal reflection. These have been removed without complication. Management of benign adenomatous polyps of the rectum and recto-sigmoid presents few problems. Simple polypectomy of the surgeon's choice is sufficient. Subsequent interval examinations are essential as the possibility of developing other adenomas exists.

The evaluation of transitional and carcinomatous adenomas requires a careful correlation of both clinical and histologic study [1]. The following important features of the polyp are noted; its size and appearance, whether it is pedunculated or sessile, mobile or fixed, and, if fixed, whether it is deep or superficial fixation. If carcinoma is present histologically, it is to be noted whether it is a frank carcinoma, which would be a killing cancer, or a carcinoma in situ.

In the 439 cases of polyps, 340 or 77.4% were benign, 41 or 9.3% transitional, and 28 or 6.8% showed areas with malignant change either in the tip or stroma considered in most cases to be carcinoma in situ. None of these showed pedicle or base invasion. 30 or 7% showed them to be replaced by frank carcinoma. The patients [69] with polyps having transitional and areas of frank carcinomatous change were not hospitalized. Removal was done as an office procedure with the electro-surgical snare followed by coagulation of the base. These have been followed for a period of 12–20 years without local recurrence or evidence of metastatic disease.

To amplify the importance of polypectomies in toto versus biopsy, I wish to report that rectal adenomas had been biopsied elswhere in 4 of the 28 patients and the polyps had undergone malignant change. Based on the histologic study of the biopsy, an abdominal perineal resection was indicated. 3 are alive and well 12 years after polypectomy. 1 died after 10 years from primary lung carcinoma confirmed by surgery and autopsy with no evidence of metastatic disease from the rectal polyp.

It is logical to believe also that a biopsy taken from a benign area could lull one into a sense of false security when a more radical procedure would be indicated.

A resection, either abdominal perineal, low anterior or "pull-through", was performed on the 30 patients having polyps with complete malignant replacement and base invasion.

The "pull-through" procedure may be done where technical and anatomic problems preclude a secure anastomosis [2]. We have found it most helpful in the resection of large benign villous papillomata which may leave only a small rectal cuff when resected.

A "pull-through" may be done which requires no perineal or anal surgery. The complete sphincter mechanism remains intact with several centimeters of rectal cuff which is most essential for proper bowel control and function of the defecation reflex.

Following low sigmoid and rectal resection, a 38 French straight Pezzer catheter is sutured into the proximal segment of colon by a "purse-string" suture. It is then passed through the rectal segment to the first assistant, who temporarily leaves the immediate operative field (Fig. 1).

Care is taken by the operating surgeon to avoid torsion over the pelvic brim which would jeopardize the marginal circulation. Three or four interrupted silk sutures are used to secure the serosal and muscular layers of the rectal cuff to the taenial bands of the "pulled through" segment.

The stoma matures just the same as it does on the abdominal wall (Fig. 2). It requires the same local care, namely, frequent dilatations, until it has completely matured and retracted to the edge of the rectal cuff. By the time this occurs, there is a firm anastomosis.

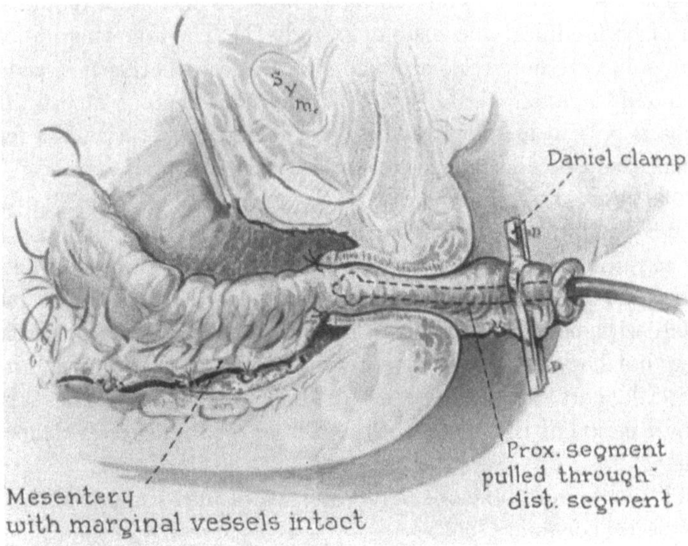
Daniel clamp
Prox. segment
pulled through
dist. segment
Mesentery
with marginal vessels intact

Fig. 1

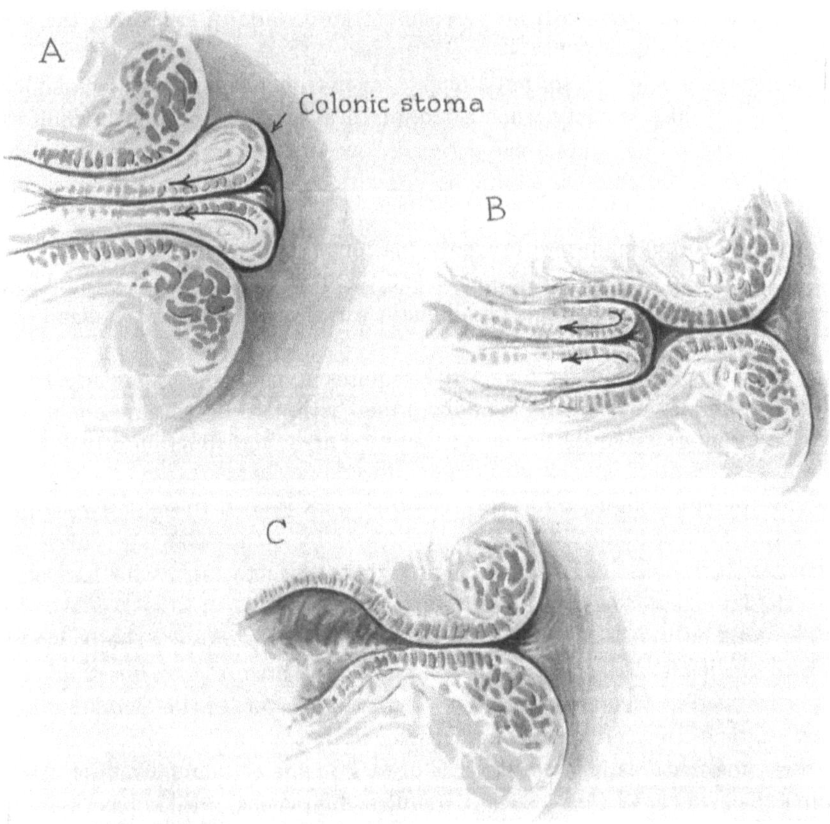
A
Colonic stoma
B
C

Fig. 2

Proximal decompression is *most* essential. A tube type cecostomy is adequate. A right angle 34 F–36 F de Pezzer catheter is the one of choice with a double purse string suture about the cecal fenestration. If there is adequate pre-operative colon preparation and there is little or no fecal content, gas accumulation and subsequent pressure are responsible for increased edema and "leaks".

Routine para-rectal or transperitoneal drains are not essential and may often be hazardous as they may transform small collections, otherwise absorbed or spontaneously drained into the bowel lumen, into chronic fistulae.

A sump type drain through the inferior pole of the abdominal incision left for 28 hours is adequate to remove any excess serosanguinous accumulations.

It must be emphasized that the cecostomy must be kept open during the maturation period of the "pulled through" stoma. Otherwise obstruction most likely will occur.

If one elects to remove polyps, benign or malignant, from the recto-sigmoid or lower sigmoid by laparotomy, coloscopy of the left, transverse and ascending colon should be done. With the lower mortality and morbidity rates from resections, resection of the recto-sigmoid rather than colotomy and polypectomy is the procedure of choice in all patients under 50 regardless of the histologic picture. This removes the segment which has the highest incidence of both benign and malignant neoplasms of any area in the colon.

Conclusion

It is not the intent of this presentation to minimize the value of radical surgery for the cure of malignant lesions of the recto-sigmoid and prevention of metastatic disease in any way nor to endorse "small operations" for small and "big operations" for large lesions. However, I do endorse the compassionate surgeon whose interest in his patient as a human being is greater than in a statistic, and who will carefully evaluate transitional polyps in the rectum and recto-sigmoid, both gross and histologic, before making a decision as to the proper surgical procedure. If abdominal perineal resections were done on the cases in which simple polypectomy is adequate, the five year survival rate for these resections would, of course, be higher, but every patient with preserved colonic continuity is not only a happier patient but a most grateful one.

Bibliography

1. Morgan, C. N.: Treatment of Cancer of the Rectum. Amer. J. Surg. **115**, 442 (1968).
2. Bernhoft, W. H., and B. A. Portin: Low Rectal Anastomosis. Arch. Surg. **90**, 1 (1965).

Problems in the Histological Diagnosis of Polyps of the Colon

K. ELSTER and K. ARNOLD, Erlangen, Germany

MORSON's proposal that every intestinal polyp be classified in accordance with its anatomical configuration or its histological picture, is nowadays largely complied with. In spite of this, problems not infrequently arise in respect to the therapeutic consequences. This difficulty results from the fact that the clinician expects a "yes or no type" of statement from the pathological-anatomical diagnosis that is, the diagnosis shall indicate unequivocally whether a benign or a malignant process is being dealt with.

On the other hand, histological findings are provided that do not allow this type of statement to be made. The classical example of such an "uncertain" finding is provided by the polypoid adenoma, in which the degree of dedifferentiation of the epithelial cells of individual groups of glands varies. Speaking from the cytomorphological point of view, sections of such an adenoma can correspond in appearance to the degree of dedifferentiation of a carcinoma. If the only certain criterion of invasive growth, namely – the penetration of the muscularis mucosae ist not determinable –, then we speak either of a carcinoma-in-situ, or of an adenoma which has become malignant. For pathological-anatomical reasons, we consider the former designation to be incorrect. The carcinoma in situ is characterized by a cellular atypia within an epithelial layer and is thus no real neoplasia, while, on the other hand, the polypoid adenoma represents an already fully-developed neoplastic process.

However, this terminological problem is only of secondary importance, when compared with the problem of the clinical diagnosis of such a histological finding. Whether or not such a finding should be followed up with the same therapeutic measures as an invasively growing carcinoma, is then generally left to the discretion of the surgeon.

A more precise delimitation, and thus an objectification, of these findings is said to be possible by means of the process of "grading" (BRODERS). Here, however, a certainty of diagnosis is often only simulated, for the determined degree of differentiation is neither free from the subjective attitude of the investigator, nor is it, in the majority of cases, representative of the whole of the tumour.

Our own catamnestic enquiries, carried out with WUNDISCH on patients with polyps have indicated that the degree of differentiation is an extremely uncertain basis for the prognostic evaluation of the polyps. Of a total of 266 patients with rectal polyps, 88 i. e. a third, of the investigated cases showed a carcinoma. Of these, a polypoid adenoma with transition to a carcinoma was diagnosed at the first biopsy in 10% of the cases, while in 62 patients (23%) a carcinoma was first discovered catamnestically (Fig. 1). Our "grading" of the polyps (which is to be considered as a working hypothesis) in the patient group with subsequently established carcinoma indicates that there is no relationship between the degree of differentiation and the frequency of subsequent carcinoma development. It is also noteworthy that there is a high percentage of carcinomas in the group of polyps with signs of great differentiation (Table 1). Of course, the conclusion must not be drawn that the development of a carcinoma was observed in every case where we had first detected a polyp and then characterized it with a certain degree of differentiation. The high degree of carcinoma danger of patients with a polypoid adenoma has been unequivocally documented with this result, however.

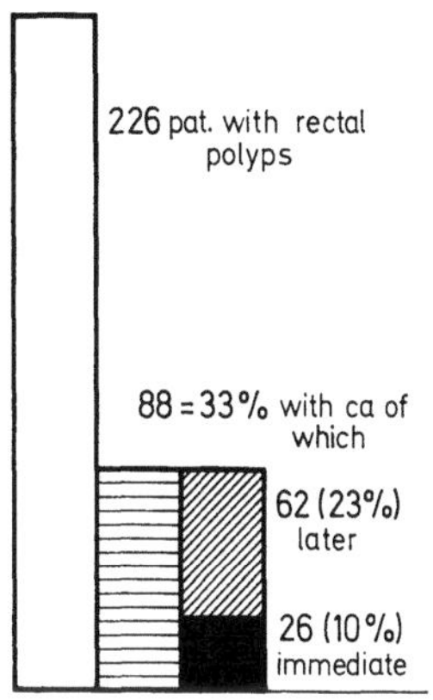

Fig. 1. Percentage of the carcinomas established (catamnestically) earlier or later in patients with polyps

Table 1. Degree of differentiation of the polyps in relation to the number of carcinomas subsequently established

Groups of polyps	Patients: total	with rectal carcinoma later	%
Group I	37	15	40.5
Group II	69	8	11.5
Group III	92	29	31.3

In a further series of investigations with FELKEL, the question was examined as to whether the "uncertain" findings characterized earlier, could lead to an unequivocal diagnosis if further excisions were carried out. Here it was shown, admittedly on investigation material which is still limited in volume, that intermittent excisions can lead to the discovery of a carcinoma. The uncertainty factor, however, remains, whether a negative result excludes the presence of a carcinoma or not (Table 2).

Table 2. Number of multiple excisions which led to the discovery of a carcinoma in initially diagnosed "polypous adenoma"

Diagnosis endoscopically "polyp" histologically after first biopsy	final diagnosis	final diagnosis by biopsy 2nd	3rd	4th	5th	6th
26 adenomata	12 carcinomas	9	2	—	—	1
	14 non-malignant					

In addition to histo-cyto-morphological problems in the diagnosis of neoplastic processes of the intestine, there are, not infrequently, also problems of method. This includes incomplete excision, which misses the actual process. Such "marginal excisions" can, however, as has already been shown in the stomach, allow the recognition of structural changes which can serve as an indication for the presence of a "localized process". Our measurements carried out with Elles on 1,700 rectal biopsy preparations, showed an average thickness of the mucous membrane of just on 0,5 mm. No noteworthy deviations were observed when the material was separated into groups according to age; a difference between the sexes was not noted either. In the immediate neighbourhood of both the carcinoma and the polypoid adenoma, an increase in the thickness of the mucous membrane of about 100% could be determined. This is based on a lengthening of the crypts as a result of hyperplasia of the epithelium. This thickening, which can be recognized by the practised observer even without the exact determination of measured data, should at least indicate to him that the finding needs to be subjected to further diagnostic investigations (Fig. 2).

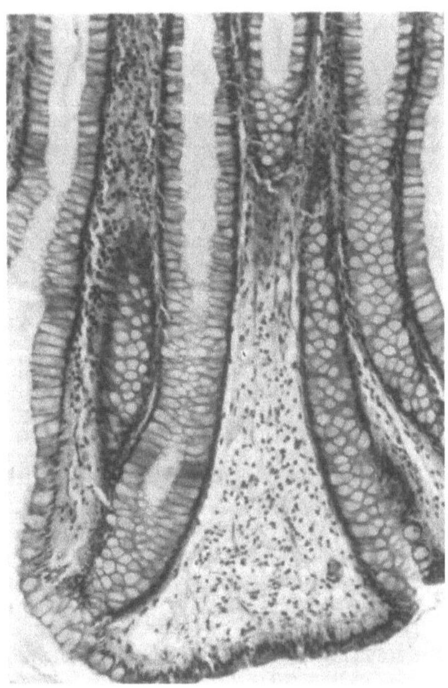

Fig. 2. Hyperplasia of the crypts with a mucosa thickness of up to 1.25 mm in the marginal area of a carcinoma (magnification 140 ×)

The problems associated with the histological diagnosis of polyps of the colon are mainly a consequence of the dynamics of biological processes. The static, instantaneous picture of a histological section should thus be a constant reminder to us of the limits of morphology. The value and significance of a histological finding are, however, not diminished if a co-operative form of attack develops from a realization of the problems.

Bibliography

BRODERS, A. C.: Grading of carcinoma. Minn. Med. 8, 726 (1925).

ELLES, D.: Varianten der Schleimhautdicke des Rektums. Diss. Med. Fak. Erlangen 1968.

ELSTER, K., u. G. WÜNDISCH: Morphologische Wertung der Rektumpolypen. Langenbecks Arch. klin. Chir. **311**, 41–63 (1965).

MORSON, B. C.: Precancerous lesions of the colon and rectum. Classification and controversial issues. J.A.M.A. **179**, 316 (1962).

Classification and Therapy of Colon Polyps

H. SCHAUDIG, Bad Mergentheim, Germany

In both, diagnosis and therapy of polypous diseases of the colon, special importance is attached to the skillful examination. The general practitioner will palpate only 16 per cent of all polyps localized in the rectum. The rectoscopically trained physician is able to visualize 80 per cent of the lesions. By means of biopsy we can determine the nature of the disease and undertake the appropriate treatment (Fig. 1).

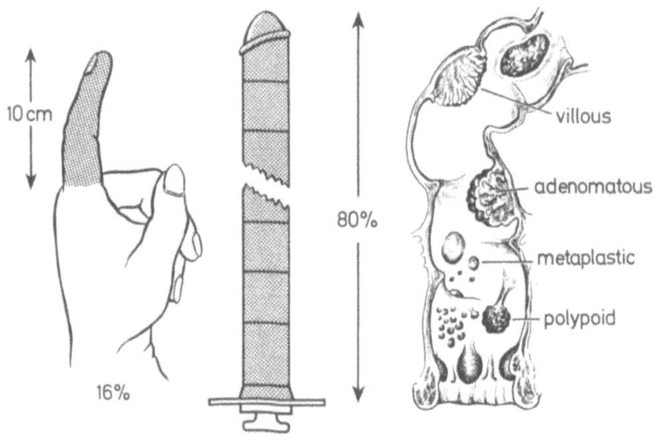

Fig. 1

Classification

A concise and therapeutically useful classification of the various polypous diseases is difficult, but it will be attempted here as follows (Table 1):

Table 1. *Polyps of colon – hamartomas*

Single Polyp	Most without symptoms
PEUTZ-JEGHERS	to be found in colon in 50%. Most without symptoms
Polyposis PEUTZ-JEGHERS	to be found in colon in 50%. Most without symptoms
Juvenile Polyp	Bleeding
Juvenile Adenoma	spontaneous amputation before the 20th year
Retention polyp	
Cystic mucous polyp	
Juvenile Polyposis	Symptoms before the 10th year. Other malformation in 50%

Peutz-Jeghers Type of Polyp

It can be found as an isolated malformation of the muscularis mucosae in any segment of the colon and at any age.

Juvenile Polyp

Its pedicle is weak, it contains no muscularis mucosae, its contour is smooth and roundish. Often it falls off spontaneously. By this self-amputation the disease will be healed in up to the twenty-year-olds in almost all cases.

Peutz-Jeghers Polyposis

A clinical appearence inherited as a dominant characteristic, affecting men and women. Every part of the digestive tract can be attacked by polyps. The polyps are not arranged like a bed. They are distributed as single polyps in great numbers throughout the colon. Most of the time, one will find darkbrown to black, melaniferous, perioral, perinasal and buccal pigmentation of the mucous membrane.

Juvenile Polyposis

Is hard to define as a clinical picture as such. It will always occur before the tenth year of age. The polyps are shed, resulting in continuously reappearing bleeding from the rectum. The benignity of the disease is proved by the histological examination. However the heredity of the disease requires the examination of all members of the family since one member possibly suffers from adenomatous polyposis.

A sharp line must be drawn between the benign development of polypous diseases and the new growths originating from the colonic epithelium some of which can be an early stage of a malignant tumor (Table 2).

Table 2. *Polyps of colon – epithelial neoplasmas*

Metaplastic Polyp	Hyperplastic Polyp	Often and benign
Adenoma	Adenomatous Polyp Polypous Adenoma Pedunculated Polyp	Benign neoplastic growth ↓
Papillary Adenoma	Papillary Polyp Papillary Adenoma Papilloma	Growing up to malignancy
Villous Adenoma	Villous Adenoma	
Polyposis familiaris	Adenomatous Polyposis Polyposis diffusa adenomatosa	Early begin of malignancy
Gardner-Syndrom		Praecancerous illness with osteomas

Metaplastic polyps (hyperplastic polyps) are found very frequently. They are up to 0.5 mm in size, and are directly attached to the walls of the enteric canal on a broad base.

Adenomas in colon and rectum are better supplied with blood. They have a granulated almost smooth surface. They feel compact. A great deal of prolonged observation has shown, that these polyps remain benign as a rule. Their inclination to grow, however, cannot be calculated with certainty. After remaining inactive for years they may grow invasive all of a sudden, and become a metastasizing cancer; on the other hand we know cases which have remained stationary and even grew smaller while under observation for years. An important hint for judging the malignity of a polyp is its size. Only in 0.5 per cent of all observations were adenomas with a diameter of less than 0.5 cm found to be malignant. Meanwhile adenomas with a diameter of more than 1.2 cm developed into malignant tumors in 24 per cent of the cases.

Papillary Adenomas and Villous Papillomas

are spread on a broad base over the intestinal mucous membrane. The surface is soft. The examining finger may easily push the villi aside. Malignity exists in about 30 per cent only. The villous electrolyte-losing adenomas are also classified in this group.

Adenomatous polyposis is a rare disease inherited as a dominant trait with a bedlike distribution of the adenomas and villous papillomas throughout the whole colon. A carcinoma develops 10–15 years after the occurrence of the first symptoms.

The Gardner Syndrome is also an adenomatous colonic polyposis occuring together with osteomas or mesenchymic tumours. Only few cases have been recorded.

Therapy of colon polyps (Table 3) depends on their localisation. Contrast roentgenography of the colon must employed before any therapeutic measures are undertaken. The barium enema with a picture of the mucous membrane is not sufficient for refined diagnostics. A smaller polyp would fail to be visualised. The double contrast method improves the diagnostic result by 50 per cent. Despite the best technique, however, polypous manifestations less then 1.2 cm in diameter cannot be recognized with certainty. Since polyps below this measurement reveal an inclination to malignant modification in 0.9 per cent only, the diagnostic value of double contrast roentgenogramm is an indispensable and relatively certain method.

Polyps within rectoscopic reach even benign ones are removed radically on principle. In most cases they can be amputated as far as 25 cm beyond the anal ring. *Small metaplastic tumours* of multiple appearence may be removed by the diathermy needle in situ if the benign aspect of one or two of the excrescences is histologically confirmed.

Pedunculated adenomas can be nipped off by slipping over a diathermic sling and performing a constriction at the base of the pedicle with simultaneous coagulation.

Sessile, villous, papillary adenomas require extraordinary care as to their rectoscopic amputation. Up to 20 cm they can be removed by the operating proctoscope under general anaesthesia.

Less than 10 cm beyond the anal ring a direct extirpation is possible after adjustment with specula. If the pedicle does not reveal a malignant infiltration, a pedunculated polyp with malignant modifications in the head only is radically removed. This indication is also valid for sessile adenomas and villous papillomas.

Three-dimensional total extirpation in a healthy patient is very difficult in these cases. In cases of sessile polyps, one must therefore perform an operative exposure.

If the rectum is affected by polyps and in case of evidence of a polyp in the upper colonic parts, the histological diagnoses can be made by exploratory rectoscopic excision. If a harmatoma is found, the higher polyp may also be classified as such and remain in situ. To my knowledge the literature does not report any case where a patient showed harmatomatous and adenomatous colon polyps at the same time (Table 3).

Table 3. *Polyps of colon*

Diagnosis		Therapy	
Biopsy Rectum	X-Ray Colon	Rectal Excision	Abdominal Resection
Hamartoma	–	+	–
Hamartoma	+	+	–
Adenoma	–	+	–
Adenoma	+	+	–
Adenoma	+	+	+
–	+	–	+

Colon polyps detectable by roentgenography must be removed by operative treatment if epithelial new growths are found in the rectum.

Lesions more than 25 cm proximal to the anal ring require laparatomy for extirpation. Should the extirpation fail in the healthy patient, then the colonic segment must be exstirpated by segmental resection, hemicolectomy or colectomy, in accordance with the strict rules of cancer surgery.

In familial polyposis a certain death by cancer can only be prevented successfully by colectomy. With little effect on the rectum, the polyps can be removed from the lower 15 cm of the mucous membrane and an ileo-rectal anastomosis can be performed after colectomy. Thus the patient is spared the anus-praeter. Lifelong rectoscopic control, however, is necessary since polyps or even carcinomas may occur in the remaining rectum.

Polyps visualised exclusively by roentgenological examination in the face of a rectoscopically free ampulla are adenomatoid formations when the patient is more than 15 years old. Adenomas have rarely been detected before the age of 15. They are of potential malignity and indicate operation. Adenomas before the age of 15 have rarely been observed. Considering the small operative risk, however, colotomy is justified if the symptoms of a hamartomatous disease are absent.

Polyp bearers reveal a remarkable disposition to colonic carcinamos. Therefore all patients with colon polyps require long-term re-examination by the physician especially trained for this disease.

Bibliography

ATWATER, J. S., and J. A. BARGEN: The pathogenesis of intestinal polyps. Gastroenterology **4**, 395 (1945).

ACKERMAN, L. V.: Tumors – Adenomas. S. Louis: C. V. Mosby Comp.

BAKER, J. W., and H. W. JONES: The malignant potentiality of the Colorectal Polyp. Controversy in intern. Med. Ingelfinger – Retmann-Finland: Saunders 1966.

BACON, H. E., and A. R. PEALE: Appraisal of Adenomatous Polyps of the Colon. Ann. Surg. S. 9–18 (1956).

BARTHOLOMEW, L. G., D. C. DAHLIN, and J. M. WAUGH: Intestinal Polyposis Associated With Mucocutaneous Melanin Pigmentation (PEUTZ-JEGHERS-Syndrome). Gastro-Enterology **32**, 434 (1957).

BOCKUS, H. L., V. TACHDJIAN, L. K. FERGUSON et al.: Adenomatous Polyp of Colon And Rectum: Its Relation To Carcinoma. Gastro-Enterology **41**, 225, 225 (1961).

CALABRO, J. J.: Hereditable Multiple Polyposis Syndromes of the Gastrointestinal Tract. Amer. J. Med. Vol. XXXIII, 276 (1962).

CHAPMAN, I.: Adenomatous Polyps of Large Intestine. Ann. Surg. Vol. 157 (1963).

CASTLEMAN, B., and H. KRICKSTEIN: Carcinoma Arising in Adenomatous Polyps of the Colon Is Greatly Exaggerated. Controversy in intern. Med. Ingelfinger-Retman-Finland: Saunders 1966.

CRAMER, L. M.: Gardner Syndrome. Plastic a. Reconstructive Surgery. Vol. **29**, 402–407 (1962).

DUKES, C. E., and H. E. LOCKHARDT-MUMMERY: Familial Intestinal Polyposis. S. Clinics N. Am. **35**, 1277 (1955).

DICKSEN, TH.: Polyposis Coli and Gardner Syndrom. Ned. T. Genessk. **105**, 276 (1961).

ELSTER, K., u. G. WÜNDISCH: Morphologische Wertung der Rektum-Polypen. Langenbecks Arch. klin. Chir. **311**, 41–63 (1965).

ENQUIST, I. F.: The Incidence and Significance of Polyps of Colon and Rectum. Surg. Vol. **42**, Nr. 4, 681–688 (1957).

GORDON, D. L.: Polyps of the Colon in Children. Arch. Surg. **75**, 90 (1957).

GRINNELL, R. S., and N. LANE: Benign and Malignant Adenomatous Polyps and Papillary Adenomas of The Colon and Rectum. An Analysis of 1,856 Tumors in 1,335 Patients. J. Abstracts of Surg. Vol. **106**, 519 (1958).

KNOX, W. G., R. E. MILLER, C. F. BEGG, and H. A. ZINTEL: Juvenile Polyps of the Colon. Surg. **48**, 201 (1960).

LOCKHARDT-MUMMERY, C., and H. J. R. BUSSEY: The Surgical Treatment of Familial Polyposis of the Colon. Brit. J. Surg. Vol. XLIII, Nr. 81 (1956).

LOCKWORD, R. A., u. H. J. BETZLER: Anorektale Entartungen. Stuttgart: F. K. Schattauer Verl. S. 205–211.

MORSON, B. C.: Der feingewebliche Bau intestinaler Polypen. M.M.W. **108**, 310 (1966).

— Some Peculiacities in the Histology of Intestinal Polyps. Diseases of the Colon and Rectum, Vol. 5 Nr. 5 (1962).

REICHEL, P., u. M. STAEMMLER: Die Neubildungen des Darmes. Neue dtsch. Chirurg., 33. Bd. Stuttgart: Ferd. Enke Verl. 1933.

REIFFERSCHEID, M.: Der Dickdarmpolyp. Vorträge aus der prakt. Chirurgie, 54. Heft. Stuttgart: Ferd. Enke Verl. 1959.

—, u. H. BREUER: Zur diagnostischen Erfassung und prospektiven Deutung des Dick- u. Mastdarmpolypen. Med. Kl. **13**, 560 (1959).

— DMW **42**, 1896 (1967).

SPRATT, J. S., L. V. ACKERMAN, and C. A. MOYER: Relationship of Polyps of the Colon to Colonic Cancer. Am. Surg. **148**, 682 (1958).

STREICHER, E.: Das wasser- und elektrolytverlierende villöse Dickdarmadenom. Dtsch. med. Wschr. 91. Jg. (1966).

STALEY, C. J.: Gardners Syndrome. Arch. Surg. **82**, 110 (1961).

TURELL, R., and J. D. HALLER: A Re-evaluatius of the malignant Potential of Colorectal Adenomas. Surg. Gyn. Obstet. Okt. 1964.

— Diseases of the Colon and Anorectum. Philadelph. a. London: Saunders Co. 1959.

WHEAT, M. W., and L. V. ACKERMAN: Villous Adenomas of the Large Intestine. Ann. Surg. Vol. 147, 476 (1958).

QUENN and LANDEL: Benign Villous Tumor. Rev. Chir. **1** (1894).

Hypersecretory Villous Tumor of the Colon

I. Degrell, Zalaegerszeg, Hungary

Recently many publications have reported a peculiar tumor of the colon associated with electrolyte disturbance, due to its papillous – villous structure. Beside the well – known tumor symptoms, the clinical picture is characterized by unrelievable diarrhea, which leads to disturbances in electrolyte and water metabolism.

The clinical picture is associated with the peculiar structure of the profuse secreting tumor: periodical diarrhea with tenesmus and mucous discharge. Later, excessive thirst, fatigue, then the well-known symptoms of disturbances in water and electrolyte metabolism appear: delirium, meteorism, emesis etc. In our cases we observed all these symptoms in the period 1964–1968; we have observed two patients with the "brutal disturbance" of electrolyte and water metabolism, cited by Debray, at the preparation for rectoscopy.

The treatment of the hypersecretory villous tumor of the rectum is exclusively surgical; of course the complicating fluid and electrolyte imbalance should be corrected prior to operation. Surgical treatment is radical or more or less "conservative". There are autors who perform hemicolectomy or abdomino-sacral, abdomino-perineal resection respectively; others prefer partial resection when they know the biological nature of the tumor.

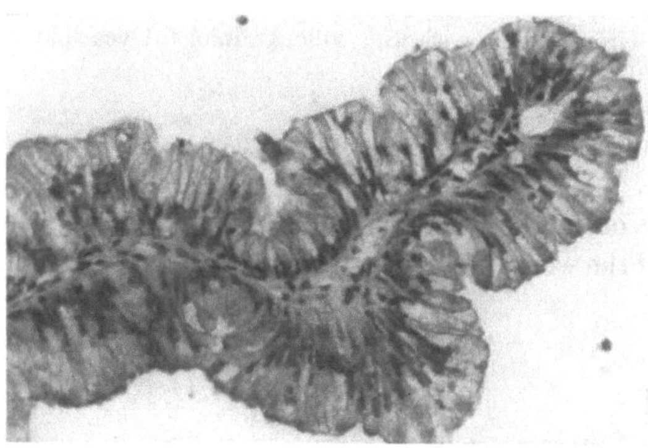

Fig. 1. Photomicrograph of the prolapsed villous adenoma; no atypical changes (100×)

Our youngest patient was a 44-year-old female, the oldest was 75 year old (Fig.1). The predilective location of the tumor were the sigmoid colon and rectum (3–3 cases). On account of malignancy, we performed a successful abdomino-sacral amputation of the rectum in three patients, in two patients a Whitehead operation was carried out. A 75 year-old-woman, who was brought in a very severe condition, "in extremis" – she was completely exsiccated in addition to having a good palpaple villous tumor of the rectum – died after 16 hours (Fig. 2).

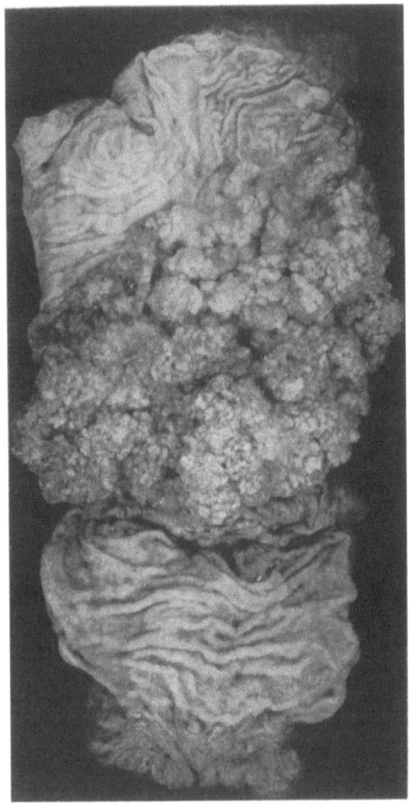

Fig. 2. Gross specimen showing villous tumor (51-year-old women)

The control investigation revealed that all five patients are symptom-free and in good condition.

Villous tumors occur rarely in Hungary compared with other countries, according to the data of the world literature. In Hungary the first publication was reported in 1964.

Bibliography

Quénu, E., and G. Laudel: Rev. Chir. Gynec. Obstet. **111**, 95 (1899).
Miles, W. E.: Rectal Surgery, London 1939.
Gabriel, W. B.: The Principles and Practice of Rectal Surgery. London 1948.
Bacon, H. E.: Anus, Rectum and Sigmoid Colon. Philadelphia 1949.
Ewing, M. R.: Ann. roy. Coll. Surg. Engl. **6**, 413 (1950).
McKittrick, L. S., and F. C. Wheelock jr.: Carcinoma of the Colon. Springfield, Ill.: **1**, 61 (1954.)
Fitzgerald, M. G.: Brit. med. J. **1**, 831 (1955).

FRAZIER, H. M.: J.A.M.A. **160**, 774 (1956).
HOFFMAN, E.: Amer. J. Surg. **98**, 99 (1959).
FINDLAY, C., and T. F. O'CONNOR: J.A.M.A. **176**, 404 (1961).
DAVIS, J. E. etc.: Ann. Surg. **155**, 806 (1962).
WHEAT, M. W., jr., and L. V. ACKERMAN, Ann. Surg. **147**, 476 (1958).
HINES, M. O., P. H. HENLEY, and R. SCHRAMEL: Sth. med. J. **48**, 891 (1955).
JANTSCHEW, W. B. and KRASTEW etc.: Z. inn. Med. 629 (1962).
BAJZIK, E., and K. RAJKOVITS: Orv. Hetil. **15**, 701 (1964).
DEBRAY, CH. et al.: Presse méd. **71**, 223 (1963).
DEGRELL, I., u. E. GIMES: Brun's Beitr. klin. Chir. **212**, 3, 320 (1966).
PRADEL, E. etc.: Arch. Franc. Mal. Appar. Dig. **56**, 5 (1967).
GOLIGHER, J. C., and N. G. GRAHAM: Arch. Mal. Appar. Dig. **56**, 51 (1967).
PARKS, M. A. G.: Arch. Mal. Appar. Dig. **56**, 89 (1967).

Malignant Transformation of Diffuse Polyposis of the Colon

GY. BARADNAY, G. PETRI and V. VARRÓ, Szeged, Hungary

The genetical aspects of diffuse familial polyposis of the colon, its pathology and clinical picture are now well known and its principles of treatment are accepted thanks to the work of LOCKHART-MUMMERY, DUKES, THOMPSON and others. A few years after the first, still acceptable description of the disease (CRIPPS, 1882). HANFORD demonstrated that polyps can undergo carcinomatous transformation in 1890.

According to the findings of DUKES, carcinoma of the colon develops by the 30th year of age in 50% of the patients. The results of a collection of literary data by WILLIAMS and co-workers show that carcinoma was found to be associated with polyposis at surgery in 43% of the cases. Out of 12 cases. MCLACHLIN demonstrated the malignant transformation in a 19-year-old patient. We think that the results of the examination of our two cases and their family members are remarkable because they illustrate in an extreme form partly the early malignant transformation of familial polyposis of the colon, partly its appearance in the shape of a harmless disease, more exactly in the shape of ulcerous colitis, till late in life.

Case 1. A 41-year-old male; for 6–7 years had had watery-slimy, later bloody diarrhea. In his youth his father had had a similar disease which was later cured and had caused no complaints now for several decades. Rectoscopy showed normal conditions. Irrigoscopy showed an undamaged mucosa. In the following three years the patient was under medical control several times with the above mentioned complaints. Diarrhetic and normal periods alternated. His complaints could be influenced with Prednisolon instillations and tranquillizers. Rectoscopy findings from 1964 onward: proctitis haemorrhagica on several occasions. The bloody, slimy, diarrhetic stools became more frequent, so we came to the conclusion that the patient had gradually worsening colitis ulcerosa. At the end of 1965 the findings were: poor condition, moderate anemia, severe hypalbuminemia (1.6 gr%), new clinical admission. Irrigoscopic picture: irregular mucosa outlines with sporadically adhering spots and a polypous picture. In a bleeding-free period we measured the enteral protein loss with Cr 51-labelled albumin (Hoechst). We found 8.33% of the Cr 51-labelled albumin given in the stool which was proof of increased enteral loss of protein (normal upper limit: 1%). The serum electrolyte value was found to be normal on several occasions. The last irrigoscopy at the beginning of 1966 showed a picture suggesting diffuse polyposis in the area of the sigmoid flexure and the descending colon, but knowing the clinical findings, we thought it to be pseudo-polyposis. Because of his tormenting colics the patient did not agree to rectoscopy at this point. After this ileostomy was performed at the Surgical Clinic in January 1966 upon which his complaints did not become much milder, yet during the three months he gained 12 kg in weight. In April 1966 total colectomy was performed leaving the ileostomy. With the exception of the mucosa of the rectum and the cecum, the whole large intestinal mucosa was covered by a forest of long-stalked polyps (Fig. 1–2). There were no ulcers on the mucosa. Histologically the polyps were typical adenomatous polyps. There were no signs of malignant transformation. On the fifth postoperative day the patient became mentally confused, developed ever worsening icterus, and on the ninth postoperative day he died. Among the autopsy findings we should like to mention particularly the very severe diffuse acinocentral necrosis of the liver lobes and the severe extensive subarachnoidal hemorrhage of the occipital lobe of both cerebral hemispheres and of the cerebellar hemispheres. The patient's 76-year-old father is even now free from complaints. On irrigoscopy diffuse polyposis could be demonstrated on him in the area of the descending colon. The patient has no brothers, his children are quite young, so we have not been able to make further investigation of the family.

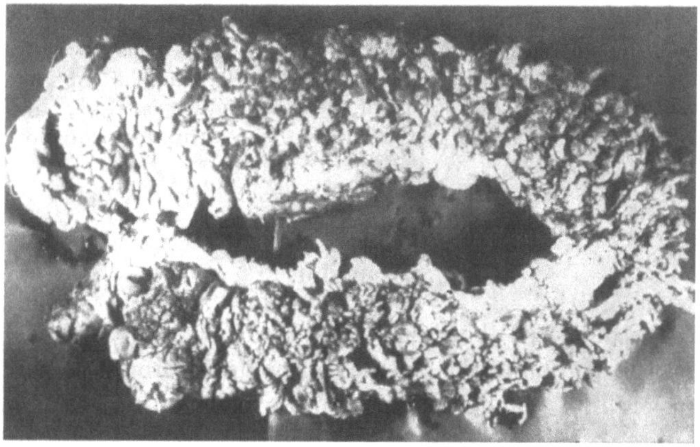

Fig. 1

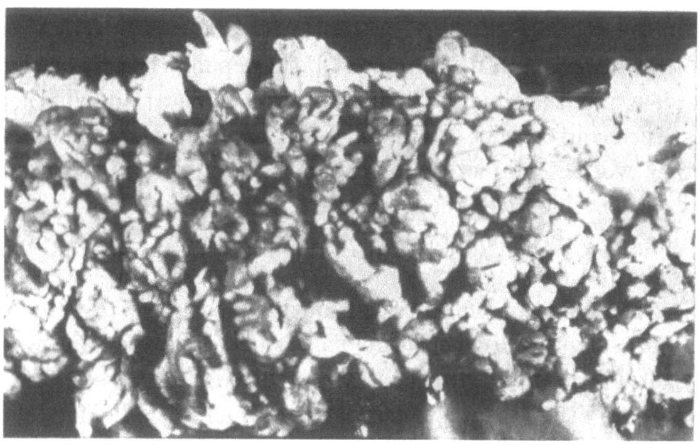

Fig. 2

Case 2. 23-year-old male. Was first examined by us in May 1966. Complaints: diarrhea for three years, colics and melena. Recto-sigmoidoscopy findings: up to about 30 cm on the mucosa of the rectum and the sigmoid flexure one found a host of lentil- or bean-sized polyps. Findings on histological examination: polyposis adenomatosus. Irrigoscopy findings: all over the area of the large intestinal tract from the cecum to the rectum, countless round shadows indicating polyps. Rectoscopic examination of the patient's mother and two sisters was negative. At this time the patient did not agree to the operation recommended, and on repeated control examinations carried out in the course of a year we found no essential change in his condition. In October 1967 he was admitted to a provincial hospital with the picture of an abdominal catastrophe which had developed in a matter of hours and was operated upon. On laparotomy, diffuse purulent peritonitis was found, but there was no intestinal perforation. In the postoperative days, an infiltration developed in the pelvis minor; a few days later, simultaneously with its absorption, the development of a bladder-to-intestine fistula was observed and ascertained by cystography. In later weeks he developed ileus. It was then that he was taken to our clinic. Here an ileostomy was made. Although the patient's intestinal passage started again, his colics did not cease. Of the laboratory examinations we may mention hypoalbuminemia and besides the normal result of other liver function tests the BSP retention exceeded 40%. In January 1968 the total colectomy was performed leaving the ileostomy. In the course of the operation, we found a sigmoido-vesical fistula under which there was total obstruction of the large intestine. We closed the bladder after excising the wall of it. Countless adenomatous polyps were demonstrated on the surgical specimens by both macroscopic and microscopic examinations. Tissue proliferation around the large intestine-bladder fistula which caused complete obstruction of the bowel turned out to be an invasive adenocarcinoma. After the operation, the patient had an uneventful recovery, and control cystoscopy showed normal conditions.

Discussion

The two cases described above prove that no definite conclusion concerning the malignant transformation of the disease can be drawn from the manifestation of the symptoms of diffuse familial polyposis of the colon or from the duration of the complaints

On the basis of already existing polyposis the starting time of the carcinoma is capricious and incalculable. Our first case with its family history proves that familial polyposis does not transform itself malignantly even after five decades. Our second case on the other hand, draws attention to the rapid carcinamatous transformation of the disease. Thus it is obvious that it depends largely on the physician's or surgeon's view, i. e. the time of the indication for operation, whether the doctor or the disease turns out winner of the contest between the treatment and the carcinoma. In other words, complete cure can be expected only if surgery is performed as early as possible after recognition of the disease.

Establishing the indication for total colectomy is chiefly the task of the physician who first sees the patient.

In our cases the result of the so-called routine laboratory tests made before the operation did not suggest a liver insufficiency which developed and was verified by histological examination. In our second case, the high BSP retention suggested a liver lesion. We think the urgency of surgical treatment is indicated whenever there is danger of malignant transformation as well as chronic bleeding, loss of protein, inflammation and the resulting liver lesion. There can be hardly any doubt that the operational risk of total colectomy performed after prolonged duration of the disease is greater than that of an early operation.

Bibliography

Dukes, C. E.: Familial Intestinal Polyposis. Ann. Roy. Coll. Surg. Engl. **10**, 293 (1952).
— Cancer Control in Familial Polyposis of the Colon. Dis. Colon & Rectum **1**, 413 (1958).
Lockhart-Mummery, H. E.: Intestinal Polyposis: The Present Position. Proc. Roy. Soc. Med. **60**, 381 (1967).

McLachlin, A. D.: Familial Intestinal Polyposis. Arch. Surg. **79**, 393 (1959).
Róth, M.: Teljes vastag és végbél kiirtása analis ileostomiával colon polyposis miatt. Orv. Hetil. **95**, 299 (1954).
Thompson, H. R.: Polyposis Intestini. Proc. Roy. Soc. Med. **51**, 241 (1958).
Williams, R. D., and J. C. Fish: Multiple Polyposis, Polyp Regression and Carcinoma of the Colon. Amer. J. Surg. **112**, 846 (1966).

Familiar Polyposis Coli

K. Arnold, G. Kemmerer, and R. Zitzmann, Erlangen, Germany

Among the various appearances of colonic polyposis, familial polyposis coli (f. p. c.) is a rare and well defined disease: it is characterized by the development of a large number of adenomatous polyps from the colonic and rectal mucosa, by their malignant degeneration at an early age and by dominant inheritance.

The polyps are not present at birth, they develop during childhood and early adult life and cause no discomfort. At about 20 years of age the first symptoms appear, the patient will be seen in the out-patient department with uncharacteristic symptoms (Fig. 1). Blood in the stool, diarrhea, abdominal pain, and loss of weight are the most common complaints. The extent of the signs and the progression of the disease often show no coincidence. In the differential diagnosis we should think of colitis, diverticulitis and carcinoma.

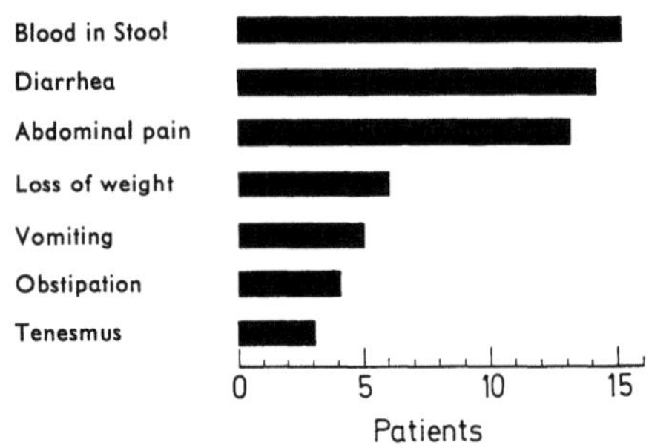

Fig. 1. Symptoms of 18 of our patients with familiar polyposis coli

The examination begins with rectal palpation. During this procedure small polyps may not be detected in the ampulla but in the case of a massive polyposis of the rectum, the palpating finger seems to glide over a bed of algae.

Familial polyposis coli can be excluded by sigmoidoscopy alone in this disease, the rectum and the distal part of the sigmoid colon always bear the greatest number of polyps becoming fewer towards the caecum. If there are no polyps within the range of the sigmoidoscope (30 cm) then no more colonies can be expected in higher parts of the colon.

When we see a dense mat of polyps in the scope, we may verify our diagnosis through biopsy of one or more adenomas, and exclude pseudopolyps after colitis, juvenile and Peutz-Jeghers-polyps.

At the time of the manifestation of the disease, i. e. about the age of 15 years, nodules of the size of peppercorns appear, they are histologically metaplastic polyps. They continue to grow and become peduncular or sessile adenomas and thus precancerous tumors. The development of carcinoma usually begins at the top of the polyp, spreading over the peduncle towards the bowel wall. So the progression to carcinoma is quicker in sessile than in peduncular adenomas. We do not know when or at what size an adenoma becomes carcinomatous. But we do know that a great number of adenomas can undergo malignant transformation early and with great certainty.

The diagnosis of diffuse adenomatosis of the large bowel is an alarm signal and forces us to use therapeutic methods. Repeated biopsies, to establish the presence of a carcinoma in an adenoma, are both false and fatal for the patient.

After the diagnosis has been asserted by sigmoidoscopy and biopsy, x-rays will inform us of the extent of the adenomas and possible narrowings of the lumen due to carcinomas. When polyposis is suspected, we immediately use the double-contrast method. Through this we not only obtain the most impressive pictures but we can also detect even the smallest polyps.

This x-ray picture (Fig. 2) shows a honey-comb relief that extends from the rectum to the caecum; the sacculations of the colon are preserved. The special view showing the border between rectum and sigma reveals not only a narrowing of the lumen with irregular contours but also barium-free areas that are so typical for malignant processes. In an additional x-ray picture of the specimen obtained at operation (Fig. 3), also using the double contrast method, the honey-comb relief is now seen to be a multitude of polyps the size of peppercorns to hazelnuts. This was what we found macroscopically in the dissected specimen too.

If the diagnosis of diffuse adenomatosis coli has been firmly established and the extent is known, then the only effective and certain method of treatment is the excision of the whole large bowel, i. e. total procto-colectomy with an ileostomy. This radical operation must be performed if a rectal carcinoma is already present or if the adenomas in the rectum are so dense that after electro-surgical removal one can expect the development of a stenosis with certainty. Often the patient is shocked at the idea of having an ileostomy for the rest of his life. Especially the young patient with familial polyposis coli who has relatively few complaints will seldom consent to a procto-colectomy.

As an alternative operation, there is the colectomy with ileorectal anastomosis which preserves the natural bowel passage. On the other hand, there is persistent danger that new adenomas may arise and become malignant. Therefore we should use this risky method only with intelligent and disciplined patients who would surely come to follow-up examinations every three months.

The second therapeutic problem is the investigation and constant observation of families with polyposis coli.

Thanks to the work of DUKES together with BUSSEY at the St. Mark's-Hospital in London the dominantly inherited character of this disease was revealed and a truly outstanding index of families with familial polyposis coli in England was set up.

Figure 4 shows a most characteristic family tree from our case histories of 9 families with 28 patients. Through remarriage of the carrier of the gene, two branches of the family with familial polyposis coli inherit the disease.

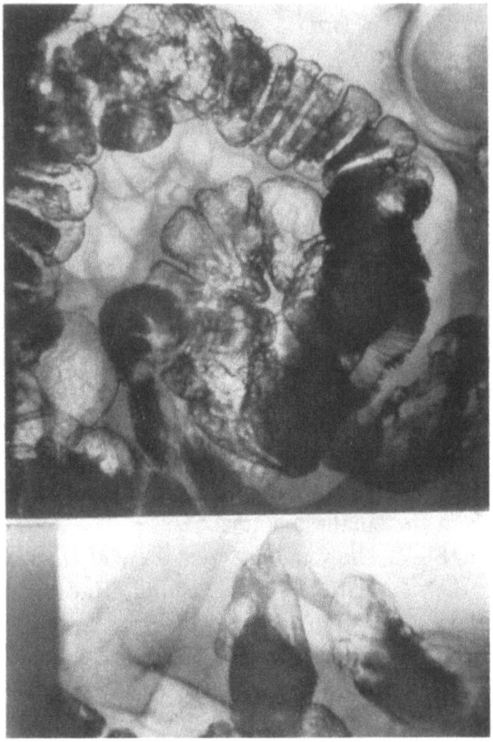

Fig. 2. X-ray picture (double contrast method) showing honey-comb relief of the large bowel above and border between rectum and sigma with carcinoma below

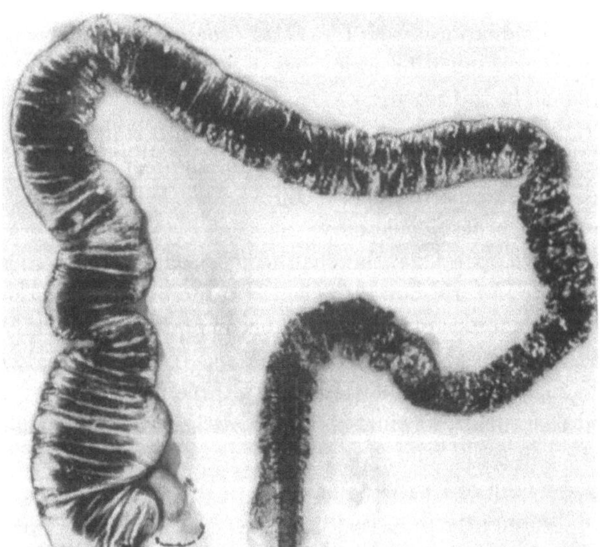

Fig. 3. X-ray picture (double contrast method) made of a specimen showing multiple polyposis

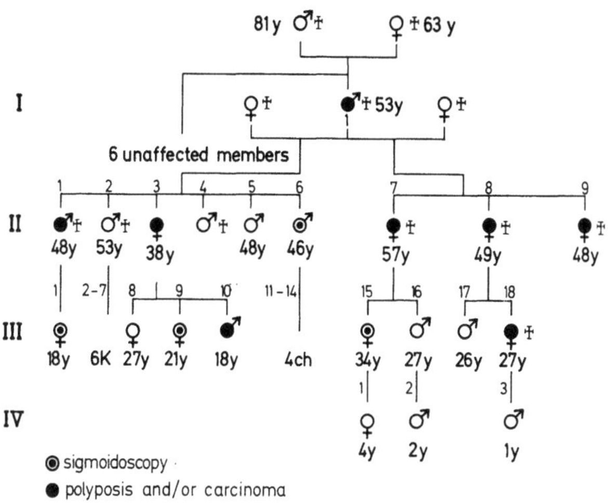

Fig. 4. Family tree with familial polyposis coli, re-marriage of I, causing two affected branches of family

The difficulties of an effective family observation lie not only in the indolence of the individuals but also to a large extent in the fear of being labelled "polyposis family" with all the therapeutic and lethal consequences connected with this disease.

The chart (Fig. 5) of our case histories of 9 families with 28 ill members so far shows 3 refusals of operation and illustrates part of our sad experience.

9 Families with Familial Polyposis coli

28 affected members

7 patients treated in our clinic

Therapy

procto-colectomy	IRA	operation refused
3	1	3

Fig. 5. Chart of case histories of the Surgical Univ. Clinic Erlangen of 9 families with 28 affected persons

Inspite of all this, it is our purpose to continue examining all members of such polyposis families and to discover and operate sufficiently all affected individuals around the 20th year of life, i. e. the time at which malignancy has not as yet been truly established.

VI. Cancer

Social Acceptability of the Colostomy – the Surgeon's Task and Duty

K. Denecke and R. Hellbach, Fürth, Germany

A statement of Leriche: "Surgery is in danger of losing her soul". It must not lose it. Where does this danger come from? The tasks of today's medicine, the multiplicity and magnitude of surgical interventions, the amplification of surgical indications and the huge work load, leads the surgeon into danger of being only an executor of medical decisions.

Already today, patients are operated by surgeons who have not examined them personally. Frequently there is no time for reciprocal confidence to arise. All patients are frightened, especially of the unknown events of the operations to which they are submitted. And only confidence in the surgeon is able to dissipate these fears. Whereas most surgical procedures we perform do not lead to external disfiguration, this is different for the abdomino-perineal amputation of the rectum. This operation alters one of the most important functions of the human body. The responsible surgeon attempts to avoid a definitive colostomy whenever possible by performing a sphincter saving resection.

Before the operation the patient must be throughly informed about what he has to expect afterwards. He must become persuaded that his situation will be tolerable. And I think this will be more so if the colostomy is not completely out of the patient's control. Otherwise the loss of control over faeces and flatus is a very high price to pay for regained life expectancy. Such a colostomy interferes with personal and matrimonial life, social and professional activities. It can destroy a marriage and be an argument for divorce. In court, colostomy has already been accepted as an ailment causing aversion.

Thus it follows, that even after a successful operation, the surgeon has to provide patients with guides for the return to social and professional life.

Already during the first decades of bowel surgery, many surgeons were engaged in these problems. But all intents to improve continence by operative means failed completely A. better management of colostomy was provided by Goetze's "run over". But his method did not have wide acceptance. I still regard it as a good method for terminal ileostomy.

Of course something can be reached by systematic training of the bowel for rhythmic evacuation. In the past, Schmieden said somewhat optimistically: "The intelligent patient soon learns what is important: bowel activity must be regulated so that faeces accumulate once or at most twice a day and are then evacuated".

In our experience this is the exception rather than the rule. In spite of prolonged efforts we have made no real progress in the care of these patients.

Generally we had to accept the fact, that patients with a colostomy, when discharged from hospital were left alone with their problems. The solution of these problems depended primarily on the intelligence of the patient, his own experiences with colostomy devices and his interest in being reintegrated in social and professional life. But the result was not entirely satisfactory.

For more than 10 years we have approached the problem in another way. We regulate defaecation with enemata.

The colon is like a tube into which faeces are continuously pushed in a distal direction. When total evacuation of the colon is achieved, replenishment is gradually accomplished, commencing proximally in the region of the ileo-caecal valve.

Complete evacuation of the colon can be achieved with high enemata. This can be demonstrated by x-ray, when giving an enema with a thin barium suspension. After the enema has induced evacuation, the bowel immediately relaxes.

Although we have used this method for many years, we have never seen signs of bowel irritation. In this regard it is to be mentioned that we use only warm tap water without any additions like soap or glycerine.

The volume of the enema is individualized and varies between 500 and 1500 ml. Evacuation occurs between 10 and 45 min after instillation. Thereafter the colostomy remains completely clean for 2–3 days. This procedure is performed every 2 days.

A follow up evaluation of 100 patients, half of whom used this method, was carried out by my co-worker HELLBACH some years ago. This study showed that approximately 50% of the patients who had performed enemata, were free of any colostomy appliance. They simple wear a Kleenex or a piece of gauze supported by a belly bandage. The rest used the appliances only to cover the colostomy in some way and protect it from clothes, or to guard against occasional surprises. The following details are essential for the success of this method:

1. The colostomy should be very small and narrow and should lie below the level of the skin. The latter is achieved by excision of a wedge of subcutaneous fat. The colostomy is anchored to the abdominal wall by sutures holding skin, fascia, peritoneum and bowel wall with one stitch.

2. To permit an easy and deep introduction of the irrigator tube, the course of the residual sigmoid and descendent colon must be straight. The latter is achieved by a generous resection of the sigmoid colon.

3. The most important prerequisite is proper selection of patients. A certain degree of intelligence must be present. Very old and clumsy individuals should be excluded.

4. Before discharging the patients, they should have a through training in the method given by competent nursing personnel.

Occasionally we have had to lament a perforation from the tube. This is an accident able to cause disrepute of the method. Patients must be informed about this danger and must be instructed that the introduction of the tube has to be performed very cautiously. Failures are possible in patients with irritable colon and a tendency to diarrhoea. Other causes of failure are dietary errors and incompetence of the ileo-caecal valve with reflux of bowel contents into the ileum. In these latter cases, the enema is followed by an immediate emptying of the colon with subsequent evacuation of small intestine contents (refluxed material) over many hours.

Caeco-ileal reflux may be very pronounced. We have seen a patient vomit 17 liters after a subaquatic bowel bath performed for another indication.

The enema is carried out in the following manner: the previously measured volume of liqiud is slowly pumped into the bowel by means of a "Darmklyse". Emptying is allowed to occur into a plastic urine bottle for women.

In some cases there are difficulties with flatus. An appropriate diet but also chlorophyll or bags with animal coal covering the colostomy, can contribute to the mitigation of this problem.

It is surprising to see, how patients learn to manage their own particular problems; more so, how as time goes on and based on the knowledge we have given them, they elaborate their own individual method with multiple little refinements, which finally render life worthy to be lived.

With this possibility in mind, we can try to dissipate the patient's fears and anxieties before a challenging but frequently lifesaving operation.

Violaine says: "For the suffering, the consolations of the cheerful are of little value, his ailment is not the same for us as it is for him". It is much better if such a patient says at his discharge: "Doctor I believed everything you said before, but I never thought I would get along so well".

Bibliography

Bayer: Zbl. Chir. **27**, 752 (1897).
Carl: Beitr. Brun's klin. Chir. **86**, 177 (1913).
Goetze: Chirurg **3**, 163 (1950).
Lichtenstein: Lehrbuch d. Darmchirurgie, 1962, S. 356.
Schmieden: Zbl. Chir. **18**, 641 (1910).
Hellbach: Inaugural-Dissert., Der Anus praeter und seine Pflege, Med. Fakultät Nbg.-Erlangen.

A Plea for Primary Hemicolectomy in Perforated Cancer of the Right Colon

C.-A. Muller, Lausanne, Switzerland

The simultaneous occurrence of carcinoma of the colon and perforation of the same represents a double threat for the patient's life; the second being the more dangerous. Whether complicated by an abscess or by diffuse peritonitis, it is the perforation that determines the state of emergency.

Perusal of the literature shows that perforation of a cancer of the right colon is rather infrequent. According to Crowder and Goligher, this complication occurs in about 1,3% of all cancers of the large intestine. It is then understandable that whenever he is confronted with this kind of emergency, the general surgeon may be faced with untoward difficulties in selecting the right operative procedure. The following case report is intended to illustrate some of these.

Case Report

On the 11th of November 1967, a 57-year-old man was caught by violent abdominal cramps localized in the right flank and in the right iliac fossa. He was nauseated but did not vomit. During the next 48 hours, the abdominal cramps became more frequent and more severe. A diffuse swelling developed in the right flank. The patient was examined by the physician on duty who referred him to his own surgeon. Another 48 hours elapsed before the patient was examined by this colleague. By now, the swelling was as large as a water-melon. It was very tender at palpation and suggested the diagnosis of localized abscess. The patient was admitted to a private hospital and operated 24 hours later. Transperitoneal incision and drainage of the abscess was performed and a Miller-Abott tube was brought down to the level of the second duodenum. It was left there, apparently on grounds of technical difficulties.

The abdomen was closed in the usual manner, over a cigarette drain (Table 1). Three days later an adynamic ileus developed, which was soon aggravated by a complete wound disruption and a first fecal fistula which appeared through the path of the penrose drain. Nine days after the operation, peristalsis had still not returned but the abdominal wall had been badly burnt by hot moist packs, originally meant to stimulate bowel movements.

On the last day of November, a large intestinal hemorrhage took place. Two days later a second massive melena followed, bringing the patient's hemoglobine value down to 50%. Three weeks later, a second fecal fistula opened in the right flank. On the same day, a barium enema revealed a malignant stenosis of the first portion of the ascending colon as well as both fecal fistulas (Fig. 1). On the 10th of December, the patient was referred to us. At that time it seemed obvious that the badly burnt abdomen together with the considerable degree of disturbance of blood, electrolyte and protein values prohibited any kind of surgical procedure. All the more since the skin was the site of a heavy infection.

Taking psychological advantage of the Yule time, we started to treat the abdominal burns with massive applications of sulfisomidin geol and proceeded to correct hemoglobine, electrolyte and protein deficits.

At the beginning of January 1968, the patient's condition had improved dramatically. We were then able to perform a right hemicolectomy with simultaneous excision of both fecal fistulas. Intestinal continuity was restored with an end-to-end ileo-transverse anastomosis. The specimen showed a very tight stenosis, the internal opening of the second fistula and remnants of the hemorrhages that had repeatedly occured above the upper margin of the tumor.

Table 1

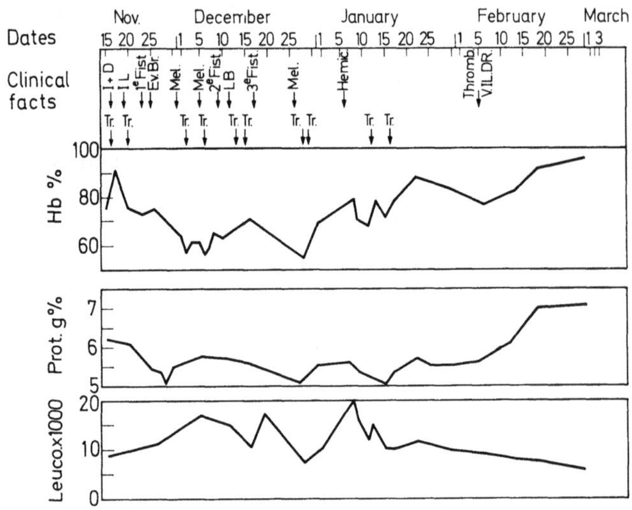

I + D: Incision and drainage – Il.: Ileostomy – Ev.: Evisceration – Brûl.: abdominal burns. – Mel.: Melena – L.B.: Barium enema – Tr.: Blood transfusion

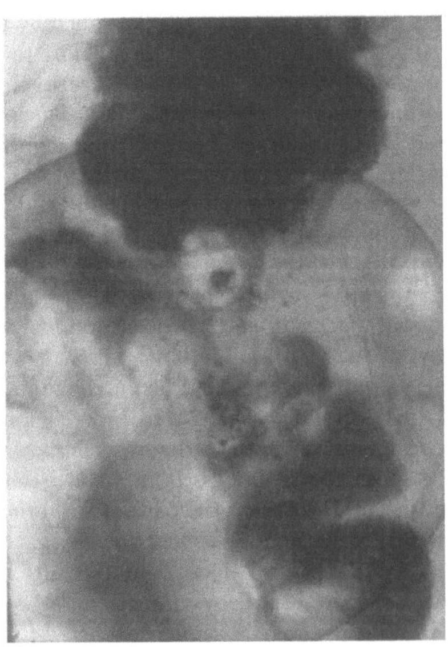

Fig. 1. Malignant stenosis of the first portion of the right colon, with fecal fistula

Immediate post-operative course was uneventful. However, on the 12th postoperative day a skin disruption occurred at the lower end of the abdominal wound. Owing to the preoperative skin condition, this was really expected, and it healed spontaneousely within the next three weeks. On February 5th, one month after the second operation, the patient developed a thrombosis of the right iliac vein. He was given adequate doses of anticoagulants and was discharged from the hospital on March 3rd, still under the protection of these drugs. This was the aspect of the abdomen 4 months after the operation.

Discussion

GOLIGHER has shown that perforation of a cancer of the large intestine occurs in about 13% of all cases and that it is equally distributed between the left and the right colon. Independently of its anatomical location, perforation occurs much more frequently at the site of the tumor than ahead of it, the rate being approximately 6–1.

Perforation of the left colon is accompanied much more frequently by diffuse peritonitis than by a localized abscess, on the right side, the situation is reversed, since we have about 8,4% of these cases with abscesses against 3,1% with diffuse peritonitis. This discrepancy is attributed to the fact that in the right colon symptoms of cancer develop much more slowly than in the left colon and this, mainly on account of a larger diameter of the intestine, the fluidity of the fecal content, and the relatively slow invasion of the intestinal wall, which results in the formation of multiple small fecal fistulas readily walled-off by surrounding tissues.

The differention between inflammatory and malignant lesions of the ascending colon may be extremely difficult and since it is impossible to rely upon elements of certitude in cases of emergency, one is forced to base one's judgement upon the probabilities. Perforation of an isolated diverticulum or of a simple ulcer of the cecum is rare. So, having excluded the diagnosis of perforated appendicitis, one must remember that in the ascending colon and in patients aged 50 or more, cancer is most likely to be the cause of the perforation and one must be technically prepared to meet this probability. The choice of the operative procedure is then much simplified. Most authorities agree that radical excision gives more chances of immediate survival to the patient, since it readily suppresses a source of contamination and suppuration. When it comes to cancer, this principle appears even more true since radical excision eliminates possible sources of malignant seeding. In addition, leaving the diseased organ in place promotes the deterioration of a patient who has already sustained important physiologic and metabolic alterations. Recalling CRILE's words, we can say: "It is the disease, not the operation that more often kills the patient".

Consequently, one should always try to shun simple drainage procedures and whenever feasible avoid drainage with internal diversion, for it is established that the most economical operation hardly ever modifies the natural course of the disease for which it was meant.

Exteriorization cannot be recommended since experience gained during the second World war and in the Korean war has shown the poor results to be expected from this technique, mainly because of the fluid and electrolyte depletion that it produced.

Moreover, in order to exteriorize the colon it is necessary to mobilize the intestine to just about the same extent that would be required by a radical resection.

Last but not least, in the presence of cancer, exteriorization is bound to considerable risk of malignant seeding, both within the abdominal wall and on the skin.

This leads us to the principle of emergency resection. Admittedly any perforation in the large intestine must be considered as a focus of intoxication or even as a dangerous foreign body which should be erradicated. Now, since cancer of the ascending colon is much more frequently complicated by perforation than by obstruction, it can be anticipated that in most cases both terminal ileum and transverse colon will show evidence of normal morphology and will prove readily suitable for a sound anastomosis. In the rare instances when perforation is accompanied by a certain degree of obstruction and when, in addition, the ileo-cecal valve is incompetent, then the terminal ileum may indeed show signs of acute dilatation. In these cases however, it also is true that early tube decompression will allow the small gut to regain its normal tonus during the course of the operation, thus facilitating a sound anastomosis at the end of it.

The safety of an anastomosis not only depends upon the availability of sound intestinal tissue but also upon the quality of the environment, and it is well known that any kind of infection within the abdominal cavity will jeopardize the anastomosis by favoring anastomotic leaks, probably resulting in an inflammatory stenosis. Until quite recently all these reasons would have strictly precluded the idea of an end-to-end anastomosis in presence of diffuse peritonitis.

Table 2. *Results of Emergency Hemicolectomy in Perforated Cancers of the Right Colon*

Authors	Years of observation	Number of cases	Complications: Abscess Localized peritonitis	Complications: Diffuse peritonitis	Emergency Hemicolectomy	Operative Mortality: Absolute	Operative Mortality: Per cent
MERRILL and VAUGH	1906–1946	3	3	0	3	0	0
GOLIGHER	1938–1943 and 1947–1955	21	15	6	21	5	23.8
MILLER	1947–1956	13	11	2	13	1	7.7
CROWDER and COHN	1948–1956	11	10	1	4	1	25.0
HERRINGTON	1955–1965	4	4	0	4	0	0
COLE F. R.	1965	2	0	2	2	0	0
Total		54	43	11	47	7	14.9

However, it has been demonstrated that in presence of diffuse peritonitis, generous peritoneal lavage reduces postoperative complications to a considerable extent. In this regard we are very much indebted to the work of PRICE, THOREK, SHUMER, BURNETT and others, who gave the surgeon the oppqrtunity to become more "radical" in their emergency procedures. In addition, the development of more powerful and diversified antibiotics radically changed the classical theories pertaining to the safety of immediate intestinal anastomosis in presence of diffuse peritonitis (Table 2). Careful scrutiny of some of the largest series of perforations of the right colon at the site of the tumor shows that since peritoneal lavage and intraperitoneal instillation of broad spectrum antibiotics have entered current surgical practice, radical surgery of the large-intestine has been used more liberally even in presence of a septic environment with a much lower operative mortality. In accordance with most surgeons, I would therefore recommend emergency hemicolectomy as the treatment of choice in perforated cancer of the right colon.

Bibliography

Burnett, W. A. et al.: The treatment of peritonitis using peritoneal lavage. Ann. Surg. **145**, 675 (1957).

Crile, G., jr.: Dangers of conservative treatment in abdominal surgery. Surgery **35**, 122 (1954).

Crowder, V. H., and I. Cohn, jr.: Perforation in cancer of the colon and rectum. Dis. Col. Rect. **10**, 415 (1967).

Goligher, J. C., and F. G. Smiddy: The treatment of acute obstruction or perforation with carcinoma of the colon and rectum. Brit. J. Surg. **45**, 270 (1957).

Herrington, J. L., jr., et al.: Colon resection with primary anastomosis performed as an emergemcy and as non planned operation. Ann. Surg. **165**, 709 (1967).

Madden, J. L.: Primary resection and anastomosis in the treatment of perforated lesions of the colon. Amer. Surg. **31**, 781 (1965).

Miller, L. D., et al.: An analysis of 284 patients with perforative carcinoma of the colon. Surg. Gyn. Obst. **123**, 1212 (1966).

Poth, E. J.: Neomycin intraperitoneally. Amer. J. Surg. **108**, 755 (1964).

Schummer, W., et al.: Peritoneal lavage in post-operative therapy of late peritoneal sepsis. Preliminary report. Surgery **55**, 841 (1964).

Witowski, J. L.: Primary hemicolectomy for perforated lesions of the right colon. Arch. Surg. **74**, 741 (1957).

Carcinoid Tumours

W. F. W. Southwood, Bath, Great Britain

The term carcinoid was first coined by Oberndorfer (1907) to indicate a lesion which had the histological appearance of a carcinoma without all its malignant attributes. In 1928 Masson showed the tissue of origin to be the argentaffin cells at the base of the crypts of Lieberkuhn. These cells secrete 5-hydroxy-tryptamine into the circulation, which produce diarrhoea as a result of excessive small bowel motility, skin flushing with patchy cyanosis and telangiectases, respiratory stridor and later valvular lesions on the right side of the heart. These features of the carcinoid syndrome were described by Thorson in 1954, yet a very accurate and detailed clinical description of all of them had been given by Sir Maurice Cassidy.

The carcinoid tumours, other than those which occurred in the appendix, have been reviewed for a 10 year period from the records of the United Bath Hospitals and the United Bristol Hospitals. 13 cases occurred altogether, 4 in men and 9 in women; their average age was 58 years.

The commonest presenting symptoms (Table 1) were diarrhoea, weight loss, and colic. Three of the patients with these symptoms had advanced primary tumours which had partially occluded the bowel lumen, as well as nodal metastases.

Table 1. *Clinical presentation*

Diarrhoea, weight loss, colic	4
Bleeding per rectum	2
Carcinoid syndrome	1
Dysphagia	1
Abdominal pain and vomiting (Infarcted bowel)	1
Incidental finding	4
(to haematemesis from G.U.)	
(to gastric polyposis)	
(to N.G. caecum)	
(to ileal obstruction after A.P.E.)	

No case had liver involvement, yet two had a raised excretion of 5-hydroxy-indol acetic acid. These symptoms may in part be due to stenosis of the bowel lumen, but the direct effect of serotonin on the small intestine must be partially responsible for the symptoms of at least two of the patients.

Rectal bleeding occurred in only two patients. One of these was found to have a mass in her right iliac fossa, which proved to be a carcinoid tumour 2 cms proximal to the ileo-caecal junction associated with a large mass of mesenteric nodes. The other had no abnormal physical signs, and no lesion was seen at sigmoidoscopy or proctoscopy to account for her bleeding. A barium meal and follow-through was therefore performed, which was reported to be normal except for the rapid passage of barium to the hepatic flexure within half an hour. Laparotomy revealed a small nodule in the terminal ileum, 4 ft. proximal to the ileo-caecal valve; this was resected and she remains free from symptoms 10 years later.

Only one patient presented with all the classical features of the carcinoid syndrome. The liver was found to be extensively replaced with metastases, yet no primary tumour was found, despite a through search. Primary tumours are often small, and can be microscopic in size with distant metastases. This patient had complained of flushing and breathlessness for 10 years, and his 24 hour excretion of 5-hydroxy-indol acetic acid was 116 mgms.

One patient, who complained of dysphagia and who had lost about 7 kg in weight during the previous year, was found to have a filling defect at the oesophago-gastric junction. Oesophago-gastrectomy was performed for an annular tumour in the region of the cardia, and pathological examination of the specimen showed it to be a carcinoid tumour with lymph node metastases. This patient lived for a year after his operation, and died from liver metastases.

One patient, who was admitted as an emergency with abdominal pain and vomiting of 9 days duration, was found to have signs of peritonitis with abdominal distension and rigidity in the left iliac fossa. Immediate laparotomy revealed a gangrenous segment of terminal ileum, approximately 8 inches long. A nodule was noted in the bowel wall, and an enlarged mesenteric node was present. Resection and anastomosis was performed and the patient made a good recovery. This mode of presentation is unusual, and is thought to be due to the release of serotonin from the mesenteric metastases into the circulation, and the powerful vaso-constrictor effect of this substance. In this instance there was evidence of recent thrombosis in a mesenteric vein, but no arterial occlusion could be demonstrated.

Four other tumours were found, incidentally, during the course of other operative procedures. None of these was associated with any lymph node metastases, and in each case the tumour seems to have been detected at an early stage.

The site of these tumours (Table 2) can be anywhere in the alimentary canal, but it is most common in the region of the terminal ileum and appendix. Colonic and rectal carcinoids are described, but only one occurred in the present series.

Table 2. *Site of tumours*

Stomach	1
Jejunum	2
Ileum	7
Multiple in small bowel	1
Ascending colon	1
No primary found	1

Diagnosis

In the absence of the carcinoid syndrome, the pre-operative diagnosis is extremely difficult, if not impossible. Symptoms found in the present series were not in any way specific, and no abnormal physical signs were found in the absence of advanced disease. Barium follow-through examination would be unlikely to demonstrate such small tumours, and was inconclusive in the two instances in which it was performed. It is not surprising, therefore, that the only patient in whom a correct pre-operative diagnosis was made, manifested the classical features of carcinoid syndrome.

Treatment

These tumours are believed to be of low grade malignancy, and local removal is probably adequate in the majority of instances. This has been practised in 51 examples of carcinoid tumour of the appendix which occurred in Bath during this ten year period. None of these, however, had infiltrated to the base of the appendix and there is no evidence to show that any extension of tumour occurred subsequently. One patient had a small nodule in the terminal ileum, which was found during the course of emergency appendectomy; it was not recognized as a carcinoid tumour by the registrar who performed the operation, and local removal alone was undertaken. Despite this, she remains well and free from symptoms 4 years later.

Even though local removal is probably adequate, the majority of surgeons would prefer to carry out a wide excision including the lymphatic field. This, of course, is obligatory when regional nodes are involved (Table 3).

Table 3. *Metastases at operation*

None	5
Nodes only	6
Liver	2

Liver metastases, when present, are usually found in both lobes and are associated with features of carcinoid syndrome. Some authors have advocated palliative resection of large masses of liver tissue, in order to reduce serotonin production and to relieve symptoms. No resection of this sort has been practised in the present series, and it hardly seems justifiable to attempt such a hazardous procedure for a slowly growing tumour when the symptoms of carcinoid syndrome can be controlled to some extent by drugs. No operative mortality in this small group.

Bibliography

Cassidy, M. A.: Proc. Roy. Soc. Med. **24**, 129 (1930).
Masson, P., and L. Bergen: C. R. Acad. Sci. **176**, 1748 (1928).
Oberndorfer, S.: Frankfurt. Z. Path. **1**, 426 (1907).
Thorson, A., A. Biorck, G. Bjorkman, and J. Waldenstrom: Amer. Heart J. **47**, 795 (1954).

Situation of Endorectal Irradiation in the Curative Treatment of Rectum Cancer at the Outset

J. Papillon, Lyon, France

By tradition, cancer of the rectum remains an essentially surgical problem. The operation is always broad and systematic, even when the tumour is of small size and at an early stage.

The arguments, which seem to justify extensive surgery and the absence of x-ray treatment, are two in number:

- the generally admitted notion, that rectal carcinoma is extensive
- the preconceived notion that this tumour is radio-resistent.

In fact, in the greater part of the cases, cancer of the rectum does not evolve rapidly. In many operable patients, questioning them reveals that their troubles may date back several months; at times, more than a year. The long survival of patients with pelvic recurrences, confirms that this form of cancer evolves slowly.

One of the principal arguments, which seems to justify the extensive surgery, even for small cancer, is the frequency of recurrences on the stump, formerly understood to be evidence of unsuspected sub-mucous extension of the carcinoma.

In fact, for Löfgren and many other authors, these recurrences are more often than not, due to self-grafts in the course of operation.

The danger of lymph node invasion constitutes a more valid argument which deserves to be analyzed in the light of recent papers.

Surgical experience, among others, that of St. Mark's Hospital, London, with more than 2000 cases, has shown that rectum cancer is indeed a localized disease, in the early stages it does not spread and the rate of lymphatic invasion lies between 5 and 10%, as long as the tumour has not passed beyond the rectal coating, though it reaches up to 58% when perirectal tissues are affected, and the tumour loses its mobility (Gabriel, Morson).

It must be admitted that the ganglionic risk is almost non-existent at stage A of Duke's classification.

Under these conditions, it may be asked whether the extent of the operation is not out of proportion with the actual extent of the lesion, and whether a bloodless and less mutilating therapy would not be better in cases of tumour found at an early stage (Duke's A or B stages).

It has been proved that some of these cancers can be healed in the early stages with a simple local excision or electro-coagulation (Todd, Poirier).

In comparison to these 2 techniques, endorectal irradiation offers appreciable advantages. It has a more selective action, since it is able to destroy tissues that are sensitive to x-rays, leaving healthy structures undamaged. Furthermore it affects the surface of the tumour as well as its depth at the level of implantation without risking perforation if the technique is sufficiently accurate.

At the same time CHAOUL of Berlin (1936) and LAMARQUE of Montpellier (1944) demonstrated the good radio-sensitivity of rectal carcinoma and the remarkable resistance of the rectal coating to endorectal irradiation, even at high dosages.

For the past 20 years, we have treated 125 patients with rectal cancer in Lyon by endorectal irradiation on this principle.

One hundred observations date back more than 3 years. We are presenting the analysis of the results we obtained.

Out of the 100 patients, 82 were treated by contact only, and 18 by radium puncture, usually in association with contact-therapy. Radium was preferred when an infiltration at the base of the tumour risked not being sterilized completely by contact-therapy, or when the tumour being situated near the anus was not suitable for radiotherapy by contact.

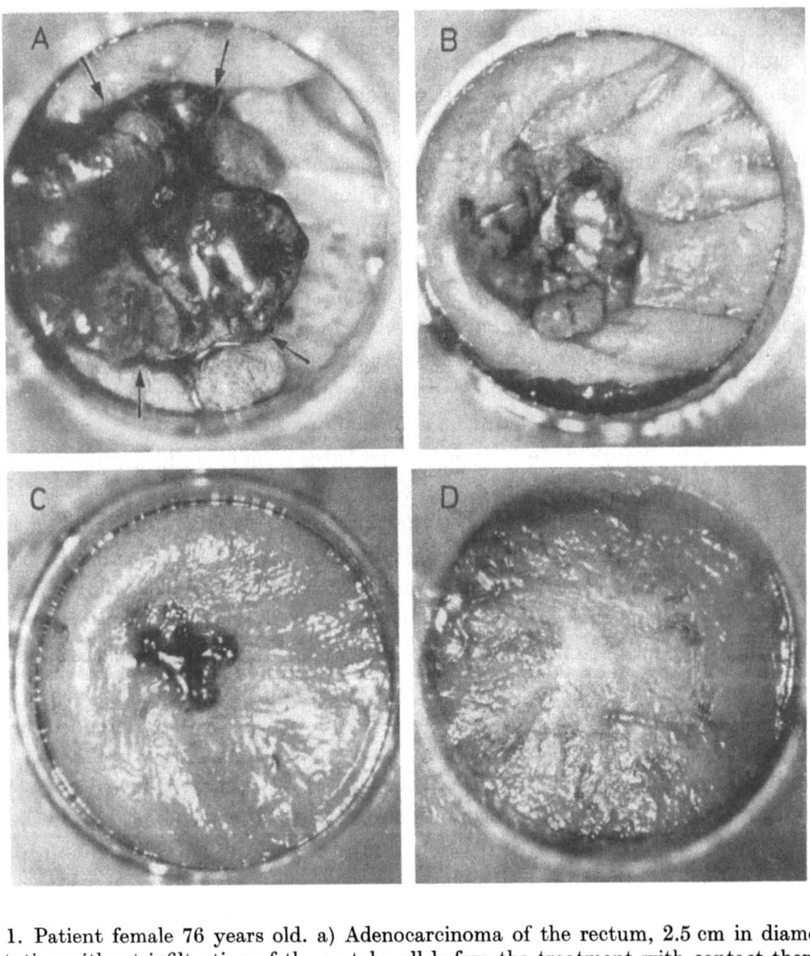

Fig. 1. Patient female 76 years old. a) Adenocarcinoma of the rectum, 2.5 cm in diameter, vegetating without infiltration of the rectal wall before the treatment with contact therapy. b) same case 1 week later after the 1st sitting. c) same case 2 weeks after the start, 1 week after the 2nd sitting. d) same case at the end of the treatment (4 sittings), the mucosa has kept a subnormal aspect. This patient is cured for five years without any trouble

Histological types were as follows:

– 93 tumours were typical adenocarcinomas,

– 5 of them were anaplastic carcinomas, the evolution of which conformed to that of adenocarcinomas.

2 of them were colloid carcinomas, whose generally admitted high malignity found expression in precocious recurrences and rapid metastasis.

Irradiation by contact has involved an average of 4 treatments, spread over 1 month; radiumpuncture in two treatments was sometimes performed. A preliminary colostomy was never performed.

The melting of the tumour is rapid and spectacular (Fig. 1). Within a few weeks, one can see the tumour sag, while at same time the adjoining mucous membrane first reacts and then regenerates rapidly. The functional tolerance is good, and a moderate rectitis is noted in one third of the cases only.

If the technique was rational, no necrosis is observed during the weeks which follow the irradiation. The mucous membrane maintains a subnormal or whitish aspect with limited subjacent fibrosis and without any retraction ordiminution of intestinal function.

Healed patients do not have any trouble with defecation and can lead a normal existence, free from any infirmity in connection with the treatment.

The slow evolution of the 82 patients, observed for 5 years, appears in the following table:

Causes of death under 5 years

Metastatic or regional, local cancerous evolution	12
Second cancer	4
Intercurrent disease	9
Post-operative complications	3
Total	28

The statements which we have been able to make, regarding the ganglionic problem, confirm that rectum cancer in its initial phase is little adenogen.

We have observed 6 only cases of adenopathy:

– 3 of these patients are dead.

– 3 others are alive for more than 5 years (one after amputation; two others after radium puncture,

The cardiac condition of those patients makes any operation out of the question.

Total results are as follows:

Survival (no evidence of disease)

	at 3 years		at 5 years	
without Surgery	72	77/100	50	54/82
with Surgery	5		4	66%

When appreciating these results, one fact must be taken into consideration: a number of patients could not be operated or operated under restriction only, in view of their age or general condition.

These results could only be obtained at the cost of a very strict selection at the first examination.

Only the following are within the province of endorectal irradiation:

– cancers that are easily approachable, i. e. the upper pole of which is at less than 14 cms from the anus.
– cancers whose dimensions do not exceed 5 cms in length and 3 cms in width,
– finally and above all, cancers whose morphology is essentially vegetating with a tiny infiltration of the implantation base.

In this manner, it is the appreciation of the pliability of the tumoral base, which constitutes the essential factor when choosing between endorectal irradiation and high surgery.

Contrary to certain dogmas that seem firmly established, rectum cancer is radio-sensitive (treated in the endorectal way) and radio-curable.

Within the frame of indications we have specified, this method is able – in a high percentage of cases – to have a curative action on the tumour, while keeping the integrity of the sphincter function. It is realized without any intestinal derivation and can be applied, even to aged or weakened patients.

Bibliography

Papillon, J., M. Dargent, A. Pinet et J. L. Chassard: Le traitement des cancers ano-rectaux par la radiothérapie de contact. Paris: Masson Editeur 1960.

—, J. F. Montbarbon, L. Dutou et J. L. Chassard: L'irradiation à visée curative et conservatrice dans le traitement du cancer du rectum (à propos de 85 observations traitées par radiothérapie de contact [78] ou par radium [7]). Arch. Mal. Appar. dig. **55**, nº 3, 177–196 (1966).

—, —, J. L. Chassard, L. Dutou, M. Croisille et G. Alziary de Roquefort: Place de la Radiothérapie dans le traitement du cancer de l'anus au début (A propos de 58 observations). Arch. Mal. Appar. dig. **57**, nº 1, 57–73 (1968).

Some Consideration on the Operative Treatment of Cancer of the Rectum

B. Krestev, St. Kirov and Zl. Dudunkov, Sofia, Bulgaria

The operative treatment of cancer of the rectum, compared with the other visceral localizations of malignant tumours, is one of the most successful [3, 4].

We maintain that the indications for the operative treatment of this disease ought to be extended as much as possible; sometimes they must include combined resections going as far as the evisceration of the pelvis.

We are also of the opinion that both methods – that of sacrificing or of preserving the sphincter – are to be applied for certain indications only. Cases of tumour located at distances over 6 cm from the anus allow the preservation of the sphincter. To be more specific, we assume that these operations concern only circumscribed tumours located at distances 6–8 cm, for *T 1–2* forms and at 8–10 cm for *T3* forms.

Tumour invasion into adjacent organs, regardless of tumour height indicates exstirpation methods.

The various sphincter preserving operations in cases of tumour localization are applied as follows:

anterior resection – 10–12 cm

abdomino-anal resection (Babcock-Bacon) – 6–10 cm.

Abdomino-sacral method as well as Toupet's operation have not been practised often, their application being limited to cases where the bowel lenght does not permit transanal reposition.

We have analyzed the results of 986 cases operated at various clinics all over the country in the period 1952–1961. Of these:

59% underwent operations according to Babcock-Bacon

37% – Miles

3% – abdominal resection; and

1% – abdomino – sacral resection.

Those data approach our own indications closely enough, as far as the height of tumours is concerned:

64% – 6–12 cm.

28% – up to 6 cm.

8% – over 12 cm [1].

Up to 1958 the most widely used method was that of exstirpation (68%).

From 1961 on the operations preserving the sphincter are predominant – 59% [1].

We have assessed the results of 280 cases operated on at our clinic. 166 of these were treated in the period 1952–1961 and 104 after 1964. 52 of these cases were treated by our "ablastico-antiblastic" method, which is in itself a variation of some standard methods applied so far [2].

In the main this method consist of the following:

a) Ligation of the vascular pedicle where the venous flow is completely interrupted before the mobilization of the bowel in order to prevent haematogenous dissemination (Fig. 1).

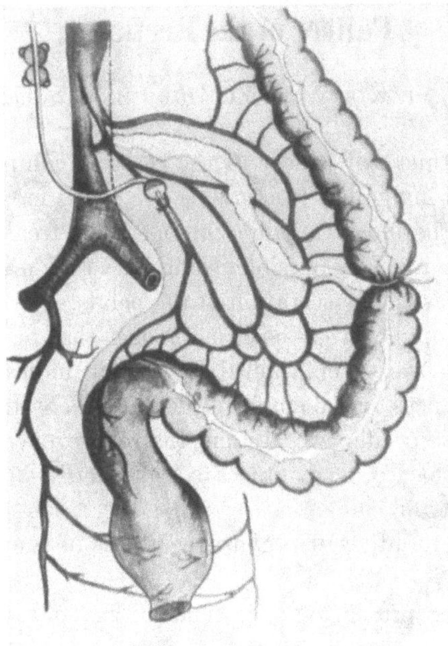

Fig. 1

b) Injection of trenimon (0.6–0.8 mg) into the superior rectal artery.

c) Closing the lumen of the bowel, superiorly and posteriorly, in order to prevent the outflow of tumour cells into the operative field (Fig. 2 and 3).

d) Frequent bathing of the presacral area in physiological saline solution.

To assess the results of the operative treatment, we divided our material into three groups:

Efficiency of method applied

Groups	Number of cases	Percentage of four year survival
I	52	97
II	52	55
III	166	51

Group I – treated by ablastico-antiblastic method. Group II – conventional methods after 1964. Group III – conventional methods for the period 1952–1961.

The ratio *T2* to *T3* in groups 1 and 2 is 57% to 43%.
Data on the ratio in group 3 are not available.
The post-operative death rate was 8.5%.

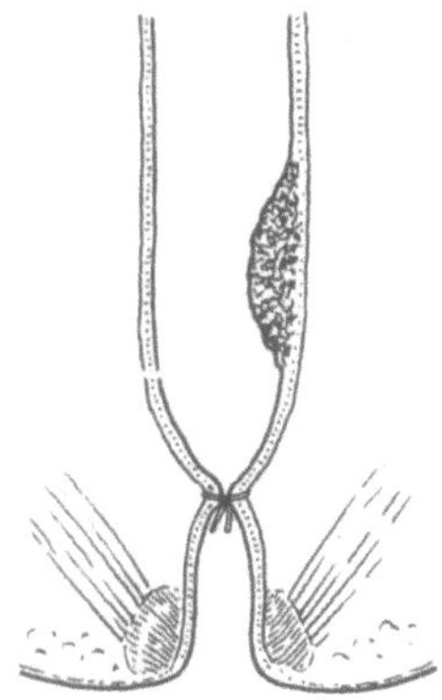

Fig. 2

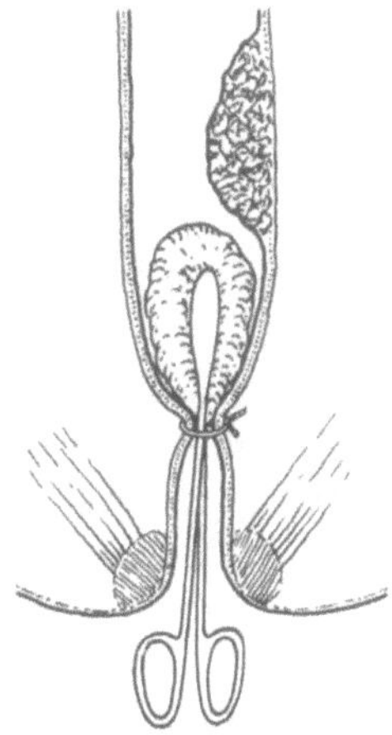

Fig. 3

Reoperations because of recurrence are an important feature of rectum cancer treatment on the whole. 22 reoperations had been performed in the period 1961–1967. Five patients died post operatively. The two year follow up of the reoperated patients showed 44% free of recurrence. The operative procedures applied at reoperation were:

Exstirpation of the neo-rectum – 18 cases
Exstirpation of recurrence in the perineum – 2 cases
Inguino-femoral lymph node dissection – 2 cases.

We therefore believe that the "ablastico-antiblastic" method applied by us has proved rather encouraging and we do think that it should be continued in order to amass more experience.

Bibliography

1. Krestev, B., Sl. Dudunkov: Verkhy lechenieto na kartsinoma na rektuma v Belgaria sa perioda 1952–1961. Oncologia **1**, 9 (1965).
2. —, S. Kirov, Sl. Dudunkov: Verkhy njakoi momenti ot ablastika i antiblastikata pri operativnoto lechenie na raka na pravoto chervo. Chirurgia **2**, 96 (1967).
3. Kholdin, S.: Slokachestvennije novoobrasovanija prjamoi kishki. Moskau 1965.
4. D'Allaines, F.: Die Chirurgische Behandlung des Rektumkarzinoms. Leipzig 1956.

VII. Colitis, Diverticulitis, Proctitis

The Surgical Treatment of Ulcerative Colitis

F. Gall and J. von der Emde, Erlangen, Germany

As the etiology of ulcerative colitis is still unknown, no causal treatment has as yet been found. A rigid conservative therapy leads to success in only 75% of the cases, whereas in about 25% the disease takes such a dangerous turn that only the excision of the entire colon offers a prospect of saving the patient. Considering that the selection of the right moment for surgery greatly influences the operative mortality, the surgeon is particularly interested in knowing the criteria which impose the necessity for operative treatment. Here we wish to deal with these criteria in the light of our experience gained with the operative treatment of 80 patients suffering from ulcerative colitis.

Acute fulminant colitis soon leads to extreme prostration of the patient due to severe diarrhoea with pus, mucus and blood in the stool, heavy losses of albumin and electrolytes as well as intoxication accompanied by high fever and tachycardia. Only $^1/_3$ of these toxic diseases can be alleviated by conservative measures, the primary mortality being 50%. Patients under 20 are more frequently affected by fulminant colitis, and the mortality rate is higher than in adults.

In our cases of acute colitis, 7.9% were due to fatal perforative peritonitis, 5.6% to toxic megacolon with a mortality of 75% and copious bleeding was found in 10% with a fatal issue for 50 per cent of the patients. This was attributed to an excessively rigid compliance with a fixed time limit set for the conservative therapy attempt. In 14 patients out of 31 with acute fulminant ulcerative colitis, proctocolectomy had to be carried out on account of such acute and dangerous complications. The operative mortality was 59%. In the case of acute fulminant ulcerative colitis we regard immediate surgery in the form of proctocolectomy as indicated whenever acute abdominal pain is experienced in response to palpation, or if there is excessive meteorism (toxic megacolon), leucocytosis above 10,000, continuous high fever and a high pulse rate, and after conservative therapy for 10 days has failed.

Most frequently, ulcerative colitis takes a chronic intermittent course. Intractable rebound relapses are the rule. The danger of acute exacerbation constantly threatens the patient. If an attack persists for more than 6 months, remission is unlikely to occur, and in about 26% of the cases, chronic continuous colitis develops.

In the chronic form of both intermittent and continuous ulcerative colitis cumulative mortality after 3 years of illness exceeds the primary operative mortality during the interval. Therefore the following arguments speak in favour of early surgery in chronic colitis. Patients suffering from colitis are unable to work and are ill for half the time the disease persists, and only 10–15% of the patients are free from relapse for longer periods. If the colon is extensively infected, healing can hardly be expected to occur. The frequency of local and systemic complications increases and the risk of carcinomatous degeneration may rise to as high as 40% the longer the disease persists.

Seen from this point of view, an operation appears indicated between 2 attacks of chronic recurrent ulcerative colitis. The operative mortality of our 20 colectomies and segment resections was 4.5%. A recent follow-up examination showed that all surviving patients had remained healthy and completely fit for work ever since the operation.

The operative procedure also depends on the extent of the ulcerative involvement. In 49% of the cases the entire colon is involved, in 25% the left colon is affected, in 60% the involvement takes a course ascending orally, in 7% there is an isolated infection of the rectosigmoid and in about 5–15% the right colon only is involved.

For understandable reasons, patients with ulcerative colitis again and again express the wish that the surgeon establish a relieving fistula. The temporary exclusion of the colon by ileostomy or caecostomy must be refused, because many concurring observations show that it is a dangerous and useless roundabout way. Earlier, 22 colitis patients received such a relieving bowel fistula in our clinic. Nevertheless, half of them died of typical complications, 5 of them from carcinoma.

Prior to 1955, we performed a left-sided hemicolectomy with terminal transversalis-anus in 7 patients with ascending colitis on the left side, because the right hemicolon seemed to be uninvolved from the outside and by X-ray.

This procedure failed to yield good results because 4 patients developed colitis in the right hemicolon only a few months later. The results in 5 patients with proctosigmoiditis and the establishment of an anus praeter on the left side, was even less encouraging. In 75% of these patients, we noted an ascent of the ulcerative decomposition of the mucosa of the anus praeter after a couple of weeks. Such failures with left-sided ascending colitis can be avoided only by primary proctocolectomy.

Resections in continuity and preserving the organ of continence are possible only in rare cases of right-sided descending colitis. For such procedures, an intact rectum with normal mucosa is required as a primary condition. Multiple scar formations or an atrophic mucosa of the rectum point to a previous proctitis and rule out right-sided descending colitis. Whenever right-sided colitis is diagnosed with certainty, the exstirpation of the diseased colon should be performed early and as radically as possible because the progressive involvement of the rectum by the descending course of the disease appears to be only a matter of time. Even when the process is macroscopically confined to the ascending colon and to the right transverse colon, colectomy with ileorectal anastomosis is recommended, as quite frequently a new colitis process has developed in the left colon after right-sided hemicolectomy.

Aylett [1] generally treats colitis by colectomy with ileorectal anastomosis in all his patients. He believes that after the elimination of large resorptive surfaces and the amelioration of toxemia, the rectal ulcers will heal spontaneously and the mucosa will regenerate. Only in 5% of 259 patients he operated on, did he later have to establish a terminal ileostomy. Using the same procedure in KRONBERGER's [6] 93 cases of ileorectal anastomosis however the incidence of secondary rectum amputation was 72%. Even our own experience gained with 19 resections in continuity have indicated a need for caution. Three patients died post-operatively from local complications caused by suture dehiscence and another three from general complications. Anastomosis was carried out in macroscopically uninvolved sections of the bowel. But the histological examination showed that the colon was also involved microscopically. Of the surviving 13 patients, 7 are completely free from complaint and the other 6 suffer from slight colitic symptoms at times.

Proctocolectomy with terminal ileostomy offers the best guarantee for a permanent cure of ulcerative colitis. Nowadays the operative treatment has given way to single proctocolectomy, which is also resorted to in emergencies. Especially in critically ill patients with fulminant colitis there is an urgent need for proctocolectomy performed in one operation in order to prevent life-endangering complications likely to be caused by the resorption of toxins and massive bleeding – which occured in our clinic in 7 cases – and to prevent extensive phlegmonae in the sacral area from developing after colectomy where the diseased rectal stump remains. The operative mortality subsequent to proctocolectomy was 35% in our patients. This high mortality rate can be attributed to the large proportion of free perforations, excessive bleeding and toxic megacolon with an operative mortality of 59% after proctocolectomy, whereas no patient died when the operation was carried out between two attacks. These figures clearly speak in favour of early surgical intervention in the case of fulminant colitis.

Complications as a sequel to ulcerative colitis developed in 68.5% of our 89 patients, 53 were local complications and 76 were of a general nature.

Secondary systemic diseases can hardly be influenced by conservative measures, but the exstirpation of the toxin-absorbing diseased colon leads to spontaneous healing of such disorders.

Free perforation occurred in 7.9% of our patients in the acute stage of colitis. Single or multiple covered perforations with faecal abscesses were found in 3 patients. In 4 patients, the free perforation gave rise to a diffuse peritonitis which had a fatal issue in 3 patients after proctocolectomy. With one exception, all patients suffering from a perforation were given corticoids over a protraced period of time.

Heavy bleeding was observed in 10.1%, but only in 2 cases of fulminant colitis did it occur prior to surgery. Postoperatively we have seen 7 profuse life-endangering hemorrhages accompanied by severe shock which originated from the rectal stump after colectomy was carried out in two sessions, or after resection which preserved continence. Despite immediate rectum amputation effected as an emergency procedure to control bleeding, 4 of the already seriously affected patients died from the consequences of this postoperative hemorrhage. This experience forces us to carry out a single-stage proctocolectomy even when the case of fulminant colitis has taken an extremely acute course.

Toxic megacolon developed in 5.6% of our patients. The high internal gas pressure favours perforation of a frequently inflammed colon or a migrating peritonitis develops, owing to excessive wall dilatation. Therefore, in the presence of fulminant ulcerative colitis, toxic megacolon is an urgent indication for immediate surgery.

Post-colitic carcinoma were observed in 5 patients. In patients with ulcerative colitis, carcinoma threatens to develop in 3.4 to 3.8% as was confirmed by comprehensive statistical records compiled by SLANEY et al. [9] and REIFFERSCHEID [8] who evaluated 9,469 cases and 22,456 cases respectively reported in the literature. DUKES [5] found an incidence of 5.2% during the histological examination of 153 consecutive colectomy specimens. However, this percentage drastically increases when the factor of time and the course of the disease are considered. COLCOCK [3] observed malignant degeneration after 8 years in 25% of the patients, CATTELL [2] in 33% after 9 years, and LYONS et al. [7] as well as COUNSELL et al. [4] in 43–45% after 12 years. Juveniles are especially exposed to this risk if they were 16 years old at the outbreak of the disease.

The prognosis is particularly unfavourable in cases of colitic carcinoma. With the colon carcinoma nowadays a life expectancy of 5 years can be attained in 60%, but when a cancer develops after colitis the percentage drops to 2.8%. In many cases the colitis carcinoma is not detected early enough because its symptoms are similar to those of the underlying main disease which induces the physician to interpret the cancer falsely as a recurrence of colitis. Even the roentgenological findings are not conclusive because the carcinoma grows almost exclusively intramurally. But any stenotic condition is highly suspicious of carcinoma.

In young patients the risk of cancer and the poor prognosis of the postcolitic carcinoma are indications which justify an early prophylactic proctocolectomy. The same holds for chronically recurring or continuous ulcerative colitis and for a total involvement of the entire colon.

Bibliography

1. AYLETT, S. O.: Three hundred cases of diffuse ulcerative colitis treated by total colectomy and ileo-rectal anastomosis. Brit. med. J. **1**, 1001 (1966).
2. CATTELL, R. B.: Surgical treatment of ulcerative colitis. Gastroenterology **10**, 63 (1948).
3. COLCOCK, B. P.: Complications of the surgical treatment of ulcerative colitis. Surg. Clin. N. Amer. **37**, 725 (1957).
4. COUNSELL, P. B., and C. E. DUKES: The association of chronic ulcerative colitis and carcinoma of the rectum and colon. Brit. J. Surg. **39**, 485 (1952).
5. DUKES, C. E.: Prognosis in ulcerative colitis. The Medical Press, April 16 (1958), Vol. 239, Nr. 6206, 357.
6. KRONBERGER, L.: Fate of rectal stump in ulcerative colitis. Arch. Surg. **91**, 967 (1965).
7. LYONS, A. S., and J. H. GARLOCK: Ulcerative colitis. Gastroenterology **18**, 170 (1951).
8. REIFFERSCHEID, M.: Darmchirurgie. Klinik, Indikation, Technik, Prognose. 2nd ed., p. 224.
9. SLANEY, G., and B. N. BROOKE: Ulcerative colitis. Lancet **2**, 694 (1959).

One-Stage Proctocolectomy with Anal Ileostomy
Report of 50 cases

S. Drobni, Budapest, Hungary

There are two different tendencies in the surgical treatment of colitis ulcerosa and familial polyposis. The representatives of the first one emphasize the radical surgery above everything else and sacrifice the sphincter muscles, thus eliminating all hope of restoring continuity. The second tendency gives preference to maintaining continuity even on the charge of radicality. The followers of the first tendency accomplished the proctocolectomy with an abdominal ileostomy, those of the second one made an ileorectal anastomosis before performing the colectomy. As a result of the first intervention, the usually young patients became invalids. After the latter operation they were exposed to different complications – recurrence, carcinotic transformation, ligature insufficiency, ascending of the disease. However, their sphincter function was adequate.

At the same time an endeavour was made to perform radical surgery, i. e.: the removal of the mucous membrane of the colon, as the bearer of the disease, was connected to restore of continuity. As you know, no one followed the unique surgical intervention of Nissen carried out in 1933 for a long time. Later it was Ravitch who discarded his own ingenious method, worked out for two teams, saying that it was not adequate in the management of ulcerative colitis. This statement was supported by such well known experts as Bacon, who possesses perhaps the largest material in the world on the surgery of the colon.

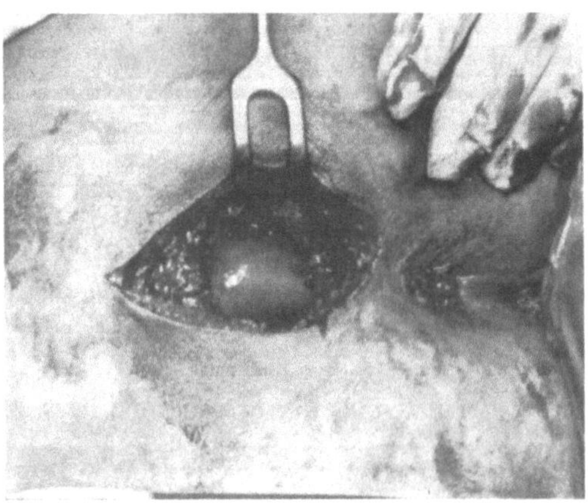

Fig. 1. Terminal portion of ileum is pulled through

Having carefully considered the possibilities and eliminating the weak points in the method of RAVITCH, we elaborated a new procedure which is carried out by a single team complying entirely with the above requirements. Essentially, this procedure is a one-stage proctocolectomy with a pull-through of the small intestine and with anal ileostomy carried out from an abdomino-perineal exposure (Fig. 1).

From September 1960 to September 1968, I performed this operation in 50 cases and had 6 deaths. Instead of discussing the statistical data, I wish to emphasize the fact that the results obtained with this technique have proven that this procedure can be carried out routinely in cases of colitis ulcerosa as well as in familial polyposis. Thus, the opinion of RAVITCH which has influenced numerous authors is obviously in error. As the mucous membrane not only of the whole colon but also of the entire rectum as well as of the sphincter canal is removed, this procedure meets the requirement of radical surgery. Furthermore it conserves the lower third of the muscular rectum wall and the sphincter apparatus. By pulling through the terminal portion of ileum the continuity is restored and the patient can continue his life as a full member of society.

After the proctocolectomy has been carried out with anal ileostomy the following questions arise: what is the continence like? what is the number of daily stools? is there a necessity for the administration of opiates or other drugs? – In general it can be stated that in 76 per cent of cases, the number of daily stools varies between 2 and 4 – without the support of drugs, using only a diet. The sphincter function of the patients is excellent; they are able to distinguish flatus from stool. The environment of the anal ileostomy was intact in 84 per cent of the cases and after the removal of the coccyx, no complications occurred. The patients are now able to carry out more than sitting work. There is a tractor driver who is ploughing 16 hours a day, or another patient, who is a motor-cycle rider and in spite of his post-colectomy state, he could not be saved from prison where he had to sit 6 months for speeding (Fig. 2).

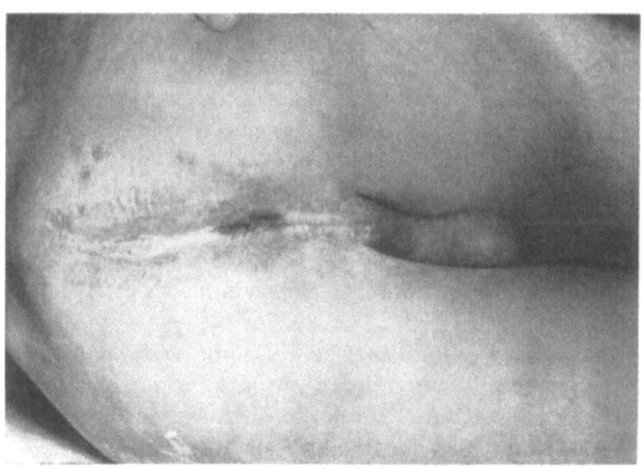

Fig. 2. Anal ileostomy two months after colectomy

Surely, it can be stated, that no patient would willingly exchange his anal ileostomy against an abdominal one.

On the basis of 8 years it was possible to modify the operative technique. Today we accomplish the resection of the rectum at a level 3 cm beyond the levators during the abdominal phase of the operation, at the same time we place the terminal portion of the ileum in the sacral cavity. Finally, after total peritonealization, the abdominal wound is closed in layers. – In the perineal phase of the operation, we insist on the reliable removal of the mucous membrane based on the method of WHITEHEAD. Then we attach the small intestine pulled through the sphincter, in three levels to the upper and lower margine of the sphincter and to the skin. The fluid content accumulating in the rectum during operative mobilization will be removed by flushing. For this purpose we have constructed a special instrument to be used in course of our anterior resection operations as well. Its most important advantage is the viability of the pulled-through intestine which can be observed immediately and constantly through the perineal "window". Only once did we observe the small intestine to become necrotic and because of this as well as for other complications in three cases we have repeatedly performed the pull-through of the small intestine: in two cases we operated 6 months and or 1 year after the original surgical procedure with full success. The third patient died as a result of peritonitis.

It is advantageous to draw the small intestine over the anal margin. Thus it becomes possible to remove a one to two cm wide superficial ring under local anaesthesia whithin 2 to 3 weeks after the adhesion. With a view to the success of the operation, the most indispensable factor is an adequate elongation of the terminal ileum. For this purpose, a good choice of the ligation site is very important. On the basis of our experience it can be stated that the length of the small intestine is regarded as adequate for the pull-through when it reaches beyond the symphysis pubis after being drawn over the abdominal wound. Soiling of the abdominal cavity must be prevented by thorough isolation and a great care must be taken not to injure the sphincter fibres in the course of removing the mucous membrane.

Bibliography

AYLETT, S. O.: Ulcerative colitis treated by total colectomy and ileorectal anastomosis: A ten-year review (abridged). Proc. Roy. Soc. Med. **56**, 183 (1963).

BACON, H. E., and H. D. TRIMPI: The selection of an operative procedure for patients with medically intractable ulcerative colitis. Surg. Gynec. Obst. **91**, 409 (1950).

DEVINE, J., and R. WEBB: Resection of the rectal mucosa, colectomy, and anal ileostomy with normal continence. Surg. Gynec. Obst. **92**, 437 (1951).

DROBNI, S.: In einer Sitzung durchgeführte Colectomie mit Dünndarmdurchziehung und Erhaltung des Sphinkters bei Colitis ulcerosa. Chirurg **33**, 216 (1961).

EKESPARRE, v., W.: Radikale, kontinenzerhaltende Operationsmethode bei der Colitis ulcerosa. Z. Kinderchir. **1/2**, 156 (1964).

— Weitere Erfahrungen mit der chirurgischen Behandlung der Colitis ulcerosa. Z. Kinderchir. Suppl. **5**, 84 (1968).

GASTON, E. A.: The physiology of fecal continence. Surg. Gynec. Obst. **87**, 280 (1948).

— Physiological basis for preservation of fecal continence after resection of rectum. J.A.M.A.

NISSEN, R.: Berliner Gesellschaft für Chirurgie, Sitzung vom 14. November 1932, in der Chirurgischen Univ.-Klinik der Charité. Zbl. Chir. **15**, 888 (1933).

RAVITCH, M. M., and D. C. SABISTON, jr.: Anal ileostomy with preservation of the sphincter; A proposed operation in patients requiring total colectomy for benign lesions. Surg. Gynec. Obst. **84**, 1095 (1947).

— Anal ileostomy with sphincter preservation in patients requiring total colectomy for benign conditions. Surgery **24**, 170 (1948).

WANGENSTEEN, O. H.: Primary resection (closed anastomosis) of the colon and rectosigmoid; Including description of abdomino-anal methods for restoration of continuity accompanying excision of carcinoma of the rectal ampulla. Surgery **14**, 403 (1943).

Surgical Treatment of Nonspecific Ulcerative Colitis

I. M. MATYASHIN, Donetsk, UdSSR

Wide-spread occurrence of such a severe disease as nonspecific ulcerative colitis of the large intestine forced numerous guests to look for effective methods of treatment. Lack of reliable data on the etiology and pathogenesis of the disease makes existing methods of conservative treatment barely effective in severe forms of the disease.

Surgical management of patients in serious condition is difficult.

Our clinic has been busy with the problems pertaining to the treatment of nonspecific ulcerative colitis for over eight years. In this period 206 cases were under observation, 130 of them were treated conservatively, 76 patients were operated on. The postoperative mortality is 35.9% (27 patients died). The pattern of radical operative treatment differed depending on the patients general condition and the character of the colonic lesions. The management of patients in extremely poor general condition and with involvement of the entire colon was started with a double-barrelled ileostomy (39 cases) followed by total colectomy or hemicolectomy (57 cases). When the patients were in satisfactory condition, total colectomy or hemicolectomy was performed in one stage ending in a single-barrelled iliac fistula.

From our point of view the operation may be called the operation of choice in nonspecific ulcerative colitis. One of the pecularities of this operation is the necessity for thoroughness when separating the colon.

One must take into account that the thinned wall of the affected intestine may be easily broken through. There is great danger that the highly virulent microflora can empty into the abdominal cavity followed by the inevitable development of diffuse peritonitis with a fatal outcome in most cases.

Striving to perform the operation in one stage is also wrong. Making an ileorectal anastomosis in extremely weak patients against the background of considerable hypoproteinemia and decreased regenerative capabilities usually results in anastomosis failure followed by death. We used this procedure in two patients and death occured in both cases. Moreover, we disapprove of a single-stage ileorectal anastomosis when striving to provide the affected rectum with immobility.

Protracted rectal disconnection provides good conditions for the healing of its mucosa and it means restoration of the intestinal continuity under more favourable conditions.

The problem of restoring intestinal tract continuity by forming the ileorectal or colorectal anastomosis was solved several months later, sometimes 2–3 years after removal of the colon, depending on rectal status. Such anastomoses were made in 31 cases, in one patient colonic continuity was restored by ileo-coloplasty, bringing the colon down onto the perineum – in one patient and small intestine (ileocoloplasty) – in three cases. In all other cases, the rectum had to be removed because it was a large lesion, with the exception of four patients where we cherished the hope of restoring continuity. Observation of the patients who had undergone radical operations in connection with nonspecific ulcerative colitis does not allow us to characterize any operative methods as the most successful in the treatment of this disease. Total colectomy and even coloproctectomy does not cure patients completely.

In remote postoperative periods (2 and 3 years later) we observed two patients who died with the appearance of ulcerative colitis, large ulcerations of skin and mucosa, sepsis, cachexia.

In many patients where the rectum was left, one could see considerable inflammatory changes in the mucosa, which made it necessary to remove the rectum.

In the absence of inflammatory changes, there develops a "syndrome of the colonic absence", characterized by frequent and liquid stools, dyspeptic disorders, emaciation.

Clinico-laboratory examination revealed such changes as anemia, left shift in the white blood cell count, ESR increase, hypo- and dysproteinemia, avitaminosis with a particular decrease in the vitamin B_1 content, disturbed mineral metabolism and exchange of tracer elements.

In this connection, we consider it expedient to restrict the indications for such a traumatic and crippling operations as total colectomy and colproetectomy. The main criterion for operation has to be a distinct disturbance in metabolism rather than local changes. In the absence of such shifts, therapeutic treatment is possible in the hope of a stable and prolonged remission.

When choosing the character of the operative intervention, it is necessary to use the least stressful one (excepting especially severe forms of the disease).

Attention shoud also be paid to the study of the operation elaborated in the Soviet Union by I. E. BEREZOV and V. S. SIMONYAN – paranephrocolopexy, meant to improve the vascularization in the affected sections of the intestine. The essence of the operation resolved itself into the mobilization of the descending colon (in cases of left sided lesions) and then placing it retroperitoneally. This operation was performed by us twice and both times with favourable results. Besides from our standpoint in cases of stable rectosigmoiditis, it is possible to make a double-barrelled sigmostome (occasionally for a one-year-period and more). Practicing such surgical procedures will enable cessation of the further spread of process on the one hand, on the other hand it will assist in restoring the normal state of the mucosa of the nonfunctioning S-romanum and rectum.

Further advances in the surgical treatment of nonspecific ulcerative colitis probably lie in the search for more harmless operative procedures ensuring the patients recovery and their complete occupational rehabilitation.

Primary Syphilis of the Anorectal Region

B. SAMENIUS, Göteborg, Sweden

The regression of syphilis after the second world war mainly ceased during the years 1954–1957; since then the disease has again increased considerably throughout the whole world. According to SCHMID (1960) venereal diseases, especially syphilis must be considered as the diagnosis behind anal symptoms. SCHMID therefore stresses that primary syphilis has to be excluded before haemorrhoids, fissures, pruritus ani are treated.

The incidence of syphilis reported in thre USA has tripled since 1957 (SMITH 1963); in Sweden it has tripled since 1960. Seafaring is one source of spreading the disease, but also the increased mobility of the population. This is exemplified by the fact that in Switzerland, where every third worker is a foreigner, the frequency of syphilis has increased over tenfold since 1957 (BURCHKHARDT 1963). Nowadays homosexual behaviour seems to play an important part in the transmission of syphilis, particularly in big cities and ports as stressed by NICOL (1960). Appreciable increases in syphilis due to homosexuality have been noted during the last years not only in the USA but also in the European countries including Scandinavia.

Former surveys indicated that only 2–4% of extragenital chancres were located in the anal region. In recent years, however, homosexual contacts seem to be responsible for about 25–50% or more of primary syphilis occurring in male patients (KVORNING 1963). Reports from countries in western Europe state that the increase in the number of syphilis cases is practically and exclusively due to the increase of the disease in homosexual circles.

Homosexual men as a rule believe that they cannot contract syphilis because they regard it as a woman's disease (HERMANS and DE COCK 1963).

Even among our colleagues there are many who believe that syphilis no longer presents any problems and that venereal diseases are not transmitted by homosexuals.

Anal involvement in syphilis can sometimes be completely overlooked by the patient, as the complaints are mild and of short duration; as a rule, however, he is likely to ascribe his anal symptoms to piles: if the patient asks for medical advice, the disease will rarely be correctly diagnosed, at least not primarily; this is not due to the physician's lack of interest in rectal lesions, but to the fact that it is difficult to recognize the luetic affection of this area.

Because a venereal disease is seldom suspected, the patients are referred to a surgeon, interested in proctology, who will have the responsibility of making a correct diagnosis (SCHMID 1960, NICOL 1962).

A short review of cases of anorectal syphilis seen in Göteborg is presented. Much larger series of anorectal syphilis have been published, but it has usually been difficult to tell the true number of cases of primary syphilis as the clinical findings were not so accurate or dark-ground examination was not performed (HOLLINGS 1961) to a great extent.

Ten cases of anorectal syphilis were seen at the Out-Patient Department of the Surgical Dept. I at the University Hospital, Göteborg during the years 1958–1967.

The first case of anorectal chancre in this series was in a 31-year-old woman who had practised analism for several years with visiting sailors. She was referred from a gynaecologist as having a carcinoma of the anterior wall of the rectum; the lesion looked very much like an early carcinoma with an elevated edge and central necrosis with a diameter of about 2 cm; it was typical of primary syphilitic lesions of the rectum (WELLS et al. 1959, SMITH 1965).

The rest of the material consists of nine single men with different occupations, all admitting homosexual exposure. It is significant that 7 of them were either infected abroad or by foreigners visiting Sweden.

The difficulty of recognizing anorectal syphilis has been stressed by many authors, among them HECHT (1957) and SCHMID (1960). None of the cases in our material was correctly diagnosed at the time of referral. One case had been examined six different times by six surgical registrars at the Emergency Department of the hospital without syphilis being suspected.

There is no single finding pathognomonic of syphilis of the anal orifice. The most constant is ulceration, usually in the posterior midline, as a rule very difficult to differentiate from ulcerations produced by an anal fissure (MORSON 1964) (Fig. 1 and 2). Sometimes the ulceration consists of one or several erosions causing abundant, foul smelling discharge with secondary irritation and itching. Sometimes the ulceration has a bizarre and atypical appearance (Fig. 3).

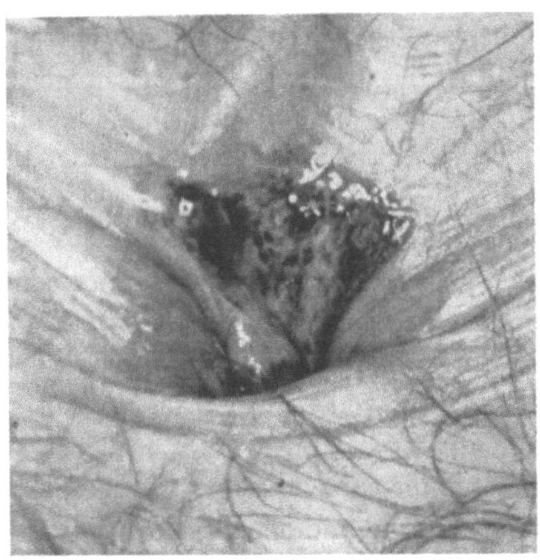

Fig. 1. Anterior anal ulceration. Dark-ground examination positive

Many authors state that ulcerations of the luetic type are practically painless and produce very little discomfort at examination. In this series, however, 8 patients complained of pain, 2 had such severe pain at night that they had to seek help as emergency cases.

Anorectal syphilis has to be diagnosed early as the local changes rapidly disappear and the lesions heal spontaneously, usually within 3–4 weeks. Even if syphilis of the anorectal region can be diagnosed solely by clinical examination, the definite diagnosis should be made by the dark-field procedure and by serological tests. Among the diseases to be considered in the differential diagnosis of syphilis of this region are anal fissures, haemorrhoids, anal manifestations of Crohn's disease, basal and squamous cell carcinoma of the anal canal and even carcinoma of the rectum.

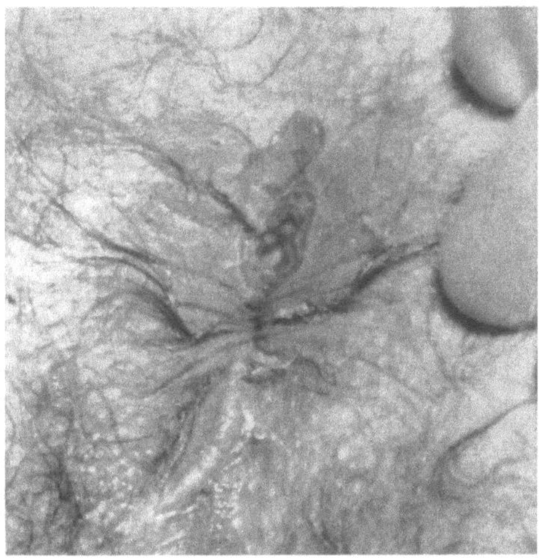

Fig. 2. Posterior anal ulceration. Dark-ground examination positive

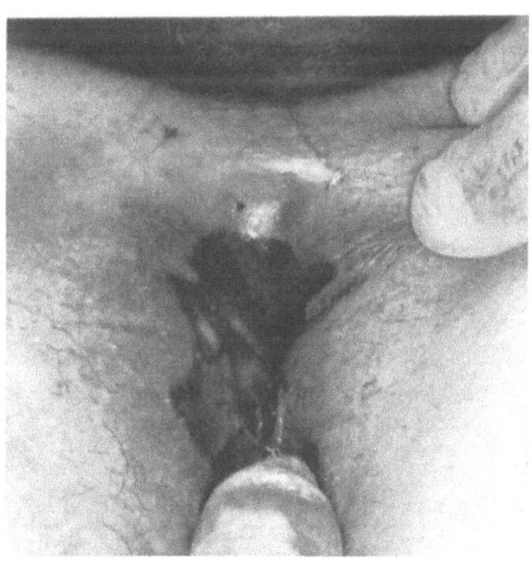

Fig. 3. Areas of ulceration completely surrounding the anal canal. Dark-ground examination positive

Syphilis must be especially suspected in all cases of ulcerations in or around the anal canal if these are associated with hard bilateral inguinal glands. This is particularly so if the patient is a single male and has the indefinable characteristics of a homosexual.

It is probable that the comparative rarity of the cases hitherto reported is more an expression of overlooking or misinterpreting the lesions than a low frequency of luetic infections in the anorectal region (Marino 1964). An improved awareness of the possibility of syphilis in this region may result in earlier diagnosis and treatment and prevent spreading of the disease (Magnusson and Otterland 1964, Vereide 1964).

Treating the patient alone does not cover the extent of our responsibility. Locating and examining persons who have had sexual contacts with infected patients is also essential for the eradication of syphilis (Tarr and Lugar, 1960).

Bibliography

Hecht, H.: Acta derm.-venereol. Stockh. **37**, 182 (1957).
Hermans, E. H., and P. de Cock: Dermatologia **127**, 278 (1963).
Hollings, R. M.: Proc. Roy. Soc. Med. **54**, 730 (1961).
Kvorning, S. A.: Brit. J. vener. Dis. **39**, 261 (1963).
Magnusson, B., and A. Otterland: Acta derm.-venereol., Stockh. **44**, 141 (1964).
Marino, M. jr.: Dis. Colon Rectum **7**, 121 (1964).
Morson, B. C.: Proc. Roy. Soc. Med. **57**, 179 (1964).
Nicol, C. S.: Practitioner **184**, 145 (1960).
— Proc. Roy. Soc. Med. **55**, 870 (1962).
Schmid, A. H.: Med. Klin. **37**, 1635 (1960).
Smith, D.: Dis. Colon Rectum **6**, 7 (1963).
— Dis. Colon Rectum **8**, 57 (1965).
Tarr, J., and R. Lugar: Calif. Med. **93**, 35 (1960).
Wells, B. T., R. R. Kierland, and R. J. Jackman: Arch. Derm. **79**, 719 (1959).
Wereide, K.: Tidsskr. norske Laegeforen. **84**, 1696 (1964).

A Case of Pseudo-Cancerous Endometriosis of the Rectal-Vaginal Wall – Radiography and Therapy

J. M. Garrigues and Y. Alquier, Montpellier, France

Rectal localization of endometriosis is unusual. Since the original description by Meyer in 1909 only about 250 cases of recto-sigmoidial localization have been reported. Only 45 of these were exclusively rectal. This localization represents only 2% of the total endometrioses diagnosed, which according to Counseller should be 25% of the cases.

It is not the exceptional character of this affection which incites us to present this observation[1], but its macroscopic aspect, its arteriographic character, and its evolution under hormone therapy which make it interesting!

The patient was a 38-year-old woman, mother of a 17-year-old son. She had had a miscarriage and had had a curettage 5 years ago and an ovariectomay for lutein cyst of the left ovary 2 months ago. When the menstrual cycle recommenced rectorrhagia was present for six days prior to menstruation. Actually, menstrual rectorrhagia had existed for many years in association with constipation, but because it was slight the patient thought it unimportant and never disclosed this sign to the doctor.

An early examination uncovered a suspected neoplasia in the rectum which corresponded microscopically to a polypous formation with no cytological anomaly.

The patient was sent to the clinic for Diseases of the Digestive Tract (Pr. Bert) in September 1967 for complementary examinations. Her general state was excellent, the rectorrhagia having stopped since the end of the menstrual period. The physical examination showed no abnormalities. A digital exploration disclosed a series of polypoid formations, very firm, mobile but planted in an indurated zone, and situated on the recto-vaginal wall. A rectoscopy showed a slighthy congested polypoid formation covered with a normal mucus on the anterior face of the rectal ampulla between 8 and 13 cms. It was sprinkled with bluish spots, whose indefinite base was indurated and resistant to pressure from the rectoscope tube. A new biopsy showed it to be a rectal endometriosis.

The barium enema revealed a single well-defined mass of polypoid aspect, slightly irregular, obstructing part of the colic lumen without inhibiting the flow of feces.

The vaginal examination confirmed the diagnosis of endometriosis.

---

[1] Already published in "Soc. de gastro-Enter. du Littoral méditerranéen" 17-WII-1967. Arch. Fr. Mal App. Digestivo 57-3-1968 p. 392.

Nevertheless, the macroscopic aspect and the fixedness of this mass to the lower levels made us fear the possibility of degeneration. Of course we know that besides the subserosal form, tumoral with tar-like cysts, and the hemorrhagic cystic form, there is also a pseudo-cancerous form, very hard, almost scirrhous, with polypoidal excrescences. This was well-described by BENZ in 1957 and is thought to be unusual. This is why we decided to perform an arteriography.

A selective arteriography of the inferior mesenteric artery showed:

1. disorientation of the superior hemorrhoidal arteries which were quartered,
2. hypervascularization of the rectal ampulla,
3. irregularity of injection of the terminal branches,
4. at a later time, numerous hypervascularized formations near the recto-sigmoidal joint.

Selective arteriography of the hypogastric artery showed:

1. very early injection of the right uterine artery which is hypertrophied and more flexuous than normal,
2. irregular and dense arterial time,
3. early and dense parenchymatous time,
4. uterine body augmented in volume and hypervascularized.

These two examinations brought to light an important hypervascularization which remains limited to the uterus and the recto-vaginal wall but without vascular disorders or neo-vessels.

This seems to eliminate the possibility of degeneration entirely.

Because of the infirmity that surgical treatment would involve, it was decided to use hormone therapy, a synthetic estroprogesterone product: METRULENE (ethinodiol acetate 2 mgr + mestranol 100 mgr by tablet dosage: 4 tablets per 24 hours).

The patient has survived one year so far. The therapeutic tolerance is good, and her general state is excellent. She has gained 3 kilos and gone back to her normal work. All the same she sometimes discharges a little rectal mucus slightly colored with blood. She had one menstrual period without presenting much rectorrhagia. Digital exploration and repeated endoscopic examinations showed no diminuation in the volume of the mass though it has become more supple, more flabby, friable, and bleeding. The histological examinations are happily more encouraging.

The first control examination, seven months after treatment was initiated, showed that a few islands of endometriosis with rather fibrous chorions still persisted. Two months later, the epitelium of the rectal paries was still intact, the glands were reduced and encircled by an extremely abundant inflammatory granuloma. No endometriosis lesions were recognizable, but on the periphery of the granuloma were found several large cells identifiable as deciduous elements. It is therefore very probable that this granuloma developed inside the cytogenous chorion made deciduous by the hormone therapy. This would explain why the volume of the tumor remained constant. This evolution confirms that the establishment of a pseudo-progestative state by progesterone hormones leads to a decidual reaction – degeneration, necrosis, and fibrosis of the endometrial foyer

(Gompel 1963). Moreover, Henson (1964) noticed that the tumor was reduced by half, but remained palpable four years later in a case of endometriosis of the rectum which was treated by castration and post-operative progesterone. All the same, Gray (1966) thought that hormonal treatment could not establish a definitive cure of this lesion. In contrast, Fradin (1965) observed the complete disappearance of intestinal and peritoneal localization after nine months of progesterone treatment.

How should the treatment be conducted, then? If the tumor has been shown to be benign, we must be as conservative as possible, especially in rectal localizations, and not consider hormone therapy as complementary therapy. It is perhaps the only exception to the rule that the treatment of an endometriosis is essentially surgical. If this hormonal treatment does not always allow a restitutio ad integrum, it will leave a cicatricial fibrosis and will thereby facilitate eventual surgery.

Colon Biopsy in Undiagnosed Chronic Amoebiasis

TH. DOXIADIS and Z. YIOTSAS, Athens, Greece

Rectal biopsy may be essential in contributing to the diagnosis of the colon diseases, since microscopic changes have been noted in cases where rectoscopy was normal.

The method has been used in the diagnosis of chronic amoebic colitis, as well as for the differential diagnosis of acute amoebic and non-specific ulcerative colitis [1, 4].

It is well-known that the detection of E. histolytica in the stool examination confirms the amoebic origin of colitis [5, 20, 22], but a negative stool examination does not exclude the presence of the disease. This fact has made us take a rectal biopsy during proctosigmoidoscopy from all the patients suspected of suffering from chronic and acute amoebic colitis as well as chronic amoebic hepatitis [2, 6, 7, 8, 9, 11, 12, 19, 21]. The rectoscopy does not require any special preparation. The rectal specimens were taken from a depth of 6–14 cm in the majority of patients (92–95%), and the specimens were obtained by means of forceps biopsy without any complications. We have never experienced a single instance of perforation, bleeding etc. despite the large number of patients examined.

The colon specimen is fixed in 96% alcohol, and then embedded in paraffin. Subsequently, paraffin sections were stained with hematoxylin-eosin and in some instances with PAS.

The described cellular elements suggesting amoebae are always positive with PAS.

In the majority of cases, these cellular formations represent unusual and atypical forms of Entamoeba histolytica with deformed nuclei and are therefore difficult to identify [3]. A very skilled pathologist is essential for the detection of these atypical forms of Entamoeba histolytica.

Perhaps the above problem will be solved by means of fluorescent microscopy. DOXIADIS and CANDREVIOTIS [10] have proved that amoebae in culture are stained orange-red in colour by acridine orange, and are thus distinctly discerned from the surrounding cells [3]. These experiments continue with the staining of amoebae in tissues and seem to us to be very promising.

Clinical Material

From July 1st, 1962, to December 31st, 1967, 20,140 patients were admitted and examined in the First Medical Department and the Gastroenterology Center of the Evangelismos Hospital. Out of these patients, 4,927 (24%) complained of gastro-intestinal disorders and symptoms from the right hypochondrium.

The clinical manifestations of these patients were mostly diffuse abdominal cramps, constipation alternating with diarrhoea, tenderness and pain in the right hypochondrium, persistent constipation, diarrhoea containing mucus and/or blood, borborygmi, fullness of the abdomen, dizziness, weakness, headache, tenesmus, low back pain, anal itching and ash, febrile psychoneurotic symptoms etc. These symptoms were taken into consideration concerning the diagnosis of the patient's disease. One hundred and eighty-one patients (3.7%) out of 4,947 examined, were admitted with an acute dysenteric syndrome i. e. severe abdominal pain, blown-up and distended abdomen, diarrhoea (7–15 times per day), profuse bleeding and fever. All the patients underwent complete laboratory tests, including liver function tests and B.S.P. They also had upper G.I. series, G.B. series, special X-ray examinations of the liver [13], barium enemas, stool examinations and culture for ova and parasites, proctoscopy and histological examinations of the rectal specimens [9, 14, 15].

In this paper we will report the results of the stool examination, proctoscopy and histological examinations of the rectal specimens.

Among 4,927 patients examined, 444 (9%) were found to have trophozoites of E. histolytica in the fresh stool preparation. Subsequently all 4,927 were submitted to proctoscopic examination and rectal biopsy. The rectoscope was introduced at least 15–28 cm from the external anal opening. The rectal biopsy was taken 6–14 cm from the anus in the majority of the patients in cases where the lesion was diffuse. When changes were noted in other parts, additional specimens were taken, if this was technically possible.

The proctoscopic observations concerned redness, oedema, granularity of the surface, presence of mucus, irritability and friability, smoothness and atrophy of the mucosa, bleeding and ulceration. With regard to inflammatory changes, the findings were classified as: *normal* (redness, slight oedema, or irritability or atrophy and smoothness), *mild* (redness, slight oedema, atrophy, smoothness and granularity of the mucosa), *moderate* (friable, painful, easily bleeding and pronounced oedematous, mucosa and presence of mucus), *severe* (pronounced and painful ulcerations diffuse or isolated, inflammation, abscesses and spontaneous bleeding).

The proctoscopic observations on 4,927 patients showed the following results: severe colitis in 181 (3.7%), moderate in 361 (7.3%), mild in 2,687 (54.5%) and apparently normal mucosa of the rectum in 1,698 (35.5%) of the patients. During the proctoscopic examination, a routine rectal biopsy was taken for histological examination and the positive number rose from 444 to 854 (17%). These cellular elements represent degenerated and atypical forms of E. histolyticae [3] (Table 1).

Table 1. *Colitis*

	Severe		Moderate		Mild		Normal Mucosa		Total	
	No.	%	No.	%	No.	%	No.	%		
Proctoscopically	181	3.7	361	7.3	2687	54.5	1698	34.5	4927	
Positive stool examination	21		41		247		135		444	(9%)
Positive rectal biopsy	41		76		468		269		854	(17.3%)

Furthermore, the percentage of correlation between the different types of colitis and the total number of 20,140 patients examined is 0.9% in cases of severe colitis; 1.8% of moderate; 13% of mild colitis and 8.4% in those with apparently normal mucosa (Table 2). The majority of the above 20,140 patients were selected because the First Medical Department is mostly concerned with patients suffering from gastrointestinal disturbances.

Table 2. *Percentage of colitis in 20 140 examined patients*

Severe		Moderate		Mild		Normal Mucosa	
No.	%	No.	%	No.	%	No.	%
181	0.9	361	1.8	2687	13	1698	8.4

It should be noted that the mucosa of the rectum in 4,746 out of 4,927 cases showed no ulcerations and that the proctoscopic findings varied from moderate or mild colitis to normal mucosa. These cases were diagnosed as chronic colitis clinically and at proctoscopy. However, 813 out of these 4,746 instances revealed E. histolytica in the rectal biopsy specimens.

The seasonal distribution of the proctoscopical findings in 4,927 cases is given in Table 3. According to this table, the exacerbation of colitis increased gradually from winter to summer; 882 cases appeared in the winter, 1124 in the spring; the number rose to 1414 in the summer and to 1507 in the fall. It should also be noted that similar findings were observed in cases with positive stool examination, as well as in those with positive rectal biopsy (Table 4), i. e., the positive cases increased from winter to summer and fall. However, we were amazed to see that the percentage of positive cases by rectal biopsy increased during the fall and winter, in relation to the number of colitis cases detected at proctoscopy. Table 5 presents 1124 cases of colitis occurring during the spring season with 186 (16.5%) positive cases at rectal biopsy and 1414 cases during the summer with 196 (14%) positive cases, while during the fall they reached 1507 with 296 (19%) and in the winter 882 instances of colitis with 178 (20%) positive at rectal biopsy.

Table 3. *Seasonal distribution of colitis*

Proctoscopic Findings	Winter	Spring	Summer	Fall	Total
Severe Colitis	29	34	57	61	181
Moderate Colitis	58	74	89	140	361
Mild Colitis	508	641	732	806	2687
Normal Mucosa	287	375	536	500	1698
Total	882	1124	1414	1507	4927

All the examined patients underwent anti-amoebic therapy only. The clinical symptoms had either disappeared or were considerably improved in about 77% of the cases with chronic amoebiasis, while in those with acute amoebic colitis the symptoms entirely disappeared in 60%.

Table 4. *Seasonal distribution of colitis*

	Winter	Spring	Summer	Fall	Total
Colitis	882	1124	1414	1507	4927
Positive Stool Examination	75	89	116	164	444
Positive Rectal Biopsy	178	186	196	294	854

Table 5. *Seasonal incidence and relation of rectal biopsy to colitis cases*

Season	Colitis	Positive Rectal Biopsy No.	%
Spring	1124	186	16.5
Summer	1414	196	14
Fall	1507	296	19
Winter	882	178	20

Discussion

The failure to establish new diagnostic procedures for amoebiasis is probably due to the fact that the majority of the physicians do not bear in mind the possibility of the existence of amoebiasis in their area. The second cause is their complacency that non-specific ulcerative colitis is much more common than acute and/or chronic amoebic colitis. This is the reason why the classical methods, such as fresh stool examination for parasites and proctosigmoidoscopy, are still used for diagnosing amoebiasis. The rectal biopsy as a diagnostic procedure for amoebiasis in such a large number of cases has been investigated by us for the first time. We have used it in all our patients suspected of suffering from chronic or acute amoebic colitis and chronic amoebic hepatitis. It has been found that the positive cases of Entamoeba histolytica rose from 444 to 854 (17.3%) out of 4,927 patients. The percentage of positive cases detected by rectal biopsy in the total number of 20,140 examined patients was found to be 4.4% and by stool examination 2.2% (Table 6). These percentage are similar to those reported by authors in other countries [5, 20, 22]. The above figures indicate that the method of rectal biopsy is more reliable than fresh stool examination for parasites.

Table 6. *Percentage of positive findings in 20 140 examined patients*

Cases	Positive Stool Examination No.	%	Positive Rectal Biopsy No.	%
20140	444	2.2	854	4.4

However, what impressed us was that 737 out of the 854 cases diagnosed by rectal biopsy were patients with mild colitis or apparently normal mucosa. This suggests that rectal biopsy should be performed not only on severe cases of colitis but also on those with findings of mild colitis, as well as with normal mucosa. E. histolytica may be found not only on the walls of the ulcers [16, 17, 18], but also in regions where no ulcers exist. The histological examination of the rectal specimens is of diagnostic value, especially in doubtful cases where rectoscopy is normal.

With regard to the seasonal distribution, we have noted that the number of colitis cases increased from winter to summer (Table 3). According to our statistics, the same thing happened in positive cases detected by stool examination, as well as by rectal biopsy (Table 4). It is remarkable, however, that the percentage of positive cases by rectal biopsy, which refers to the number of colitis patients, is increasing in reserve, i. e., it is 16.5% in the spring dropping to 14% in the summer, then rising to 19% in the fall and finally reaching 20% in the winter (Table 5). This may be due to the fact that the disease in the majority of the patients is in a quiescent phase during the winter, without any exacerbation and with negative or mild proctoscopic findings. The existence, of E. histolytica in the rectal mucosa is probable, however, and may be detected by the histological examination of the rectal specimen. Maybe the mild nature of the Greek climate, the individual reaction of the patient to the disease, the wide use and application of antibiotics, the peculiar virulence of the E. histolytica during the seasons and the nutritional factor of our country greatly modify the variety of clinical manifestations and the proctoscopic findings of the patients.

The simplicity of the method of rectal biopsy, the preservation of the slides for a long time, their availability for the identification of the disease, are the factors that make us consider the rectal biopsy of great value and reliability in diagnosing intestinal amoebiasis.

Summary

A total of 4,927 patients out of 20,140 with clinical manifestations suggesting inflammatory diseases of the colon were investigated. The factors of proctoscopical findings, the histological examination of the rectal biopsy and the fresh stool examination for E. histolytica were taken into consideration for the identification of the disease. Out of 4,927 patients examined by proctoscopy, 181 (3.7%) were found to have severe colitis; 361 (7.3%) moderate; 2,687 (54.5%) mild and 1,698 (34.5%) had apparently normal rectal mucosa. Rectal biopsy was obtained at the time of proctosigmoidoscopy on all these 4,927 patients. The histological examination of the rectal mucosa revealed E. histolytica in 854 (17.3%) cases, whereas, the stool examination detected only 444 (9%) positive cases. The importance of the discrepancy in the results obtained by the application of these two methods is emphasized in the present paper, and consequently the contribution of the rectal biopsy to the diagnosis of intestinal amoebiasis. The percentage correlation of amoebic colitis cases detected by rectal biopsy with the total number of 20,140 examined patients was 4.4% (854 cases), while by fresh stool examination 2.2% (444 cases). Furthermore, it is advisable that anti-amoebic therapy, emetine and chloroquine, should be applied preferably at the beginning, also on patients with apparent symptoms of non-specific ulcerative colitis. The factors that modify the seasonal distribution of amoebic colitis and the patient's response to anti-amoebic therapy are discussed.

The results obtained by using the rectal biopsy are compared with the results by stool examinations; the simplicity of the method of rectal biopsy and its great contribution to the diagnosis of intestinal amoebiasis, suggest that it is of great value as a diagnostic procedure.

It is advisable that the rectal biopsy be applied as a routine method, not only on patients suffering from acute severe colitis, but also on those with chronic colitis, as well as those with apparently normal rectal mucosa at proctosigmoidoscopy.

Bibliography

1. Bhathal, P. S., P. B. Brown, and W. B. Essex: A case of fulminating amoebiasis. Aust. N. Z. J. Surg. **33**, 3 (1964).
2. Bockus, H.: Gastroenterology 893–918: V1, Second Edition, Philadelphia: W. B. Saunders Co. (1964).
3. Candreviotis, N.: Chronische nicht-suppurative bzw. nicht-ulcerierende Amoebiase. Pathologic und Pathologische Anatomie **104**, 367 (1963).
4. Conway, Hugh, and Watt: Indigenous amoebic dysentery in Scotland: a case report. Scot. med. J. **6**, 520 (1961).
5. Craig, C. P.: The etiology, diagnosis and treatment of amoebiasis. Textbook. Baltimore: Williams and Wilkins Co. (1944).
6. Doxiadis, Th.: Über Amoebiase. Münch. med. Wschr. **104**, 14, 5, (1961).
7. — Chronic amoebic hepatitis. Brit. med. J. **1**, 6 (1962).
8. — Diagnostic procedures of chronic amoebiasis. J.A.M.A. **187**, March, 7, 1964.
9. —, and Z. Yiotsas: The importance of rectal biopsy in the diagnosis of amoebiasis. Amer. J. Gastro., March 1965.
10. —, and N. Candreviotis: Detection of Entamoeba histolytica by fluorescent microscopy. Brit. med. J. **1**, 6 (1962).
11. —, —, Z. Yiotsas, and F. Smyrniotis: Chronic amoebic hepatitis. Arch. intern. Med. **111**, 2, 219–225 (1963).
12. —, —, — Chronic amoebic hepatitis as a distinct clinico-pathological entity. 2nd World Congress of Gastro., Munich, 1962, 130–133, 1963.
13. —, L. Stergiou, Z. Yiotsas, and D. Tsitsanis: X-ray films in the diagnosis of chronic amoebic hepatitis. Brit. med. J. **1**, Feb. 8, 1964.
14. —, Z. Yiotsas, C. Velibassakis, and D. Christoforides: Significance of rectal biopsy for amoebiasis. Gastroenterology **44**, 6 (1963).
15. Kistner et al.: Rectoscopy and rectal biopsy in the diagnosis of colitis proctitis. Gastroenterology **103**, 47–59 (1965).
16. Juniper, K. jr.: Acute amoebic colitis. Amer. J. Med., **33**, 1962.
17. Juniper, K., V. M. Steel, and C. L. Chester: Rectal biopsy in the diagnosis of amoebic colitis. Sth. Med. J., 51, 1958.
18. McAllister, A. T.: Diagnosis of amoebic colitis on routine biopsies from rectum and sigmoid colon. Brit. med. J. **1**, 2 (1962).
19. Shaffer, J.: Discussion on Doxiadis' paper "Chronic Amoebic Hepatitis". Arch. intern. Med. **111**, 2, 219–225 (1963).
20. —, W. H. Shlaes, and R. A. Radke: Amoebiasis. p. 104. Springfield, Ill.: Charles C. Thomas 1965.
21. Sherlock, S.: Diseases of the liver and biliary system. 558. Springfield, Ill.: Charles C. Thomas, Publisher 1963.
22. Wilmot, A.: Clinical amoebiasis. Blackwell, Sci. Publications 1962.

Ulcerative or Amoebic Colitis?

Th. Doxiadis and Z. Yiotsas, Athens, Greece

"If hardly anyone seeks a disease, then few indeed will find it – especially if the disease in question is such as amoebic colitis." – Editor, *Lancet* (8th Dec. 1962)

The diagnosis of idiopathic ulcerative colitis is based on indirect clinical, radiological and proctoscopic findings. There is not one single symptom or test which could be considered as being specific. For this reason the question arises: are all patients who are diagnosed as cases of ulcerative colitis really suffering from this disease, or is another entity responsible for their illness in some of them? To answer this question we believe that the amoebic origin of such a colitis is generally ignored. If by chance the doctors do think of amoebic colitis they believe that the detection of E. histolytica in the stools is imperative for this diagnosis. Physicians forget that the negative result of the stool examination no more excludes amoebic colitis than the absence of Koch bacilli in the sputum of a patient excludes tuberculosis of the lung. This cannot be stressed strongly enough. The absence of parasites in the faeces appears to support the erroneous belief that the proctoscopic and roentgenological findings are specific for ulcerative colitis. One wonders if they are indeed specific and if their appearance is so different from ulcerations of amoebic origin. It is rarely realized that ulcerative colitis may produce sigmoidoscopic and roentgenological changes identical to those of amoebic colitis.

Clinical Material

We shall try to give the answer to the above questions from our experience with 181 patients with severe gastro-intestinal disorders such as diffuse abdominal pain, constipation alternating with diarrhoea containing mucus and blood, rectal bleeding and flatulence. At proctoscopy all were found to have diffuse inflammation and ulcerations of different size, profuse bleeding and a friable and bleeding mucosa. In addition, barium enema examination of the colon revealed loss of haustration, presence of ulcerations and marginal irregularity.

The above findings were identical with those of ulcerative colitis. All the patients were thoroughly examined to exclude other diseases.

In 62 out of our 181 patients, E. histolyticae were detected either in the rectal biopsy or [3, 10] in the fresh stool or after repeated smear examinations. These have been considered as cases of amoebic colitis simulating ulcerative colitis (Table 1).

Table 1. *Therapeutic results in 181 cases of ulcerative colitis*

Treatment		No. Cases	Results
Anti-Amoebic (1st)		181	90
Ulcerative Colitis	181 − 90 =	91	60
Anti-Amoebic (2nd)	181 − 90 − 60 =	31	18
Satisfactory Response to Anti-Amoebic Treatment: No. Cases: 90 + 18 =			108
Cases with Entamoeba histolyticae:			62
Cases without Entamoeba histolyticae:			46

As our intention was to differentiate between these two diseases, also ex-juvantibus, and although E. histolyticae were detected in these 62 cases only, anti-amoebic therapy with contact amoebicides, chloroquine diphosphate, enteric coated antibiotics, niridazone, and sometimes injections or oral administration of emetine hydrochloride, was given to all our 181 cases. A distinct clinical improvement was registered in 90 (50%) of them, including all the positive cases of E. histolyticae. In a certain number of these patients who had been treated some years previously, and in whom there has been no reappearance of the symptoms, it can be assumed that there has been a definite cure. The remaining 91 cases were subsequently submitted to the treatment of ulcerative colitis, (Cortizone, ACTH, Azulfidine, etc.). A satisfactory remission of the symptoms was obtained in 60 (33%) of these cases. There remained 31 patients, who failed to respond to the ulcerative colitis therapy and these were submitted to a second anti-amoebic therapy and 18 of them responded well with a satisfactory remission of their symptoms.

We present three cases which illustrate the result of this therapy. These patients had the typical picture of ulcerative colitis and responded well to anti-amoebic therapy.

Case Reports

Case 1: A 42-year-old man, who had been previously hospitalized on many occasions, was admitted to the Evangelismos Hospital in 1960, because of diffuse abdominal pain and bloody diarrhoea (15–20 stools daily). Temperature up to 38.5 C. Weight loss about 20 pounds. Proctoscopy up to 18 cm disclosed a granular, firable, oedematous mucosa with diffuse bleeding ulcerations. Rectal biopsy, culture and stool examinations for E. histolyticae were negative. Barium enema examination showed loss of haustration, small ulcerations and marginal irregularity (Fig. 1). Radiography showed an enlarged liver [4] reaching the iliac crest with bulging of the right dome. All other laboratory tests were negative; leucocytes within normal limits and sedimentation rate 30 mm in the first hour. The patient had been suffering from these complaints since 1951 and during his many periods of hospitalization he had been given ulcerative colitis therapy without any improvement. In our Department the patient was also given ulcerative colitis therapy for 30 days without successful results. The surgeons refused to carry out a colectomy, fearing that the patient would die during surgery. The patient's condition deteriorated; his bloody diarrhoea increased to 25 per day. The patient became emaciated and was placed in the isolation room. As this man was "in extremis" we decided that nothing would be lost if we tried a drastic measure, and we administered emetine. There was a dramatic improvement with a gradual subsiding of the symptoms. The blood ceased and the stools became semi-formed; the temperature dropped to normal and the patient slowly recovered. The therapy was continued with contact amoebicides. The patient gained 15 pounds in weight, made an excellent recovery and was discharged one month later. We have followed-up this case and to date he is well.

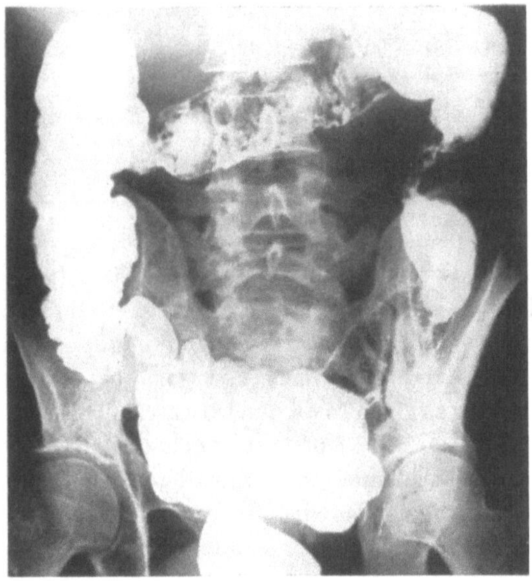

Fig. 1. Marginal irregularity, small ulcerations, no haustration

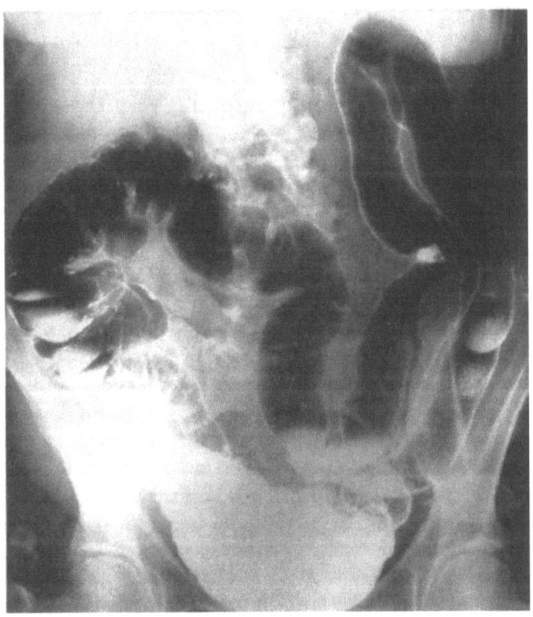

Fig. 2. Marginal irregularity, tiny ulcerations, no haustration

Case 2: In 1961 a 60-year-old woman, also repeatedly hospitalized in other hospitals, was admitted to the Evangelismos Hospital suffering from diffuse abdominal cramps, watery diarrhoea with mucus and occasional bloody stools of several years duration. Proctoscopy up to

15 cm revealed a granular, friable, oedematous and easily bleeding mucosa and pin-point ulcerations. Barium enema examination showed loss of haustration, tiny ulcerations and marginal irregularity (Fig. 2). Stool examination revealed E. histolytica. X-rays of the liver [4] showed an enlarged liver with the characteristics of amoebic hepatomegaly. Despite the similarity of the proctoscopic and roentgenological findings to those of ulcerative colitis, the detection of E. histolytica indicated that the patient was suffering from severe amoebic colitis. She was treated with emetine and contact amoebicides with a clinical and proctoscopic response. This patient also made a dramatic recovery and to date there has been no relapse.

Case 3: A 16-year-old girl was admitted with complaints of diffuse abdominal cramps, borborygmi, diarrhoea with blood and mucus, progressive anorexia and weight loss, from which she had been suffering periodically over the past four years. Repeated stool examinations for E. histolytica before and during several hospitalizations were negative. Prior to hospital admission, the patient had been treated repeatedly with corticosteroids by doctors who diagnosed her condition as ulcerative colitis. X-ray of the liver [4] showed the typical picture of amoebic hepatomegaly. This treatment produced no improvement. Physical examination revealed the patient to be well-developed but underweight with pale conjunctivae. The abdomen was slightly distended and the liver four finger-breadths below the right costal margin, soft in consistency and tender on palpation. The spleen was not palpable. Barium enema was negative. Proctosigmoidoscopy up to 17 cm showed edema, hyperemia and from pin-point up to 2 mm, bleedings ulcer of the mucosa. Rectal biopsy [3, 10] revealed a group of E. histolyticae between the intestinal glands and the muscularis mucosa; the cytoplasm was vacuolated and the nucleus small and deeply stained. The patient was given anti-amoebic therapy and both the clinical symptoms and the proctosigmoidoscopic findings vanished. A new rectal biopsy for amoebae was negative.

Discussion

In cases of chronic colitis with ulcerations and irregular stools, it is imperative, as in other diseases, to arrive at the exact diagnosis. Failure in response to the treatment is sometimes indicative of an inaccurate diagnosis. One of the diseases which is rarely taken into account, as an etiological factor, is amoebic infection, the more so as it very often masquerades as idiopathic ulcerative colitis. The literature is full of such cases.

McAllister [5] reported three cases in which typical proctoscopic and roentgenological findings of idiopathic ulcerative colitis and E. histolyticae were found. There was a rapid regression of the symptoms after specific anti-amoebic treatment.

Passarelli [7] reported that E. histolytica was found in 5 out of 18 patients whose conditions had been diagnosed as chronic idiopathic ulcerative colitis.

Paulley [8] reported that he had six cases in which amoebic colitis resembled ulcerative colitis.

Monaghan [6] found that great difficulty may be met with in those cases of chronic amoebic dysentery where diffuse ulcerative colitis develops as a result of secondary infection of the colonic mucus membrane.

Reed and Rochex [9] reported 7 out of 30 patients with idiopathic ulcerative colitis who had amoebiasis before developing ulcerative colitis.

Brown and Winkelman [1] reported 12 cases in which there were typical proctoscopic and roentgenological changes of ulcerative colitis. Those cases were diagnosed as cases of ulcerative colitis. The detection of E. histolytica in their faeces indicated the correct diagnosis. In one of the two cases of Winkelman, there was such a poor response to the treatment for ulcerative colitis that colectomy was planned for the next day. It was cancelled because E. histolytica was found.

We have met with some difficulty in differentiating between these two diseases in patients in our country. It should be noted that chronic idiopathic ulcerative colitis is encountered here, the same as in other parts of the world, and that there is not a particularly high incidence of amoebic infection in Greece in comparison with other mediterranean countries.

The numerous factors in the pathogenesis of ulcerative colitis, the unknown possible specific infections that may precipitate its appearance and the knowledge that the typical picture of the two diseases sometimes leads us astray, obliged us to liberate our minds from the notion that amoebic infection is imperatively based on the detection of amoebae in the stools and also that amoebiasis is a tropical disease.

The cited references considered all their cases to be suffering from ulcerative colitis and amoebic colitis was only diagnosed in those patients presenting E. histolytica in their stools. We think it is important to repeatedly question patients in an effort to discover if they have had any dysentery in the past, even many years ago, or if they have suffered from any amoebic infection previously; one often sees patients who refer to a past history of amoebiasis and later present pictures which are considered as being ulcerative colitis because of the absence of E. histolytica. In our series of patients, there were 46 cases that responded favourably to anti-amoebic therapy, although no E. histolyticae were detected in their stools or in the rectal biopsy. The fact that 18 cases responded only after a second therapeutic trial proves that there are cases which are initially resistant – a phenomenon which has always been found in all other chronic diseases due to "invaders", diseases such as syphilis, malaria, TB. The same is true when selecting the one or other anti-amoebic medication. Although injections of emetine hydrochloride have been rather abandoned during the last decades, or applied only in cases of amoebic abscess of the liver, we still consider it to be the best drug and it gives the best results when all other medicines have failed. This is also the case with the various chloroquine compounds, although they are only considered to be effective in amoebic involvement of the liver, and also with Niridazone.

In reality, we have here 108 cases, that is 60%, all of whom responded to anti-amoebic treatment in the end. If anti-amoebic therapy had not been administered because of the absence of E. histolytica, 46 cases would have been wrongly diagnosed with the resulting deterioration of their condition. Probably a number of them would have died or would have undergone colectomy (Table 1). Such cases are reported by BROWN and WINKELMANN. The same would have been the case if the therapy had been restricted to contact amoebicides.

Indirect findings suggesting the amoebic origin of the infection [2, 4] such as a typical radiologically detected hepatomegaly, with the characteristic bulging of the medium half of the right diaphragm and/or the elegant tongue-like elongation of the right lobe of the liver, a liver soft and tender on pressure or tap would support our decision to employ anti-amoebic therapy.

From the above-mentioned facts, it becomes clear that neither the roentgenological nor the proctoscopic picture of the colon should be considered as being highly specific for the diagnosis of ulcerative colitis. One has to be reminded that on the question of amoebiasis, the geographical, the climatic and the nutritional conditions, the virulence of the strains of E. histolytica, the individual resistance of the patient to the disease, as well as the wide and useless application of antibiotics could change the clinical and proctoscopical picture, at least in patients in Greece.

Chloroquine Diphosphate = Aralen
Hydroxychloroquine = Plaquenil
Niridazone = Ambilhar

Bibliography

1. Brown, C. H., and E. I. Winkelman: Amoebiasis and Ulcerative Colitis. Cleveland Clin. Quart. **32**, 61–67 (1965).
2. Doxiadis, Th.: Diagnostic Procedures of Chronic Amoebiasis. J.A.M.A. **187**, 7, (1964).
3. —, and Z. Yiotsas: The Importance of Rectal Biopsy in the Diagnosis of Amoebiasis. Amer. J. Gastro., March 1965.
4. —, L. Stergiou, Z. Yiotsas, and D. Tsitsanis: X-ray Films in the Diagnosis of Chronic Amoebic Hepatitis. Brit. med. J. **1**, 8 (1964).
5. McAllister, T. A.: Diagnosis of Amoebic Colitis on Routine Biopsies from Rectum and Sigmoid Colon. Brit. med. J. **1**, 362–4 (1962).
6. Monaghan, J. F.: Ulcerative Colitis. p. 549–614. In: Bockus, H. L. et al. Gastro-Enterology, **2**. Philadelphia: W. B. Saunders Co. 1944.
7. Passarelli, N.: Chronic Ulcerative Colitis: Introduction to its Study; Incidence in Brazil; General and Etiological Considerations based on 18 Cases. Arg. Brasil Med. **50**, 55–82 (1960).
8. Paulley, J. W.: Amoebic Liver Abscess in Great Britain. Brit. med. J. **1**, 462–3 (1961).
9. Reed, A. C., and F. L. Rochex: Treatment of Chronic Ulcerative Colitis Based on Thirty Cases. Northw. Med. **40**, 332–336 (1941).
10. Yiotsas, Z., and Th. Doxiadis: Evaluation of Rectal Biopsy in Colon Diseases. Amer. J. Proct. **17**, 1 (1966).

Diverticulitis, Diverticulosis Coli

P. Kyrle and R. Leitner, Vienna, Austria

We would like to report our experience with diverticulitis of the colon and first of all point out that we have found an increasing number of cases during the last 15 years in comparison to earlier years. Furthermore, severe complications were found at this time in a smaller number of cases than in our recent study. The greatly increased number of surgical cases is due to the improvement in the diagnosis, the increased life expectancy and an extended indication for operation. Our recent material is in no way selected.

Altogether we observed 318 cases. Of these 238 patients were treated conservatively and 80 patients underwent operation. Colon diverticuli and carcinoma were found in the same patient in only 9 cases.

Regarding the diagnosis, it is quite possible to make one in case of an "appendicitis sinistra", since the focus of the disease is localized in the sigmoid colon in 80% of the cases. But the diagnosis can also be difficult in this localization because of atypical symptoms. Not too rarely we have observed a congestion of the cecum with pain on the right and the differential diagnosis with appendicitis was difficult. Diagnostic problems may also arise because the symptomatology is masked by antibiotic treatment.

The diagnosis is supported and confirmed by irrigoscopy, but information about the extent of the diverticulitis is not always obtained, as some of the diverticuli may fail to fill with contrast medium. Diagnosis is easier if the diverticulitis is accompanied by a paradiverticulitis with a palpable tumor.

Hemorrhages can occur with all types and they are more frequent than generally assumed. We observed one in 15% of the cases.

Especially the complications of diverticulitis present an indication for operation. The frequency is shown in the following table.

Table 1. *Complications of diverticulitis*

1. Free perforation	7.2%
2. Permigration peritonitis + covered perforation + abscess	10.5%
3. Stenosis and ileus	7.9%
	25.6%

Beside these complications there is an absolute indication for operation, when clinical suspicion of carcinoma exists. With X-ray diagnosis a neoplasm can be difficult to detect between the diverticuli. Recently we resected a little carcinoma crater between the diverticuli of the sigmoid colon, which was covered by the surrounding mucosa in such a way, that it was almost invisible. It was not detected on the X-rays.

Furthermore the chronic cases of diverticulitis tumor, which do not respond to conservative treatment, and the chronic recurring cases are indications for operation.

Table 2. *Indication for operation*

	Number of cases	Cured	Deaths
1. Free perforation with diffuse peritonitis	24	10	14
2. Permigration peritonitis in acute diverticulitis, covered perforation and abscess formation	25	17	8
3. Stenosis and ileus	18	15	3
4. Diverticulitis chronica + carcinoma suspicion	10	10	—
5. Diverticulitis with rectovesical fistula	2	1	1
6. Liver abscess	1	—	1
Total	80	53	27

Of the 24 cases with free perforation only an emergency operation was possible in 14; all these patients died. However the 10 patients who survived the operation, were those in whom the colon could be brought to the front of the abdominal wall.

In the second group the situation was more favourable. Of the 25 cases 9 were resected and cured, in the remaining 16 a colostomy was performed 10 times. A large abscess was opened once and 5 times suture and drainage were performed. Out of these 16 patients, 8 died.

In *sigmoid stenosis with ileus*, we prefer transversostomy. In anatomically favourable cases it will sometimes be possible to bring the colon to the front of the abdominal wall.

10 cases of *chronic diverticulitis with suspicion of carcinoma* underwent operation. Here we did not lose any patients postoperatively.

In the case of a 62 year old (female) patient with a *rectovesical fistula*, the fistula was first excluded by a colostomy, then we waited for the reduction in the size of the fistulating, inflamed tumor and only after this did we perform the resection. The fistula was not seen either at the radical operation or on the specimen. After closing of the colostomy the patient is now healed.

In the individual case, the choice of operation naturally depends on the abdominal findings and on the general condition of the patient. The ideal treatment for perforation, abscess, fistula and stenosis is removal of the pathologically altered part of the bowel, either by resection or by bringing a part of the bowel to the front of the abdominal wall. Numerous authors like W. J. Mayo, H. Finsterer, and many others have suggested this and also performed it a long time ago.

In free perforation with diffuse stercoral peritonitis, a resection is frequently not possible because of the poor general condition, the advanced age and the severe peritonitis. The operation can also be technically quite difficult because of the fixation of the inflamed tumor, which M. Reifferscheid pointed out, too. In such cases one has to depend on smaller procedures like colostomy, suture, omentopexy, and drainage. We have had poor results with these emergency procedures, but in all those, who could tolerate a resection or colostomy resection, we had good results.

Table 3. *Applied operating methods*

	Number of cases		Mortality	
1. Drainage	4	45	4	25
2. Suture and drainage	3		1	
3. Colostomy	20		11	
4. Colostomy + drainage	7		5	
5. Colostomy + suture + drainage	4		2	
6. Other operations (adhesiolysis, invagination, probatoria)	7		2	
7. Resections				
a) one stage	8	35		2
b) two stages	9		1	
c) three stages	18		1	
		80		27

Out of 35 resections we lost two patients, one from an intercurrent cholangitis, the other from encephalomalacia due to hypertension.

Among the causes of death, peritonitis is found in the first place, but striking is the frequency of severe heart and vascular diseases which are mostly due to old age.

Regarding the primary one time resection it should be noted, that the sutures of the anastomosis are quite endangered by the inflammatory changes as well as by the macroscopically uncertain extent of the diverticulitis. The operation can also be quite time consuming, depending on the anatomical preparation in the inflamed tissue which is not unimportant in older patients with secondary diseases.

Therefore we usually perform a three stage operation (18 cases), starting with an axial colostomy followed by a resection under more favourable conditions 3 to 4 weeks later, when the tumor is already reduced in size. After a period of 2 to 3 months the colostomy closure is performed. X-ray examination is carried out to be certain that the anastomosis is adequate and that flushing of the anastomosis in both directions is possible.

The question of whether a repeat resection is necessary after perforation of a diverticle that was removed in an emergency procedure is difficult to answer. In our patient material, we frequently performed repeat resections and in almost all cases found a complete involution of inflammation and diverticulitis tumor. Depending on the transverse colostomy, stool retention in the diverticles could not occur and therefore the inflammation subsided. Similar considerations sometimes result from cases of chronic stenosing diverticulitis tumor, which has largely subsided after the first stage of the operation, namely the transversostomy.

There are indeed cases where normal stool passage is obtained without resection, by the decrease in inflammation alone. Yet this may be a transient state, later on a diverticulitis accompanied by all kinds of complications will occur and the repeat resection will now be necessary more than ever. Therefore it is not always easy to come to a decision for resection especially in dangerous cases.

Even if the average age of death is relatively high, one has to consider how to lower the mortality. Above all there is an indication for operation in cases of uncomplicated chronic-recurring diverticulitis if this disease causes severe pain in spite of conservative treatment. These patients, who do not yet show any acute complications, can be operated on with relatively small risk and good results, while procedures in cases of already existing complications are very risky. Therefore complications should be avoided, if possible.

Bibliography

Arfwidsson, S.: Pathogenesis of Mult. Diverticula of the Sigmoid Colon in Diverticula Disease. Acta Chir. Scand. Suppl. **342**. Stockholm 1964.

Bacon, H. E., Sherman: Amer. J. Surg. **80**, 3 (1950).

Berry, R. E. L.: Amer. J. Surg. **101**, 66 (1961).

Celio, A.: Helv. chir. Acta **19**, 93 (1952).

Cleméncon, G. H.: Schweiz. med. Wschr. **91**, 960 (1961).

Colcock, B. P., and R. E. Saas: Surg. Gynec. Obstet. **99**, 627 (1954).

Finsterer, H.: Die Chirurgie des Dickdarms. Wien-Düsseldorf: Wilhelm Maudrich 1952.

Gütgemann, A., H. F. Oester, u. H. W. Schreiber: Dtsch. med. Wschr. **82**, 553 (1957).

Mayo, W. J.: Brit. med. J. **2**, 574 (1929).

Merz, W. R.: Schweiz. med. Wschr. **86**, 1004 (1956).

Neff, G.: Ergebnisse der Chirurgie und Orthopädie **31**, 302 (1938).

Reifferscheid, M.: Darmchirurgie. Stuttgart: Georg Thieme Verlag 1962.

Ryan, P.: Brit. J. Surg. **45**, 611 (1957/58).

Waugh, J. M., and A. J. Walt: Surg. Gynec. Obstet. **104**, 690 (1957).

Wildegans, H.: Fortschr. Med. **75**, 177 (1957).

Winkelbauer, A.: Med. Klin. **52**, 1095 (1957).

Diverticular Disease of the Colon in Greece (Analysis of 350 cases)

EL. PHOCAS, N. MOSCOUTIS, D. GIANNACOS and C. NICOLAIDIS, Athens, Greece

Diverticular disease of the colon was believed to be a rare condition in Greece until 1963 (ZEUGOLATIS et al., 1963). However, our personal experience was contrary to this belief. This led us to study the barium enemas of 4,000 patients of various professions. All these patients presented gastrointestinal symptoms and had undergone laboratory tests and full radiological and endoscopic examination of the bowel.

Out of the 4,000 patients examined, 348 (8.7 per cent of the total) had diverticular disease of the colon of various localizations, extension and gravity. The age at the time of the first investigation ranged from 27 to 91 years. The distribution of age in decades is shown in Fig. 1. From this graphic representation it is evident that the greatest incidence of diverticular disease is found in the 6th and 7th decades. However, these findings do not necessarily correspond to the exact distribution, for pathological manifestations might have developed long before the patient's present admission.

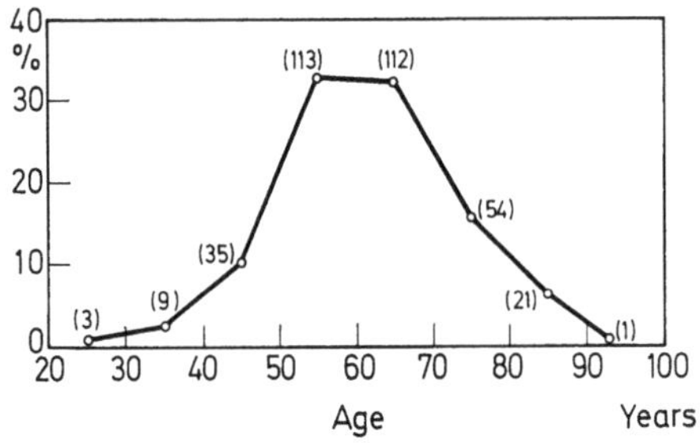

Fig. 1. The numbers in brackets represent the number of patients per decade

Special investigation of a total of 1436 barium enemas performed on children, from 0 to 15 years of age, showed only 2 cases of solitary diverticula. This data is not included in the present statistics, which concern only adult patients, in order to avoid erroneous interpretation of the results.

From the above number of 4,000 cases, 2,020 were men and 1,980 women. Out of these, 191 men and 157 women were found to have diverticular disease of the colon (9.4 per cent and 7.9 per cent respectively of the studied number of men and women) (Table 1).

Table 1. *Sex distribution in 4000 cases*

Sex	No. of Patients (barium enema)	No. of Cases	%
Male	2020	191	9.4
Female	1980	157	7.9
Total	4000	348	8.7

The regional distribution of the diverticula is shown in Table 2. According to this table, the incidence of localization of diverticula of the sigmoid and descending colon appears to be much higher than in the rest of the bowel. This is probably the reason why this condition often manifests itself with the clinical symptomatology of irritable colon.

Table 2. *Distribution of diverticula in relation to the region*

Region	No. of Cases	%
Caecum	5	1.4
Ascending Colon	12	3.5
Transverse	3	0.9
Descending and Sigmoid	107	30.8
Sigmoid	141	40.6
Diffuse	18	5.0
Disseminated	62	17.8
Total	348	100

As indicated in Table 3, about one half of our patients with diverticular disease consulted us for atypical abdominal symptoms and about one third for spastic colon phenomena. Patients with typical complications arising out of this condition were far below 1/5 of the studied cases.

Table 3. *Symptoms and complications*

	No. of Cases	%
Non-Typical Symptoms	164	47.1
Spastic Colon Phenomena	107	30.8
Acute Diverticulitis	44	12.8
Hemorrhage	23	6.6
Intestinal Obstruction	9	2.5
Perforation	1	0.2
Total	348	100

Discussion

The diagnosis of diverticular disease was essentially made by barium enema examination, except for 10 cases where it was established during exploratory laparotomy.

Nine of these cases refer to intestinal obstruction and one to a suspected ectopic gestation. No X-ray examination was possible because of the patient's critical condition at the time of admission. All nine case of intestinal obstruction were due to diverticulitis, whereas the suspected ectopic gestation proved to be a perforation of a sigmoid diverticulum.

It is to be emphasized that the limited number of post-operative diagnoses does not seem to correspond to reality, as all acute abdominal conditions are usually sent to surgical centers.

In nine other cases, X-ray examination failed to provide a correct diagnosis because of the difficulty in differentiating between diverticulitis and cancer associated with diverticula. The histological findings of the surgical specimen proved that the strictures were due to diverticulitis in five cases and to cancer in the other three (0.9 per cent of the studied 348 cases).

This low incidence of cancer, in accordance with other statistical data and in relation to the higher incidence of colonic cancer in the general population, supports the previously expressed opinion that diverticular disease is not considered to be a pre-cancerous condition.

In the presence of colonic diverticula, a thorough and careful examination of the patient complaining of abdominal symptoms is always necessary in order to exclude any other co-existing disease, when one remembers that a great number of cases of diverticulosis are asymptomatic or appear with atypical symptoms. In five of our cases, the main condition found was tuberculous adnexitis, high-grade malignancy of the female internal genitalia, thrombosis of the mesenteric artery, aneurysm of the abdominal aorta and urolithiasis.

On the other hand, diverticulitis was found to be the main lesion in patients treated unsuccessfully for other diseases until their admission to hospital. Amoebic colitis and appendicitis were the principle misleading diagnostic pitfalls. Twenty patients had undergone long-term and ineffective treatment for amoebiasis, which had been considered as the cause of their symptoms, and seventeen others were submitted to appendectomy with no positive results.

Hemorrhage is considered to be one of the principal complications or manifestations of diverticular disease. However, care must be taken not to miss other associated conditions of the bowel such as cancer, polyps or ulcerative colitis. Massive hemorrhage necessitating urgent blood transfusions was a rare complication on all encountered in eight out of the 348 cases studied (2.3%).

The association of diverticular disease with hiatus hernia and cholelithiasis, as described by Saint, was found in four cases (1.2 per cent of the studied 348 patients). This number could have been greater, as accepted in the literature (Boles and Jordan, 1958; De la Vega et al., 1964; Fagin, 1955; Palmer, 1955) if X-ray examinations of the stomach and cholecystographies had been performed of our patients.

The increasing incidence of diverticular disease in Greece, as well as in other countries, is undoubtedly due to the improvement of the radiological techniques.

Furthermore, our knowledge of specific radiological signs, such as the accordion pleating and the saw-tooth sign, (WILLIAMS, 1963), due to an abnormality of the circular muscle of the colon, (MORSON, 1963), helps us considerably in making the correct diagnosis.

In conclusion, we think that diverticular disease is among the prominent lesions of the colon. The knowledge of this fact will enable an early diagnosis which will limit complications and protect the patients from unnecessary long-term medical treatment, surgery or both.

Bibliography

BOLES, R. S. and S. M. JORDAN: Gastroenterology **35**, 579 (1958).
DE LA VEGA, J. M., J. N. GONZALES, A. PONCE DE LEON, and H. L. BOCKUS: Gastroenterology (1964).
FAGIN, I. D.: Amer. J. dig. Dis. **22**, 316 (1955).
MORSON, B. C.: Proc. Roy. Soc. Med. **56**, 798 (1963).
PALMER, E. D.: Amer. J. dig. Dis. **22**, 314 (1955).
WILLIAMS, I.: Brit. J. Radiol. **36**, 393 (1963).
ZEUGOLATIS, C., P. OECONOMOPOULOS, and G. THEODOROPOULOS: Proc. 1st Inter. Congr. for the Diseases of Colon and Rectum (1963).

VIII. Diagnostic Procedures

The Present State of Radiodiagnostics of the Colon and Rectum

J. ALTARAS and G. BARTH, Giessen, Germany

In patients with diseases of the colon, the diagnosis is based on the history, palpation, rectal examination and proctosigmoidoscopy, as well as on a radiological examination with a contrast medium. However, few patients have a radiological examination of the colon after referral from a specialist – surgeon or internist – and after a rectoscopy has been performed. Thus the radiologist is responsible for a major part of colon diagnosis, particularly of the early diagnosis of cancer of the colon. Furthermore the responsibility of the radiologist is very high for the following reason: only by X-rays is it possible to visualize the entire colon, whereas manual examination and endoscopy are limited to the rectum and sigmoid colon. Frequently changes in the large bowel are multicentric, frequently polyps or other precancerous lesions are combined with changes in the more proximal or more distal intestinal segments.

Which radiological colon examinations are customary at the present time and what information do they provide? *Visualization* of the colon by an *orally administered contrast medium* is always inadequate. Only too readily does this result in incorrect diagnosis. Since the contrast medium reaches the distal colon in a thickened condition, the shape of the large bowel cannot be assessed.

Irrigoscopy

Even though this method has the advantages of simple performance, quick survey, good visualization of large space-occupying lesions, diverticula and signs of displacement, it must be regarded as a crude examination method. Ileoscopy or a barium enema with evacuation radiograms should be abandoned since in the dense barium shadow intracavitary tumors are repeatedly submerged and covered over, whereas the evacuation radiogram in many cases cannot supplement the radiograms in which the colon is completely filled with contrast medium, since the small polypoid tumors in the folds of the mucosa of the collapsed intestine can frequently not be recognized.

The radiological symptoms of the prestenotic phase is the filling defect. It can be demonstrated best by completely filling the colon with contrast medium. However, if the filling defect is not very extensive, it is only visualized near the bowel wall. Thus its visualization depends on luck unless a large number of radiograms are obtained. Thus numerous early carcinomas are missed during radiological examination and are only diagnosed once the stenoses become visible radiologically.

The *hard-ray method* with a diluted contrast medium and penetration of the column of contrast medium by increasing the voltage, still reveals small tumors. The method is simple, rapid and inexpensive. On account of the decreased sharpness of the details and its limited resolution potential, it has not been widely accepted.

Optimum examination of the colon is only possible with the *method of double contrast* which first tightly fills all segments of the intestines with a positive contrast medium and which, subsequently allows the intestines to become an unfolded, transparent tube, by filling them with gas.

With the double contrast method the technique of radiological examination of the colon has been brought to a high level during the last decade (preparation of the patient, contrast medium, simplification of the administration of contrast medium and air), it has proved its efficacy and it has always been evaluated positively. However, the double contrast method is not just one possible method among many methods which may or may not be used as desired. It offers definite advantages which can be quite readily confirmed by statistical data on precancerous lesions and their demonstrable malignant changes. At present, this is the best method and it should no longer be withheld from the patient. However, even this method can fail if it is not carefully prepared, if the necessary instruments are lacking, if an inadequate number of radiograms are obtained, and unless really all segments of the bowel are screened by fluoroscopy. Obviously, particularly the caecum poses problems to many examiners so that they prefer to leave the caecum tightly filled with barium. The sigmoid colon is frequently difficult to evaluate because too many loops of bowel are superimposed on one another. In the caecum, the contrast medium can be uniformly distributed with a compressing balloon. In the rectosigmoid colon, free projections of the terminal bowel can be achieved by special views (Chassard-Lapinée, Altaras) (Fig. 1).

Pathological findings are frequently visualized directly in a plastic manner due to the high clarity of details and the decreased visualization of marginal contours at various depths.

In patients with extreme stenosis of the large bowel, the double contrast method may produce excellent results since, it permits air to enter the proximal segment even in cases with severe stenosis. Thus the entire length of the stenosis can be visualized.

Only the double contrast method permits visualization of the typical changes in the bowel wall and mucosa in patients with intestinal complications after gynecological radiotherapy. Small tumors, particularly of the posterior and anterior wall of the rectosigmoid colon are frequently missed at standard irrigoscopy. Double contrast visualization very beautifully and almost plastically demonstrates the villous adenoma (Fig. 2). Polyps of various sizes and shapes become covered with a thin layer of barium and show up as small protrusions into the intestinal lumen. Polyps are mainly found in the rectum and in the sigmoid colon.

Ulcerative colitis is a rewarding examination field for the double contrast method. Ulcerative colitis can also be demonstrated with other methods, but it is visualized particularly well by the double contrast method since in addition to an assessment of the ulcers according to the marginal contours it is also possible to

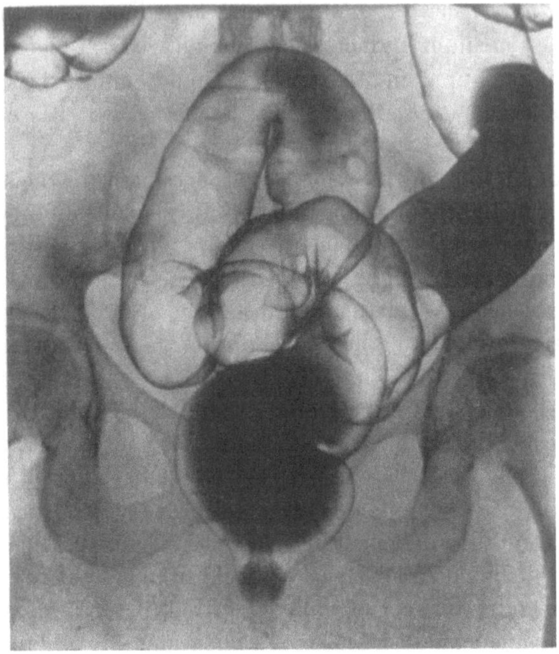

Fig. 1. Free projection of the whole recto-sigmoid

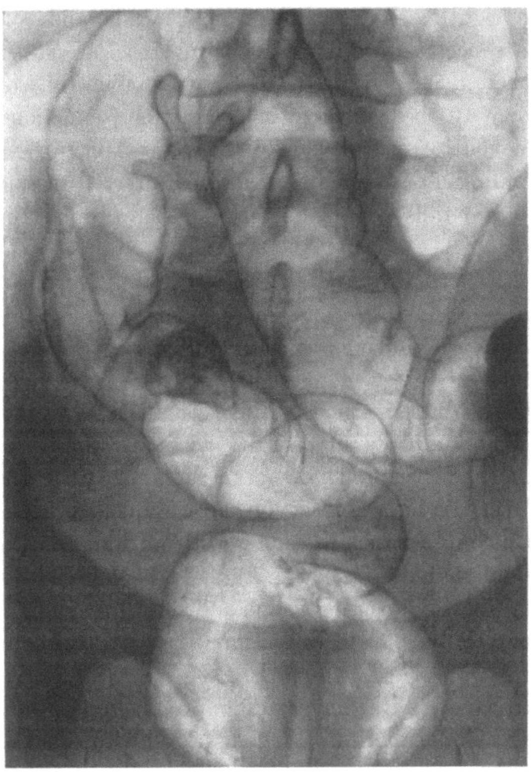

Fig. 2. Villoma of the sigmoid

examine the mucosa with a direct view and to obtain a comprehensive survey of the extent of the changes. According to our knowledge, the granular type of ulcerative colitis can only be demonstrated with the double contrast method.

Discussions or even opposing opinions as, for example contradictory statistics on the malignant change of various excrescences of the colon prior to operation or biopsy, as vehemently as they may be conducted are useless unless we offer our best radiogram of the colon to the clinician. Only then can he establish the objective basis for such studies and analyses.

With the double contrast method, a qualitatively good radiogram of the colon has been achieved. These advantages of the double contrast method by far outweigh the disadvantages which are a certain degree of technical difficulty, the "training" which is thus required, the somewhat higher cost, and the loss of functional analysis of the colon.

Bibliography

ALTARAS, J.: Röntgen-Bl. **8**, 376–380 (1968).
— Med. Welt **40/67**, 2392–2393 (1967).
ANDREN, L., S. FRIEBERG, and S. WELIN: Acta radiol. **45**, 201–208 (1955).
BELL, J. C.: Radiology **55**, 20–21 (1950).
CIMMINO, C. V.: Med. Radiogr. Photogr. **30**, 44 (1954).
ECKMANN, L.: Ciba Symposium **8**, 23 (1960).
ETTINGER, A., and M. ELKIN: Amer. J. Roentgenol. **72**, 199 (1954).
FIANDESIO, G., and G. D'AGATA: Minerva med. **49**, 3213 (1958).
GIANTURCO, C. A., and G. A. MILLER: Radiology **60**, 496–499 (1953).
LEVENE, G., and S. A. KAUFMAN: Amer. J. Roentgenol. **78**, 685 (1957).
MORETON, R. D.: Radiology **60**, 510 (1953).
—, E. M. COOPER, and E. F. FOEGELLE: Radiology **56**, 214 (1951).
PIQUET, E.: Arch. Mal. Appar. dig. **46**, 45 (1957).
ROBINSON, J. M.: Amer. J. Roentgenol. **77**, 700 (1957).
ROOT, J. C., and CH. M. GREENWALD: Radiology **63**, 241 (1954).
RÜTTIMANN, A.: Bibl. radiol. Vol. II, 77–95 (1961).
— Schweiz. med. Wschr. **90**, 807–812 (1960).
SWENSON, P. C., and R. WIGH: Amer. J. Roentgenol. **59**, 108 (1948).
WEBER, H. M.: Amer. J. Roentgenol. **25**, 577 (1931).
WELIN, S.: Fortschr. Röntgenstr. **82**, 341 (1955).
— Münch. med. Wschr. **100**, 1142 (1958).

Scintigraphy in the Preoperative Diagnosis of Rectal Carcinoma

K. KEMINGER, Vienna, Austria

In literature we find numerous investigations and observations on the lymphatic system (GERTEIS, KAINDL et al., BOBBIO et al., FUCHS et al., REIFFENSTUHL, WALLACE et al.).

KINMONTH (in 1952) was the first to describe a simple method for the direct introduction of a contrast medium into the lymphatic vessels of humans. Since then this method has been applied to the classification of various pathological problems.

However, direct lymphography has the essential disadvantage of involving technical difficulties, as well as the fact that this examination causes considerable discomfort to the patient. SCHEER and z. WINKEL have recently developed a method that may be described as scintigraphy of the lymphatic vessels.

We know from nuclear medicine that radioactive colloids with a particle size of 5–15 mμ injected subcutaneously are carried off primarily through the lymphatic system. Together with the intercellular fluids, the isotope is carried into the lymphatic vessels so that these vessels do not have to be exposed.

The *technique* is extremely simple. We used 100 microcuries of radioactive gold 198 together with 75 units of Permease and a 2% solution of Novocain. The injection was carried out intradigitally between the first and second toe, para-anally and into the region of the tumor. 3 to 4 hours later the scintigram was made.

A mechanical stress on the lymphatic system, such as occurs in direct lymphography because of the comparatively large amounts of contrast medium and the surgical exposure, does not occur in isotope lymphography. It is not expected that radiation damage would be incurred, since the amount of radiation involved is comparable to that of an X-ray. In addition, the use of an isotope probe will permit us to measure radioactivity and to search for lymph nodes even during the operation; thus, we are in a position not only to carry out comparative measurements before and during the operation but we may also check on the completeness of the removal of the lymph nodes intraoperatively. This fact constitutes an essential contribution to tumor surgery which, as we know, should realize the exstirpation of all lymph nodes far into healthy tissue.

In a normal scintigram performed after injection into the dorsum pedis, we visualize the inguinal, iliacal and para-aortal groups of lymph nodes. The isotope is carried into the general circulation by way of the thoracic duct and is finally stored in the liver. Unfortunately, in direct lymphography the lymph nodes which have been substituted by the carcinoma are not visualized.

Due to the way in which the lymph is drained, injection into the foot will not make the regional lymphatic area of the rectum – which runs in a cranial direction along the inferior mesenteric vein – visible; however, it will show groups of lymph nodes of the second and third order. Thus, an early diagnosis of metastases is not possible in rectal carcinoma. We have tried to visualize the regional lymphatic system by injecting the isotope close to the tumor. As was to be expected the regional areas were not visible after para-anal, subcutaneous or submucosal injection. Rather the isotope was drained off by way of the inguinal, iliacal and para-aortal areas, just as in the case of the injection into the dorsum pedis. However, if the test substance is injected into the vicinity of the tumor, the isotope is carried off by way of the regional grouping of lymph nodes in a para-aortal direction. Since the deposit is extensively stored in the minor pelvis, we get super positioning of the lymphatic areas on the record so that an evaluation of the areas we are interested in becomes impossible. However, with an improvement in the technique, it should become possible to examine the local lymphatic area.

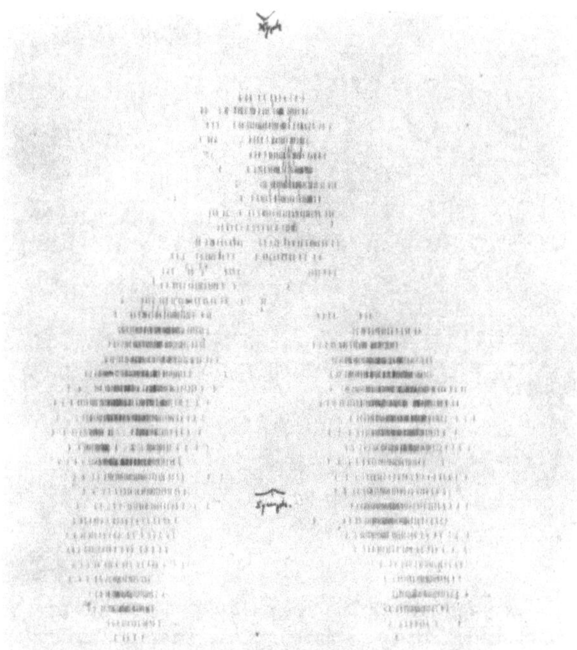

Fig. 1. Preoperative scintigraphy of the lymphatic system. Isolated disappearance into the iliacal group of lymph nodes by metastases

At present a subtile evaluation of pathological changes in the lymphatic nodes themselves, as in direct lymphography is not yet possible. We may, however, conclude that the lymphatic pathways have been blocked if the drainage of the isotope is impeded or prevented (Fig. 1, 2).

Conclusion

Isotope diagnosis undoubtedly constitutes a very interesting and virgin field of endeavour, one that is particularly attractive because of the simplicity of technique and the rapidity with which information is obtained. However, in rectal carcinoma the value of the information for preoperative diagnosis is slight, because:

1. preoperative evaluation of operability is not possible and
2. the disappearance of groups of lymph nodes may be caused by metastases, but does not in itself provide positive proof.

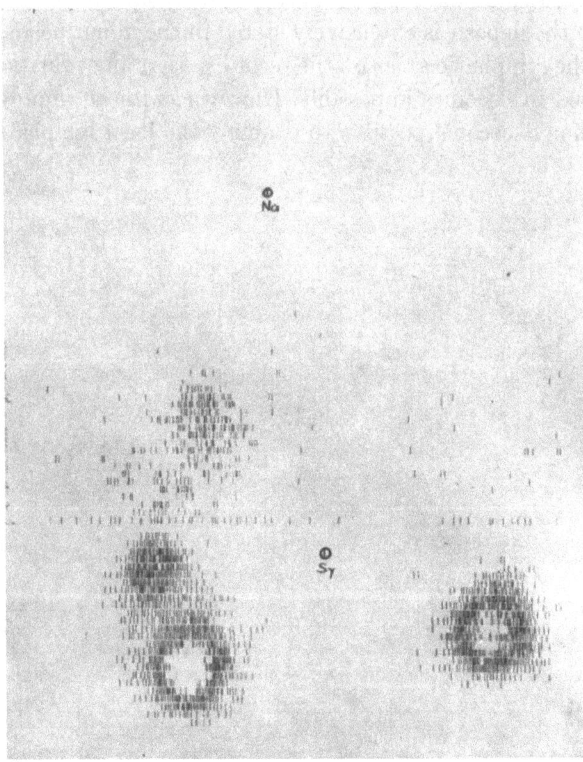

Fig. 2. Preoperative scintigraphy of the lymphatic system. Disappearance into the left iliacal groups of lymph nodes. Disappearance into the paraaortal groups of lymph nodes by metastases

Bibliography

BOBBIO, P., F. PELLEGRINO, et PERACCHIA: Ateneo parmense **32**, Suppl. 2, 3–24 (1961).
FUCHS, W., A. RÜTTIMANN, u. M. S. DEL BUONO: Schweiz. med. Wschr. **89**, 755 (1959).
—, —, — Fortschr. Röntgenstr. **92**, 608 (1960).
GERTEIS, W.: Lymphographie u. topographische Anatomie des Beckenlymphsystems. Stuttgart: F. Enke 1966.
HÖFER, R., u. K. KEMINGER: Paper, 7. Tagung österr. Ges. f. Chir. u. Traumat., Wien 1965.

KINMONTH, J. B.: Clin. Sci. **11**, 13 (1952).
REIFFENSTUHL, G.: Arch. Gynäkol. **187**, 375 (1956).
— Das Lymphsystem des weiblichen Genitale. München-Berlin-Wien: Urban u. Schwarzenberg 1957.
RÜTTIMANN, A., u. M. S. DEL BUONO: Fortschr. Röntgenstr. **97**, 552 (1962).
SCHEER, K. E., u. K. ZUM WINKEL: Nucl. Med. **1**, 219 (1960); **4**, 300 (1965).
SCHWAB, W.: Z. Laryng. Rhinol. **43**, 230 (1964).
ZUM WINKEL, K., u. D. v. KEISER: Fortschr. Röntgenstr. **100**, 90 (1964).
WALLACE, S., et al.: Radiology **76**, 179 (1961).

Scintigraphy of the Colon

A. D'ADDABBO, A. CAPURSO, M. BONOMO, G. GAETANI and M. RUBINO, Bari, Italy

Till now very little has been published on scintigraphy of the colon [1]. Therefore it is not yet possible to say whether this method is useful for diagnosing diseases of the large intestine. Only FRÈRE was able to detect tumours of the colon after intravenous injection of ^{131}I rose bengal. The rose bengal finds its way into the small intestine and into the colon together with the bile via the liver [2]. However, the link between the radio-iodine and the rose bengal molecule is relatively weak [3] and various intra- and extrahepatic factors can also influence the elimination of the dye in an indeterminable manner [4, 5]. Therefore, it is advisable to look for better test substances and a new examination technique, which meet the requirements of colon scintigraphy: low activity with corresponding radiation exposure; visualization of the colon without overlapping of the intestinal loops; uniform distribution of the radioactive material in the intestinal lumen; repeatability of the scintigram; visualization of structural lesions and filling defects; at the same time, the method should yield information on possible intestinal resorption disorders.

For the above reasons we have developed a new examination technique. Using radioactive enemas containing a dye, the large intestine can be visualized scintigraphically and at the same time disorders of intestinal permeablity recorded quantitatively. The new method was first carried out on rats, in which inflammatory and dystrophic alterations of the intestinal mucosa were produced artificially. Patients with ulcerative colitis and with colon cancer were examined during clinical testing of the method.

Methods

A) Clinical Studies

Twelve control persons, three patients with ulcerative colitis and two patients with tumour of the colon (1 tumour of the transverse and 1 of the descending colon) were examined. After a two-day preliminary treatment involving dietetic and evacuation measures [6] the enemas were carried out. Of three groups each comprising 4 control persons, the first was given ^{198}Au, the second ^{51}Cr albumin and the third ^{131}I oleic acid. All pathological cases received ^{198}Au. The liquid was introduced with a rubber canula (model W.R., Varay, Paris) and remained in the intestine for 1 hour; it consisted 1000 ml of lukewarm water containing 50 mg Evans' blue, 50 ml 2% Xylocaine (Astra, Södertälje, Sweden) and 300 μ Ci of the radioactive test substance.

The progress of the radioactive liquid through the colon was followed with the scintillation counter until the caecum was reached. The instilled volume varied with the different patients between 800 and 1200 ml. After 1, 3 and 24 hours the dye and radioactive concentrations in the plasma were determined. The activity in 3 ml serum was measured with a scintillation well crystal (EKCO) and the dye concentration with a spectrophotometer (DU, Beckman). The localization and distribution of the radioactivity were determined immediately after introduction of the enema and then after 12 and 24 hours with a scintigraph (Magnascanner III with 3″ × 2″ NaI(Tl) crystal, with a colour-recording system, a coarse collimator with 19 holes and 10 cm focal distance, Picker Nuclear) over the thorax and abdomen with the patient in prone, supine and lateral positions.

B) Animal Experiments

Two groups of 13 rats each were used; one served as the control group, the other was pretreated with a bactericide (hexadecyltrimethyl ammonium stearate, City Chemical Corp., New York). This chemical causes profound changes in the intestinal mucosa [7, 8]. Both groups were given enemas with 3 ml of a 3% Evans' blue solution under Nembutal anaesthesia. In all the animals the dye concentration in the serum was determined along with a few enzyme activities in the wall of the small intestine (succinic dehydrogenase [9], β-glucuronidase [10], aspecific esterase [11] and monoaminooxidase [12]).

Results

I. Scintigraphy of the Normal Colon

Immediately after administration of the enema, the shape and size of the colon can be easily visualized (Fig. 1, A, D). Of the test substances, ^{198}Au and ^{51}Cr albumin gave equivalent results. Visualization with ^{131}I oleic acid was poor since this was not distributed homogeneously and did not remain suspended in the enema liquid.

Taeniae and haustra cannot be visualized and the kinks at the hepatic and splenic flexures as well as in the sigmoid segment impair representation. We obtained the best scintigrams with the patient in the supine position. Independent of intra- or retroperitoneal dislocation of the different segments, a good picture was obtained of the ascending, transverse and descending colon. The form and length of the colon differed depending upon the degree of filling. 12 and 24 hours after the enema, Fig. 1, E, F show some accumulations of activity, due to the progressive evacuation of the radioactive material. After 36 hours there was hardly any radioactivity left in all cases.

II. Scintigraphy of the Pathological Colon

Scintigraphy carried out in the first hour, i. e. before the enema is discharged, exhibited in patients with colitis ulcerosa a nonuniform distribution of the radiogold colloid in the intestinal lumen (Fig. 1, B). Also there was diffuse localization of the radioactivity in the abdomen and, surprisingly, an accumulation of activity in the liver.

Radioactivity disappeared from the colon sooner than with the controls; after 12 hours the colon could not be outlined scintigraphycally. In contrast, the radioactivity in the abdomen and in the liver could still be detected after 48 hours. In all cases no radioactivity could be shown above the lungs even with repeated measurements.

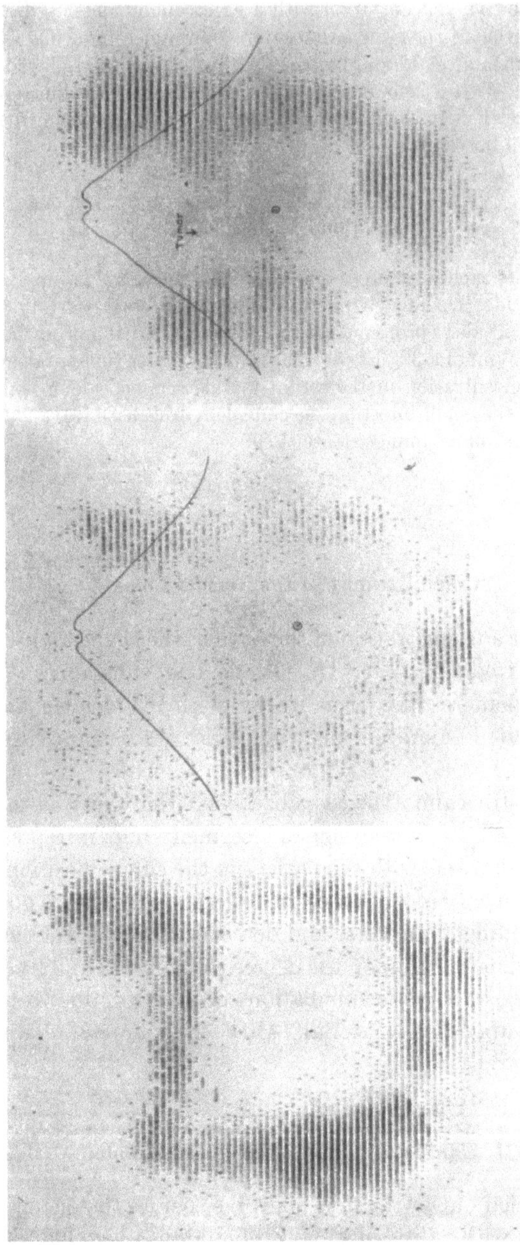

C B A

Fig. 1

In the two patients with a constricting tumour of the colon the filling defect corresponded to the localization of the tumour determind roentgenologically beforehand (Fig. 1, C). This incomplete filling zone differs from spastic filling defects in that with spasms the defect is more clearly delineated and changes shape and location in the course of a further scintigram. With tumours, the area devoid of radioactivity does not change and has blurred contours; here no accumulation of activity was found in the liver.

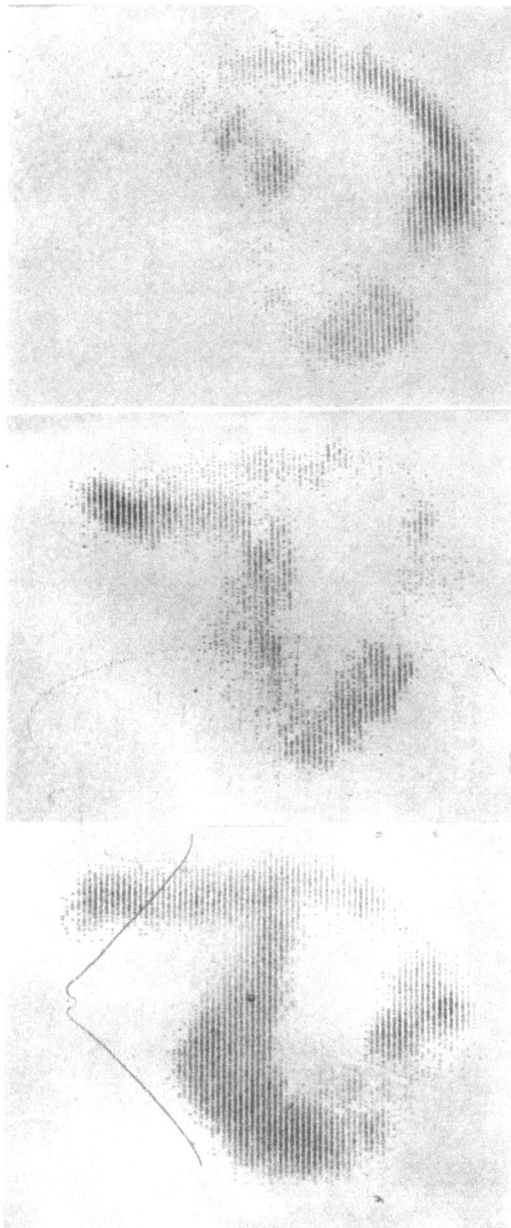

D E F

Fig. 1. Scintigraphy of the colon after enema with radiogold colloid (^{198}Au) with control persons (A, D, E, F) and pathological cases (B, C), 1 hour (A, B, C, D), 12 hours (E) and 24 hours (F) after administration of the enema

III. Resorption Studies

In the case of the rats treated with hexadecyltrimethyl ammonium stearate, about 1% of the administered dye passed into the plasma during the first hour after the start of the experiment. In contrast, in the control animals only slight traces of the dye could be detected in the plasma. The bactericide hexadecyltrimethyl ammonium stearate causes profound changes in the intestinal mucosa

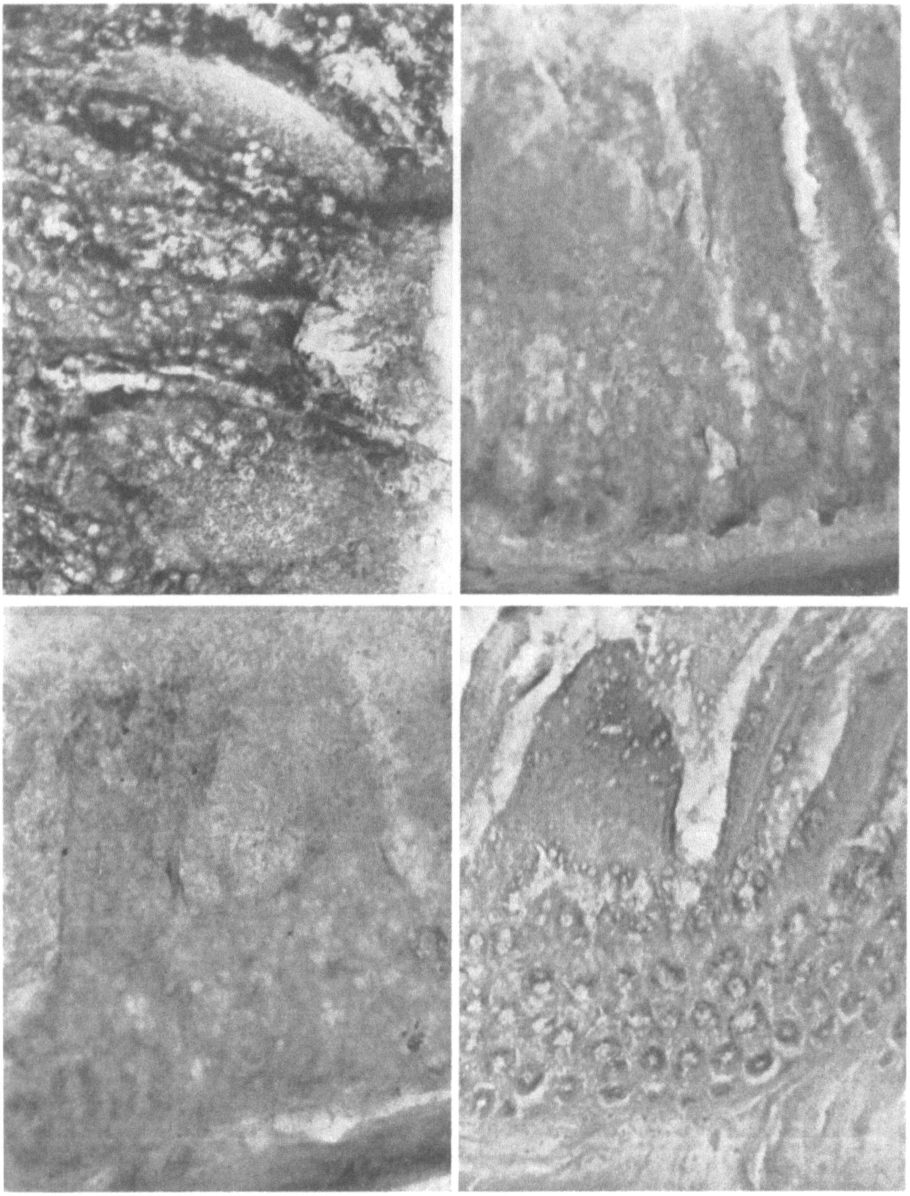

Fig. 2. Enzyme activity in the small intestine of rats after treatment with 0.6 g hexadecyltrimethyl ammonium stearate per kg weight. A) Succinic dehydrogenase activity (blue-black): hardly affected despite severe histological changes of the intestinal mucosa. B) Aspecific esterase activity (brown): preserved only in a few crypts and villi. C) Monoaminooxidase activity (blue): can only be found isolated and irregularly in the tips of the villi. D) β-Glucuronidase activity (brown): well preserved in the epithelium of the crypts and villi

[7, 8], which range from cell infiltration of the stroma to complete loss of the epithelium with ulcerations. A few enzyme activities were determined in segments of the small intestine. The β-glucuronidase and succinic dehydrogenase were

normal, whilst the alkaline phosphatase, the monoaminooxidase and the non-specific esterase were strongly reduced (Fig. 2). In the case of the patients with ulcerative colitis the Evans' blue resorption reached values between 20 and 30% of the administered dose during the first hour after the enema already. In the case of the controls and the patients with tumour of the colon this value was less than 1% of the dose.

Discussion

Scintigraphy of the colon after enema with radioactive test substances yields information on intestinal lesions and on the function of the colon. Consequently, the scintigram is a valuable adjunct to the radiograph. In the case of patients with ulcerative colitis, ^{198}Au radioactivity is not restricted to the colon, but within a short time appears diffusely in the abdomen and concentrated in the liver. Presumably the radiogold colloid is transported into the regional lymph nodes after fixation by the macrophages of the damaged intestinal wall. Our assumption, that the radioactivity would accumulate in the ulcerations of the intestinal mucosa was wrong. In order to locate ulcerations it would probably be necessary to choose other radioactive test substances and other enema retention times. The radioactivity accumulated in the liver during the first hour might is probably due to the accelerated passage of the colloid from the intestinal lumen into the blood. However, the plasma radioactivity could not be measured since the colloid has a half-life of only three minutes and disappears quickly from the blood stream [13]. It is improbable that the gold colloid is transported via the lymph channels since above the thorax, no radioactivity was found in the hilus region.

The results of resorption studies with Evans' blue in rats with experimental enteropathy speak in favour of an immediate passage of substances from the colon into the blood. The enzymatic changes in the small intestine of these animals agree well with the histological findings indicating profound alterations in the intestinal mucosa. The fact that in these animals and in patients with ulcerative colitis large quantities of Evans' blue passed into the blood despite the malabsorption syndrome, points to considerable permeability disorders of the colon.

Appendix

Radiation exposure

Assuming that 1 litre of ^{198}Au colloid solution is distributed homogeneously throughout a colon measuring 1.20 m in length, the total β-dose at the *surface of the mucosa* is $D_{\beta}\infty = 9$ rd. If the effective half-life of the enema should amount to 10 hours under extremely unfavourable conditions (incomplete evacuation after one hour, pathological obstipation), a radiation exposure of about 1½ rd must be assumed. However, since in reality most of the enema (presumably 80–90%) is evacuated immediately after scintigraphy, i. e. during the first hour, the effective dose can be estimated at less than 0.5–1.0 rd approximately. This applies even when during the first hour about half of the enema water is selectively resorbed so that the radioactive concentration doubles up to the moment of evacuation.

Since the *gonadal dose* arises exclusively from y-radiation, it amounts to about 50 mrd for woman and 75 mrd for men with a half-life of 10 hours; the true dose (again 80–90%

evacuation within one hour) is about 50–100 mrd for women and for men about 25–50 mrd. At the surface of the abdomen the dose can be assumed to be about 75 mrd (10 hours) and 25–50 mrd (about 1 hour).

Bibliography

1. FRÈRE, A. G.: Les isotopes a l'usage du médecin practicien. Bruxelles: Editions Arscia 1966.
2. NORDYKE, R. A., and W. H. BLAHD: The differential diagnosis of biliary tract obstruction with radioactive rose bengal. J. Lab. clin. Med. **51**, 565 (1958).
3. COHEN, Y., J. WEPIERRE, G. ENGELMANN, et O. COSTEROUSSE: Etude pharmacologique de deux composés iodés (rose bengale et diodone) utilisés dans l'exploration fonctionelle humaine. In: „Radioaktive Isotope in Klinik und Forschung" **5**, 405 (1962). München: Urban und Schwarzenberg 1963.
4. BENNHOLD, H.: Über die Bedeutung der Serumeiweißkörper für Transportvorgänge im lebenden Organismus. Pharmakokinetik u. Arzneimitteldosierung, Kolloquium, Borstel 1962. Antibiot. et Chemother. Vol. **12**, 1–28. Basel/New York: Karger 1964.
5. KAWAGUCHI, M., J. E. BERK, and A. R. SOBLE: Studies with ^{131}I-labelled rose bengal. II. Clinical evaluation of a modified technic for differential diagnosis of jaundice. Amer. J. dig. Dis. **7**, 300 (1962).
6. HETTLER, M.: Die Vorbereitung des Dünn- und Dickdarmes für diagnostische und therapeutische Maßnahmen. Dtsch. med. Wschr. **86**, 2120 (1961).
7. NISSIM, J. A.: Reduction of intestinal absorption by a synthetic chemical. Nature **185**, 222 (1960).
8. D'ADDABBO, F. DAMMACCO, A. CAPURSO u. V. DAMATO: Klinische und tierexperimentelle Studien zur Resorption von Farbstoff und kolloidalem Radiogold. Vortrag beim internationalen Symposium „Bedeutung der Eiweißvehikelfunktion", Tübingen, 13.–14. September 1968.
9. NACHLAS, M. M., K. C. TSOU, E. DE SOUZA, C. S. CHANG, and A. M. SELIGMAN: Cytochemical demonstration of succinic dehydrogenase by the use of a new p-nitrophenyl substituted ditetrazole. J. Histochem. Cytochem. **5**, 420 (1957).
10. SELIGMAN, A. M., K. C. TSOU, S. H. RUTENBURG, and R. B. COHEN: Histochemical demonstration of beta-D-glucuronidase with a synthetic substrate. J. Histochem. Cytochem. **2**, 209 (1954).
11. PEARSE, A. G. E.: Histochemistry. London: Churchill Publ. 1960.
12. GLENNER, G. G., H. J. BURTNER, and G. W. BROWN: The histochemical demonstration of monoamine oxidase activity by tetrazolium salts. J. Histochem. Cytochem. **5**, 591 (1957).
13. HÖFER, R., A. NEUMAYR, O. PARZER u. H. VETTER: Die Bestimmung der Leberdurchblutung beim Menschen. Klin. Wschr. **33**, 792 (1955).

Angiographic and Microangiographic Patterns of Colonic Lesions

P. PELTOKALLIO and T. V. KALIMA, Helsinki, Finland

In most diseases of the colon, the proper diagnosis can be made by the usual methods, but there are still many pathological conditions where the exact preoperative diagnosis is difficult or impossible to make. It can also be difficult to estimate the stage or progression of the disease.

Arteriography, although not yet in routine use, may be a valuable method in the differentiation of colonic diseases in the future. This is why we have tried to get more information on the vascular changes in different pathological conditions in the colon or ileum by making angiograms of specimens removed during operations. We have sought to find vascular patterns of the different diseases.

During the operation, we have placed a catheter into a large mesenteric artery and through it we have perfused the preparation with a radio-opaque contrast solution for 4 to 6 hours using a perfusion pressure of 130 to 150 mm of mercury. After perfusion, X-ray pictures were taken on industrial, fine-grain films. Before exposing the films, we blew air into the lumen of the gut. This made it easier to see the vessels or to estimate the thickness of the wall and to detect intraluminal changes.

We performed angiographies in 8 cases of colitis ulcerosa, 15 cases of cancer of the colon, one case of ileal cancer and two cases of regional enteritis.

In ulcerative colitis, the vascularity is increased in comparison with the normal colon (Fig. 1). The vessels are well arranged and nearly all parallel. Often the vessels are more tortuous than normal and exhibit marked right-angle branching from the arches of the mesenteric arteries. The diameter of the smaller arteries is nearly uniform (Fig. 3a).

From the vascular pattern we can determine if the colitic changes are slight (when the vascularity is only slightly increased) or if the changes are moderate in that the hypervascularity is very marked. When the colitic changes are very pronounced, blotchy hypervascularity can be seen together with large avascular spaces and so-called pseudopolyposis. The avascular spots correspond to necrosis and ulcerations in the mucosa.

In Crohn's disease or regional enteritis, it is possible to find a circumscribed tumor and often also pathological changes in the ileum. Hypervascularity is also found here, but the vessels are smaller and not arranged like they are in ulcerative colitis. There is no variation in the diameter of the vessels (Fig. 2b).

In colonic cancers, the vascularity can be much increased, but large avascular regions are also seen at the same time corresponding to the necrotic parts of the tumor. The vessels are in chaotic arrangement and vary in diameter; some are small and narrow, some very wide and short (Fig. 3b). Larger vessels are often displaced and can form a kind of arch around the tumor. The tumor, its edges and the affected lumen are often clearly visible. The size and shape of the tumor is also often easy to see. Narrowing of the lumen is obvious, and the venous system is also distinctly seen; it may reveal a number of open arteriovenous shunts.

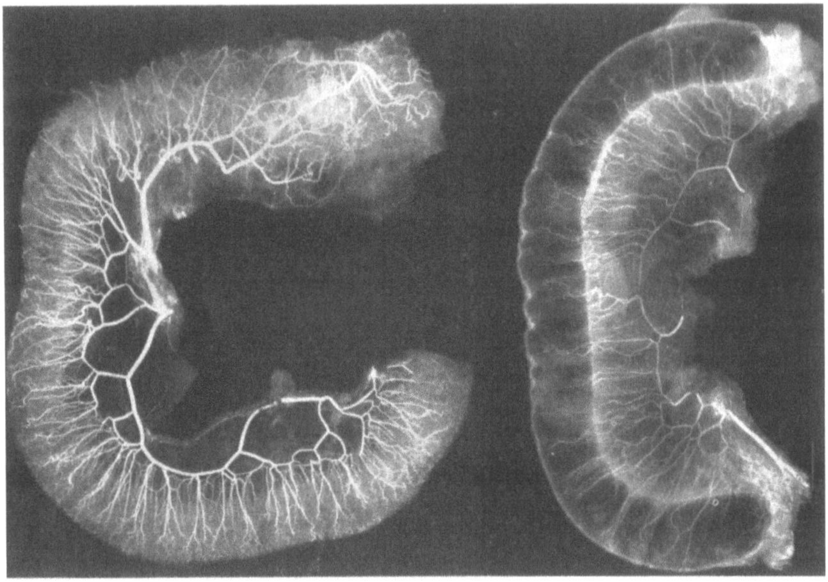

a b

Fig. 1. a) Angiography of ulcerative colitis. The vascularity is much increased and the vessels branching at right angle from the mesenteric arteries are numerous. b) Normal colon and its vessels

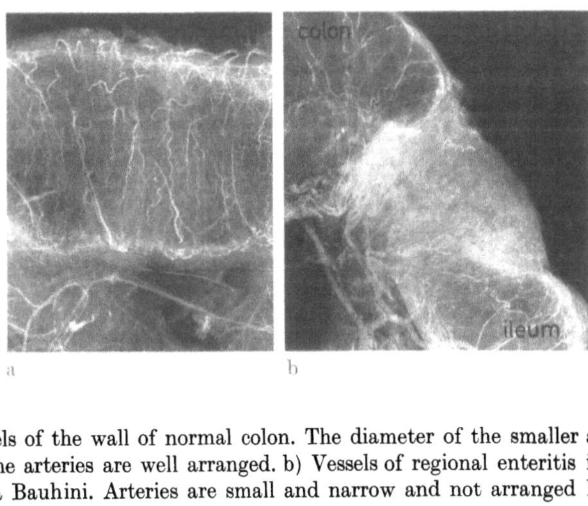

a b

Fig. 2. a) Vessels of the wall of normal colon. The diameter of the smaller arteries is nearly uniform and the arteries are well arranged. b) Vessels of regional enteritis in the region of Valvula Bauhini. Arteries are small and narrow and not arranged like in a)

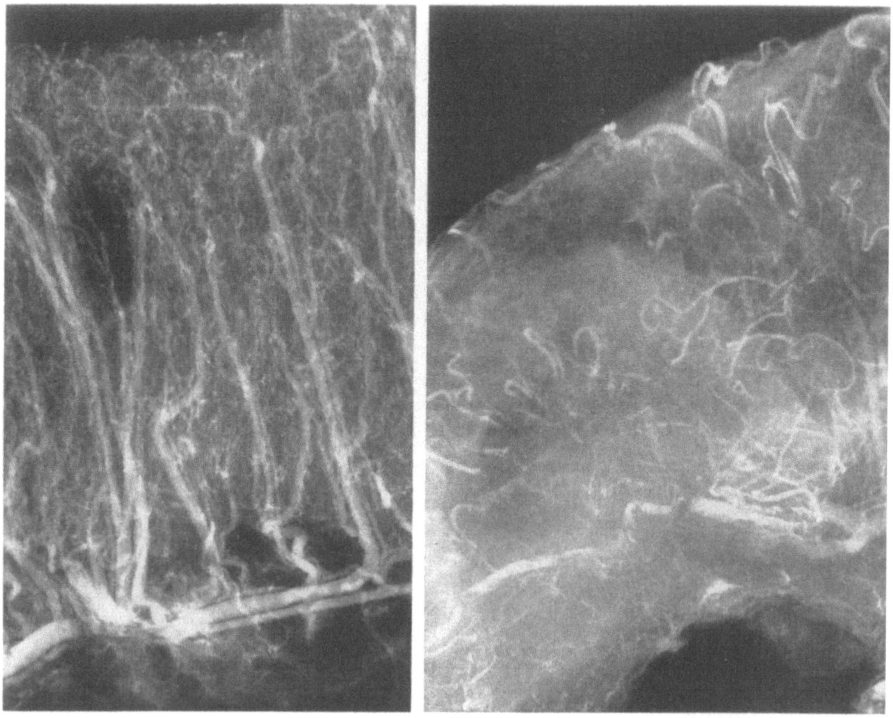

a b

Fig. 3. a) Vessels of ulcerative colitis in detail. The small arteries are tortuous and very numerous but they are in parallel order. b) A detail picture of colonic cancer. The vessels are in full chaos, vary in diameter and in length. Small avascular regions and moderate extravasation are also seen

The vascular pattern is quite typical and possible to identify in some colonic lesions and angiography gives additional information about the shape and size, severity or state of spread of the processes in the gut. Selective colon angiography in vivo is not good enough yet to present all these changes, but we hope for progress in this respect.

Bibliography

Bosniak, M. A., L. F. Williams, jr., C. A. Hasiotis, J. J. Byrne, and J. H. Shapiro: In Vivo Magnification Arteriography of the Bowel Wall. Amer. J. Surg. **114**, 359–362 (1967).

Brame, F.: Mesenteric Angiography in Regional Enterocolitis. Radiology **87**, 1037–1042 (1966).

McAlister, W. H., A. R. Margulis, P. Heinbecker, and H. Spjut: Arteriography and Microangiography of Gastric and Colonic Lesions. Radiology **79**, 769–781 (1962).

Spjut, H. J., and A. R. Margulis: Micro-Angiographic Patterns of Chronic Ulcerative Colitis. Dis. Colon Rect. **8**, 215–221 (1965).

Color Photography of the Colon with a Gastrocamera

P. PELTOKALLIO, Y. PERTTALA and U. SVINHUFVUD, Helsinki, Finland

In the diagnosis of diseases of the colon, the limitation of sigmoidoscopy is that even under favorable conditions, it permits the examination over a distance of 30 to 35 cm at the most. Roentgenography has a key position in the diagnosis beyond the sigmoidoscope range. Sometimes, however, even with roentgenography, it is difficult to detect inflammations and early changes caused by carcinoma. Even a distinct finding such as a stricture may pose great differential diagnostic problems. As a possible diagnostic aid in diseases of the colon, we have experimented with photographing the large intestine with a gastrocamera.

The camera part measured 1×3 cm and contained a lens, a flash attachment, a film holder and an air valve. The camera could be inclined 35° in either direction and turned 360°. The maximal sharpness is 2.5–4.0 cm, but the focussing range was so deep that adequate pictures could be obtained up to 10 cm. Photographs from less than 2 cm lacked detail and showed colour changes. The field of vision of the camera was 80°. Air was blown into the large intestine by a rubber ball through the holes in the camera part. The colour film used was 5 mm wide and consisted of 32 exposures.

At the beginning of the examination the camera part, the vinyl tube and the anal region were well lubricated to ease the passage of the gastrocamera. The camera lens was smeared with silicone oil to prevent dimming. Then the patients were prepared for photography in the same way as for roentgenography of the large intestine. In some cases, spasmolytics were given to prevent spasms. The camera was moved to the desired site and followed on a TV camera.

In most cases, even sharp sigmoid bends could be negotiated by turning the patient, blowing air, and bending the camera part. TV fluoroscopy showed a notch in the camera part to indicate the direction from which the photograph was being taken. Numerous exposures were taken from different directions of the site of a lesion that was roentgenologically suspect. The camera part inclined at different angles, gave a suitable focal distance.

We used a gastrocamera to photograph the colons of 41 patients. They all had roentgenologically demonstrated changes in the left half of the colon. The roentgenologic examination of eleven patients gave rise to suspicion of carcinoma, sixteen had a stricture caused by spasm or a benign process, seven had ulcerative colitis, six had polyps and one had familial polyposis. Photography failed in seven cases because the necessary focal distance of 2.5 cm, from the object could not be achieved. In three patients it was impossible to get the gastrocamera past the sharp bends in the sigmoid. It must be emphasized that there was not a single failure due to obstruction of the intestinal contents. No complications occured. Highly successful exposures were made in 29 cases. We have noticed that gastrocamera photographs of tumours are very good. In figure 1 gastrocamera photographs taken 45 cm from the anus revealed a tumour. Proximal to it a polyp and small infiltration nodes were seen. Polyps can also be seen very distinctly; figure 1 was taken in a patient with familial polyposis. On the photographs, it is possible to decide whether the polyp is benign or malignant. Changes of colitis ulcerosa can also be easily found and followed. The most aboral tumour photographed was in the upper part of the descending colon. In some cases the gastrocamera could be moved as far as the splenic flexure.

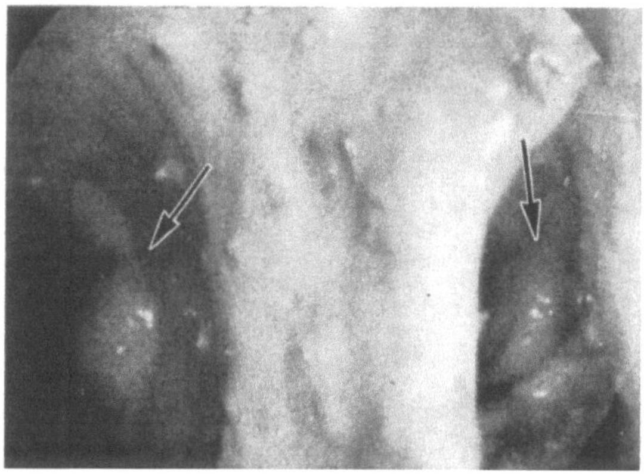

Fig. 1. Color photography taken 45 cm from anus. On the left side a polyp and on the right side a carcinoma

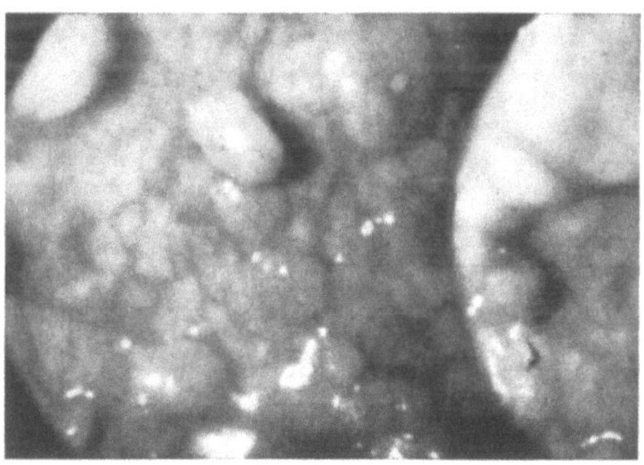

Fig. 2. Gastrocamera photograph of familial polyposis

The results of our experiments show that it is possible to photograph the colon with an apparatus of gastrocamera type. However, the gastrocamera is not the best possible apparatus for photographing the large intestine. The camera aperture should be at the front of the camera and not at the side for photographing the colon. This would make it easier to achieve the minimum focal distance to the object. On the other hand, it is an advantage in taking pictures along the length of the lumen, for the accuracy of the camera extends for a focal distance of 10 cm. Another drawback is that the camera part can be inclined no more than 35° in either direction, and even then at a sharp angle. A more suitable camera for photography of the colon would be one in which the camera part is inclined 100° in either direction, bending slightly over a distance of 10 cm.

We believe that it is technically possible to develop an apparatus – a colon camera, that would be more suitable for photographing the large bowel than a gastrocamera. This would be of greater diagnostic aid in diseases of the colon.

A Study of the Resorption of ^{131}INa from the Normal and Pathological Rectum

AD. KERESZTESSY K., A. PUPP, Z. PAPAI, E. BANCU, AM. KERESZTESSY K., T. GROZESCU and N. COMAN, Tirgu-Mures, Roumania

We have studied the resorption of ^{131}INa from the rectum on a group of patients with different diseases of the rectocolon and on normal individuals. We were led by the assumption that measurements of rectally administered isotopes, effected in time at the level of the liver, would give us information concerning the absorption of these substances from the rectum.

In the literature, we did not find any data on the resorption of isotopes from either the healthy or the pathological rectum. Authors in our country such as N. HORTOLOMEI et al., FL. MANDACHE et al., POPESCU-URLUENI, P. SIMICI et al., D. GAVRILIU as well as others have studied the problems of function and motility of the rectum.

Methods and Materials

The patients underwent clinical and laboratory controls, using the usual laboratory methods, especially in regard to hepatic functions. Those with hepatic disorders were excluded from our material.

After a preliminary evacuatory enema, a quantity of 2 ml of physiological NaCl solution, containing about 10 to 16 μCi of ^{131}INa was injected into the rectal ampulla.

The measurements were carried out with an Orion ennumerator, type 1872, coupled to a scintillometer at the level of the liver by contact. Duration 25 min.

The measured activities were expressed by impulse/minute and illustrated graphically according to the respective group of patients.

The examinations had been performed on different groups of patients as follows:

I. Normal individuals.

II. Colitis, haemorrhoids, fistula, etc.

III. Carcinoma of the rectum, carcinoma of the colon.

IV. State after rectal resection.

Results

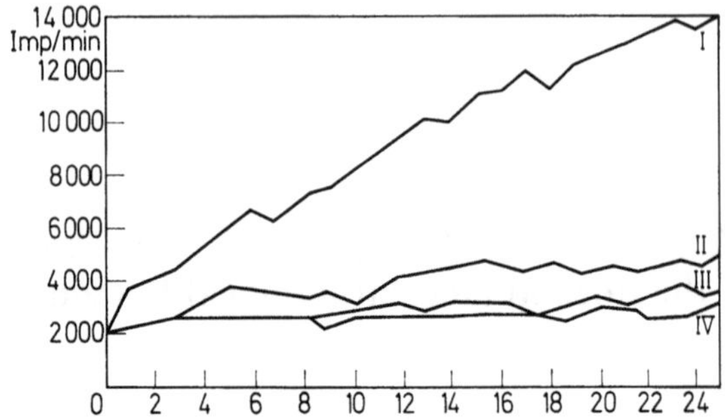

Fig. 1

Group 1. Normal (10 cases)

The fluid to be absorbed is ascending; the initial activity is doubled after 3 to 7 min and the values increase from 3 to 4 times after 20 to 25 min.

Group 2. Colitis, haemorrhoids, fistula, etc. (9 cases)

The initial activity is doubled after 12 to 25 min, however, it does not attain the values of group 1.

Group 3. Carcinoma of the rectum, carcinoma of the colon (9 cases)

Slow resorption; slackening of the rhythm, the initial value is doubled after 25 min.

Group 4. State after rectal resection (10 cases)

Very slow resorption, which does not even exceed one half of the initial activity.

Discussion

P. A. SAMPSON et al. have studied the resorption of hydrocortisone from the colon in patients with ulcerative colitis, as well as in normal individuals. The results observed by P. A. SAMPSON et al., concerning the resorption of hydrocortisone are in concordance with our observations concerning the absorption of ^{131}INa. We also found a more decreased resorption from the diseased recto-colon.

It is a remarkable fact, that although there is a hypervascularisation in malignant tumors according to recent evidence by some authors like DELARUE et al., and DEUCHER et al., there is, paradoxically, a reduced resorption in cases of granulomatous colitis. Its cause probably lies in the cellular modifications at the level of the mucous and submucous layers, which influence the resorption unfavorably.

The fact that resorptional modification is more evident after resection of the rectum, deserves attention. This can be caused by a series of factors such as:

–the modifications of the mucous and submucous layers of the anastomosed or lifted loop,

–vascular and lymphatic modifications at the level of the loop,

–cellular modifications in the liver which apparently do not influence liver function in an evident way.

M. R. VINOGRADIVA describes the infiltration of the Kupffer cells, situated around the capillaries and veins in patients suffering from colitis. V. G. YANCHEV has registered sygmographic modifications of the large intestine, observed with different disorders of the colon or rectum, and caused by emotion.

The method of measuring the resorption of ^{131}INa from the rectum by contact at the level of the liver, as well as the small number of our cases can certainly be sources of error.

Taking into consideration the above mentioned facts, we can still state that the resorption from the rectum in pathological cases as well as after rectal resection is quantitatively reduced, in contrast to individuals with a healthy rectum.

Proctosigmoidoscopy in Colon Diseases

TH. DOXIADIS, Z. YIOTSAS and T. PALEOLOGOS, Athens, Greece

Colon diseases are responsible for a very wide range of symptoms which often result in confusion when trying to arrive at an exact diagnosis.

In most colonic infections, a carefully taken history and the physical examination suggest the necessity for special examinations of the colon. Physical examination, a preliminary digital examination, stool examination and radiological study of the colon by barium enema are essential for the correct diagnosis. Yet despite these methods, a certain number of diseases of the rectosigmoid can escape detection. In patients who show signs suggestive of colonic malfunction, it is essential to carry out an examination by proctosigmoidoscopy. The method is simple and safe and does not require any special preparations. It rarely causes pain, except in the presence of active anal lesions (fissure, ulcer, acute hemorrhoids, cancer, etc.). This has the distinct advantage of assuring the correct identification of material obtained for microscopie examination. Complications are rare, occuring only in the hands of an inexperienced endoscopist, who may produce a perforation.

In our experience, the best sigmoidoscopic position is the knee-chest position. This position is comfortable for the majority of our patients; only a small number of patients (10%) in our country accept the inverted position. Sigmoidoscopy is usually applied as a routine examination, since the mucosa of the rectum or rectosigmoid is involved in approximately 75% of the symptomatic diseases of the colon [1].

The various diseases which may be diagnosed by sigmoidoscopic examination are:

1. Carcinoma and other Malignant Tumours: Sigmoidoscopy, together with biopsy, is the only positive method of making a histologic diagnosis in time. Carcinomas not fully developed may be detected by sigmoidoscopy. We have often seen patients with carcinoma of the colon who have been treated for a spastic or irritable colon, ulcerative colitis or even internal hemorrhoids. Such an erroneous diagnosis can be avoided if digital examination of the rectum and proctosigmoidoscopy have been performed.

2. Benign Polyps: The majority of "benign polyps" in the colon are located in the rectum or lower sigmoid area and are asymptomatic.

3. Diffuse Adenomatous Polyposis: These lesions are within the reach of a twenty-five cm sigmoidoscope. Their appearance is typical and their visualization endoscopically is important and necessary in the differentiation between polypoid hyperplasia of chronic ulcerative colitis and adenomatous polyposis of the colon.

4. Ulcerative Lesions: In chronic ulcerative colitis, 95% of patients exhibit characteristic changes on sigmoidoscopy, which is the only positive method of diagnosing "idiopathic ulcerative colitis".

5. Strictures: The location and character of strictures in the rectum and lower sigmoid are found best by proctosigmoidoscopy.

6. Radiation Proctosigmoiditis: The differentiation of the disease from direct involvement of the bowel mucosa by a malignant lesion is very important. Sigmoidoscopy is essential in the establishment of the diagnosis and the above differentiation.

7. Melanosis Coli: The diagnosis becomes easier by the inspection of the mucosa with the sigmoidoscope. The discoloration is striking. The colour of the mucosa varies from brown to black and the pigmentation is 2–10 mm in diameter.

8. Diverticulosis and Diverticulitis: Sigmoidoscopy is exceedingly valuable in the differentiation between diverticulitis and carcinoma of the sigmoid.

9. Spastic Colon: In some instances of neuro-muscular irritability of the colon, there are characteristic changes.

10. Megacolon: A routine sigmoidoscopy on constipated patients reveals a congenital dilatation of the lower colon. It is also useful in the differentiation of aganglionic and acquired functional megacolon.

11. Parasites: Parasites are discovered by sigmoidoscopy, and schistosomiasis is often diagnosed by rectal biopsy. Sigmoidoscopy and biopsy are also indicated for the diagnosis of chronic amoebic colitis.

In this paper we are reporting the classification of chronic amoebic colitis on the basis of proctosigmoidoscopy and the results of positive stool examinations as well as of the rectal biopsy for Entamoeba histolytica.

Clinical Material

From July 1, 1962, to December 31, 1967, 20,144 patients were examined at the First Medical Department and the Gastroenterology Center of the Evangelismos Medical Center.

Before attempting to classify the forms of amoebic colitis proctoscopically, we separated 4,927 (24%) patients with clinical symptoms that could be attributed to colonic disorders.

Patients with peptic ulcer, gastric carcinoma, gall bladder diseases, pancreatic diseases, acute appendicitis etc., were excluded after thorough observation and repeated studies.

Symptomatology

The symptomatology in the series of our patients was primarily gastrointestinal. The most frequent symptoms were diffuse abdominal pain, constipation, constipation alternating with diarrhoea, fullness of the abdomen, mucus in the stool, diarrhoea, borborygmi, rectal bleeding, right-side pain, epigastric pain, left-sided pain, dizziness, headache, weakness, anal rash and eczema, flatulence, white-coated tongue, low back pain, psychoneurotic reactions, etc. Their frequency as well as their percentage in the series of 4,927 cases is listed in Table 1.

Table 1. *Primary symptoms in 4,927 patients*

Symptoms	No.	%
Diffuse Abdominal Pain	2266	46
Constipation	1552	31.5
Constipation Alternating with Diarrhoea	1221	24.8
Fullness of the Abdomen	1064	21.6
Mucus in the Stool	1005	20.4
Diarrhoea	946	19.2
Borborygmi	887	18
Right-sided Abdominal Pain	709	14.4
Rectal Bleeding	709	14.4
Tenderness and Pain in Right Hypochondrium	689	14
Epigastric Pain	561	11.2
Left-sided Abdominal Pain	502	10.2
Dizziness	483	9.8
Headache	414	8.4
Weakness	414	8.4
Anal Rash and Eczema	374	7.6
Flatulence	295	6
White-Coated Tongue	295	6
Low Back Pain	276	5.6
Psychoneurotic Reactions	271	5.5

In addition to the above symptoms, a great number of our patients presented secondary complaints which may overshadow the primary symptoms such as anorexia, nausea, belching, vomiting, bitter mouth, red or black tongue, abdominal colic, pre-cordial pain, tenesmus, jaundice, fever, pellagra, skin rash, weight loss, myalgia, arthralgia, allergy. These symptoms are listed in Table 2, in association with the frequency and percentage in 4,927 cases.

Table 2. *Secondary symptoms in 4,927 patients*

Symptoms	No.	%
Belching	236	4.8
Nausea	236	4.8
Fever	236	4.8
Heaviness	236	4.8
Tenesmus	236	4.8
Anorexia	207	4.2
Weight Loss	207	4.2
Bitter Mouth	207	4.2
Allergy	177	3.6
Vomiting	177	3.6
Abdominal Colic	150	3
Arthralgia	150	3
Jaundice	138	2.8
Precordial Pain	128	2.6
Pellagra	123	2.5
Red or Black Tongue	118	2.4
Myalgia	98	2

A certain number of our patients were asymptomatic and diagnosis was established by proctosigmoidoscopy, by rectal biopsy and/or by stool examination [8, 9, 10].

The above symptoms were completely or partially taken into consideration for the diagnosis of the patient's disease.

The proctoscopic observations showed redness, oedema, granularity of the surface, presence of mucus, irritability and friability, smoothness and atrophy of the mucus, bleeding and ulceration.

The proctoscoping findings were classified with regard to the inflammatory changes as: *Severe* (painful ulcerations, usually diffuse or isolated, inflammation, abscesses and spontaneous bleeding). *Moderate* (friable, painful, easy bleeding, pronounced oedematous mucosa, granularity and presence of mucus). *Mild* (redness, slight oedema, atrophy, irritability, smoothness and granularity of the mucosa). *Normal* (redness, slight oedema or atrophy and smoothness or irritability) [7, 12].

The group of 4,927 patients who presented the above mentioned symptoms and were suspected of suffering from chronic colitis, was examined by proctosigmoidoscopy, rectal biopsy, as well as stool examination in addition to the routine examinations.

On the basis of the proctoscopic findings, 181 (3.7%) patients out of the 4,927, were found to have severe colitis, 361 (7.3%) had moderate colitis, 2,687 (54%) mild colitis and 1,698 (34.5%) had normal mucosa. Further study of these patients by stool examination and culture revealed E. histolyticae in 444 patients, through rectal biopsy the number of positive findings for E. histolytica rose to 854, i. e. the percentage went from 9% to 17.3% (Table 3).

Table 3. *Colitis*

	Severe		Moderate		Mild		Normal Mucosa		Total
	No.	%	No.	%	No.	%	No.	%	
Proctoscopically	181	3.7	361	7.3	2687	54.5	1698	34.5	4927
Positive Stool Examination	21		41		247		135		444 (9%)
Positive Rectal Biopsy	41		76		468		269		854 (17.3%)

We considered chronic amoebic colitis as the most possible disease on the basis of the proctoscopic findings, supported by the positive results of rectal biopsy and stool examination; however, we met with extreme difficulty in considering the group of 181 patients with severe colitis, as suffering from chronic amoebic colitis because the typical proctoscopic and roentgenographic findings were suggestive of chronic idiopathic ulcerative colitis.

It is well-known that the negative result of the stool examination and the rectal biopsy do not exclude amoebiasis. However, there are no distinct findings or criteria for differentiating amoebiasis from ulcerative colitis.

There is little doubt that severe amoebic colitis often masquerades as ulcerative colitis in temperature countries. This probably is due to the misguided complacency arising from the knowledge that severe amoebic colitis is very much less common than ulcerative colitis [2, 10, 11].

Furthermore, the wide use and application of antibiotics, the virulence of the E. histolytica during certain seasons, the nutritional conditions of the different countries and the individual resistance of the patient, might be responsible for the modification of the proctoscopical findings, as well as the clinical manifestations, at least for the patients in Greece [12].

Furthermore, we took a group of 250 patients out of the whole series of 4,927 and submitted them to roentgenological examination of the liver by a special method [3, 6], to proctoscopy with rectal biopsy and to stool examination for E. histolytica.

In 108 patients out of these 250, we noticed a characteristic hepatomegaly usually found in the cases of chronic amoebic hepatitis described by Dr. DOXIADIS and his associates [4, 5].

In 86 patients out of these 108 with hepatomegaly, E. histolytica was also detected in the rectal biopsy and/or stool examination. We noticed that 15 patients out of the 86 presented the characteristic hepatomegaly and E. histolytica in the rectal biopsy as well as in the stool examination. In 41 cases, we observed hepatomegaly and positive rectal biopsy and in the remaining 30, hepatomegaly and positive stool examination for E. histolytica.

An anti-amoebic therapy administered to these 108 patients resulted in a clinical amelioration and partial decrease in the hepatomegaly in 77 cases. A repeated proctosigmiodoscopy with a biopsy and stool examination were negative for E. histolytica in these 77 cases (Table 4).

Table 4. *Examined patients*

Examined Patients	250
Hepatomegaly	108
Entamoeba Histolytica	86
Hepatomegaly + P.R.B. + P.S.E.	15
Hepatomegaly + P.R.B.	41
Hepatomegaly + P.S.E.	30
Total	86
Response Anti-Amoebic Treatment	77/108

The above findings suggest that this simple technique of x-ray examination of the liver, followed by proctoscopy with rectal biopsy and/or fresh stool examination for E. histolytica, may be a valuable diagnostic aid in cases of chronic amoebic colitis with hepatitis [4].

Finally, the diagnosis of amoebic colitis in the whole series of our patients was suggested by the clinical picture and symptoms (Tables 1, 2), as well as by the proctoscopical findings. It was also confirmed by the results of the anti-amoebic therapy administered to these patients. There was a clinical amelioration in 77% of them with an improved recto-sigmoid mucosa in 69%.

We preferred to submit all these patients to anti-amoebic therapy at first because it is of short duration, and its response can be expected in one or two weeks time, without any risk to the patients.

Bibliography

1. Bockus, H.: Gastroenterology, Vol. **2**, 686, Second Edition. Philadelphia: W. B. Saunders Co. 1964.
2. Brown, C. H., and E. L. Winkelman: Amoebiasis and Ulcerative Colitis. Cleveland Clin. Quart. **32**, 61–67 (1965).
3. Doxiadis, Th.: Diagnostic Procedure of Chronic Amoebiasis. JAMA, **187**, 7 (1964).
4. —, N. Candreviotis, and Z. Yiotsas: Chronic Amoebic Hepatitis as a Distinct Clinicopathological Entiry. IInd World Congress of Gastroenterology, Munich 1962, **111**, 130–133 (1963).
5. —, —, —, and F. Smyrniotis: Chronic Amoebic Hepatitis. Arch. intern. Med. **111**, 219–225 (1963).
6. —, L. Stergiou, Z. Yiotsas, and D. Tsitsanis: X-ray Films in the Diagnosis of Chronic Amoebic Hepatitis. Brit. med. J. **1**, **343–346** (1964).
7. —, and Z. Yiotsas: Observations, Findings and Conclusions Regarding Proctosigmoidoscopy and Colon Biopsy. Amer. J. Proct. **16**, 5 (1965).
8. —, — The Importance of Rectal Biopsy in the Diagnosis of Amoebiasis. Amer. J. Gastro., March, 1965.
9. Kistner et al.: Rectoscopy and Rectal Biopsy in the Diagnosis of Colitis Proctitis: Gastroenterologia **103**, 47–58 (1965).
10. Juniper, K.: Acute Amoebic Colitis. Amer. J. Med. **33**, 1962.
11. McAllister, A. T.: Diagnosis of Amoebic Colitis on Routine Biopsies from Routine Biopsies from Rectum and Sigmoid Colon. Brit. med J. **1**, 2 (1962).
12. Yiotsas, Z., and Th. Doxiadis: Evaluation of Rectal Biopsy in Colon Diseases. Amer. J. Proct. **17**, 1 (1966).

IX. Proctology

Proctological Consultation

J. Gusinde, Erlangen, Germany

Since the year 1960 we have provided special consultations for patients suffering from anorectal disorders. This service quickly became increasingly popular among the patients, and as a result, as many as three residents now work a whole day once a week to carry out 50–60 proctological examinations.

Our methods of examination and treatment are based on the wealth of experience gained by the medical staff of the St. Marks Hospital, London. The instruments we used are well suited to dealing with numerous patients and correspond to those used in the London clinic. Proctoscope and rectoscope were introduced by Lloyd-Davis. We employ these aids with a bright, proximal cold-light source and are of the opinion that this innovation has greatly improved the viewing conditions. The illumination head is firmly attached on the tube by means of a slip-on cone.

For examination purposes the patient is positioned on his left side with knee and hip joints flexed at roughly 90 degrees. This helps to make rectoscopy less painful and more tolerable for the patient.

Basically, we do not prepare our patients for the ensuing examination, i. e. no laxatives or enemas are administered.

Prior to endoscopy the patients should empty their bowels spontaneously, as only then are we able to evaluate both colour and condition of the mucosa unequivocally. However, if the bowel has not been entirely cleared, we administer a clysma or a rectal lavage. Earlier, when the patients used to be prepared for rectoscopy by means of an enema, we often found the whole intestine filled with water which first needed to be soaked up with pads of cotton batting. During the examination a suction-injection pistol, built to our specifications by Storz, Tuttlingen, provides good service. This pistol allows a controlled water jet to be delivered to the mucosa being investigated and, at the same time, aspirates the fluid via a water-jet pump. With a bleeding carcinoma, this gun has proved indispensable in selecting a biopsy.

Early diagnosis of rectal carcinoma is the *most essential objective* of our proctological outpatient service. The patients, who consult us, have all types of anorectal complaints, such as anal loss of blood, pain, pruritus, burning and weeping, all of which may be symptoms of a rectal carcinoma.

We establish the *anatomical findings* by exploring the anal region, by palpation and proctoscopy, by rectoscopy up to 20–30 cm, by injecting radiopaque media into the colon or by double-contrast studies. All polyps and suspicious alterations of the mucosa are examined *histologically*. In this manner a carcinoma can be verified or precluded with a high degree of reliability. Among the 1,710 patients, who attended in 1967 we found 92 suffering from carcinoma, a surprisingly high percentage when one considers that only 124 carcinomas were established in 10,000 rectoscopic examinations performed at St. Marks Hospital.

The question may be posed as to the ambulant methods of anorectal treatment that are possible and customary?

In the case of an *extended haemorrhoidal plexus* during the initial stages 1 and 2 or a degenerated corpus cavernosum, as described by Stelzner, we inject 5% phenol in Arachis oil into the submucosus coat. For this injection we use the Gabriel syringe with a long needle. At the positions 3, 7 and 11 o'clock fluid deposits of 2–3 ml are injected, so that a glassy protrusion develops. The injection is painless if made proximal to the knot. After an average of 3 treatments carried out at intervals of 2 to 3 weeks, the knot shrinks and the treatment is concluded. In this manner we can also arrest any *haemorrhoidal bleeding* at this stage. However, once the condition had progressed to stage 3, we recommend surgery, i. e. haemorrhoidectomy after Milligan-Morgan or Parks, provided that no contraindication exists. But even in stage 3 we still use injections if the patients are advanced in years and/or in poor general condition.

Those people affected with an *anal fissure* can usually be treated on an outpatient basis. Fresh fissures with the base marked by longitudinal stripes, are treated by the regular application of dilator to normalize the blood circulation. In this way the vicious circle, inflammatory irritation, permanent contraction of the musculature or ischiamic segmental contraction can be interrupted.

Fissures of long standing with a transversely striped base and overhanging margine are excised. The flap of the skin usually presents at the distal end and the hypertrophic papilla at the proximal end of the fissure are also removed.

If an anal stenosis has developed, we dilate the anus under general anaesthesia. After excision and expansion, we continue dilating for at least 3 weeks to ensure healing by secondary intention from the wound base. We allow laxatives to be administered only at the beginning of the treatment to allay pain as otherwise there would be no physiological dilation of the anus.

Perianal, *periproctitic abscesses* are operated under general anaesthesia by making a bow-shaped incision while taking special care to keep skin open until healing of the woundbase is complete.

Patients with *anal and pilonidal fistulas* are operated on as in-patients. Outpatients are subjected to surgery only if the fistula is smooth and marginal.

Perianal haematomas are extirpated under local anaesthesia. The margin of the skin is also excised to provide a drainage route for wound secretion. We advise against the simple stab incision because of the risk of fistula formation.

In anal disorders accompanied by pruritus, we frequently find a *protrusion of the anterior wall of the rectum* with a slight secretion during the initial stage. This secretion is responsible for the pruritus. As in the treatment of haemorrhoids in the first stage, we also inject into the submucosus coat of the rectum. Frequently the patients feel greatly relieved even after a single injection.

If a hypertrophic papilla is the cause of the pruritus, it is removed surgically. If a protrusion of the anterior wall, cryptitis, a hypertrophic papilla or an anal fissure can be excluded as the cause of the *pruritus*, then the doctor has to look for such general diseases as diabetes, leukemia, or liver diseases. An oversensitivity to food or chemical substances is found in rare instances.

Corticoid ointments and suppositories are prescribed only to assist in the treatment, but whenever possible, causal therapy is the rule.

Clinical Manifestations of Anorectal Disease

G. H. Thiele, Kansas City, Missouri, USA

Proctologic patients may present a variety of clinical symptoms which neither the patient nor his physician has attributed to anorectal disease.

In order to determine a possible relationship between these symptoms and anorectal disease, an analysis was made of 225 consecutive private case records. Such symptoms were found in 70 (31 per cent) of 225 patients. When these symptoms occurred, there were generally from three to five of them associated with one another. The incidence of symptoms was tabulated from the histories. The case progress records were then referred to and the final effect on each symptom was listed under the heading of cured, improved or unimproved.

For diagnostic convenience the symptoms were classified as neurological, gastrointestinal, genitourinary and neuromuscular.

Nervous Disturbances

When symptoms representing different classifications were combined in the same patient, an incorrect diagnosis of neurosis or of functional disease had frequently been made. In this type of patient, the rectal symptoms per se are often quite mild, sometimes being manifest only as a slight discomfort after defecation, a sense of rectal weight or pressure, or of painless protrusion. When symptoms of the various classifications co-exist and have become chronic and severe, the most bizarre clinical picture may result.

I cite the following typical case history of Miß G. M., a 34-year-old stenographer.

Chief Complaint: Chills and fever; nervousness and crying; left lower abdominal pain; aching across the sacrum and down the legs; irregular menses; painful defecation.

Present Illness: For four years there has been painful defecation, almost constant aching across the lower back and down the legs, pain in the lower left abdomen, and menstrual irregularity. For the past five months daily enemas were given to prevent painful defecation, and were invariably followed by a chill and a fever of 104° to 105°, with a return to normal temperature in about eight hours. She described herself as a "nervous wreck". Three months previously she had been hospitalized for nervousness, weakness and left lower abdominal pain, and to determine the cause of the daily chills and fever. She remained at the hospital for two weeks, and was discharged as unimproved, no diagnosis having been made.

Past History: Appendectomy at 18 years. Salpingectomy three years ago at the age of 31 failed to relieve the left lower abdominal pain.

Examination, Treatment and Results: Examination revealed a posterior anal ulcer, an acute cryptitis and hemorrhoids.

The anal ulcer was excised and a papillocryptectomy and a hemorrhoidectomy were performed. The first postoperative enema was followed by a chill and a fever of 103.5°, nausea and vomiting. Her temperature returned to normal in three hours. The following day an enema was followed by nausea and vomiting but without a chill or fever. From that time on, she rapidly improved. Six weeks later she had gained eight pounds, was no longer nervous, and had had two normal menstrual periods. Nine months after operation she was perfectly well and had gained 37 pounds.

Comment

This case illustrates the widespread effect of anorectal disease on the general health of the patient. The nervousness, crying and irritability were due to reflex disturbances through the sympathetic and parasympathetic nervous systems caused by the anal ulcer and the cryptitis. The low back pain with radiation down the legs was due to bilateral piriformis muscle spasm secondary to the cryptitis and the posterior anal ulcer.

The menstrual disturbances were reflex in nature through the common sympathetic and parasympathetic innervations of the anorectum, uterus and ovaries.

I believe, the chills and fever which followed the enemas, were due to the rapid absorption of bacterial proteins through venous sinuses and lymphatics in the fresh anal wounds incident to defecation. The clinical picture of the chills and fever exactly duplicated the chills and fever which follow the intravenous injection of a vaccine. Several times a year, I have noted this reaction following the first post-operative enema.

Gastrointestinal Disturbances

A 51-year-old housewife complained of nervousness and indigestion associated with mild aching anal pain.

For one year the patient had complained of weakness immediately following defecation and lasting from one-half to one hour. Her diet had been limited to liquids because she could not tolerate solid foods without nausea and vomiting. For two years she had been nervous and irritable and had required barbiturates for sleep. A rectal examination was attempted six months before I saw her, but because of fright and pain, she would not allow it to be done. She had complained of flatulence for 15 years and had used a daily laxative for five years.

Examination, Treatment and Results: Anorectal examination revealed low vermiform fibrous anal papillae two centimeters in length which herniated into the anal canal. At the base of each papilla there was an inflamed crypt. The anus was stenosed to the degree that it would not admit the little finger even after the use of a local anesthetic.

A cryptopapillectomy was done, the perianal fibrous band was incised, and a partial sphincterotomy of the internal sphincter and the subcutaneous portion of the external sphincter was done to increase anal caliber to normal.

While the patient was still in the hospital, she was fed a general low-residue diet which she ate and enjoyed without nausea or vomiting. In two weeks, she was sleeping all night without a sedative for the first time in two years. Eight weeks postoperatively she was eating a general diet and enjoying it, and she stated that she felt better than she had for many years.

Comment

The nervousness, weakness and digestive symptoms were purely reflex through sympathetic and parasympathetic neurons. Excision of the vermiform papillae which hung down into the anal canal, removed the exciting factor of these reflexes. The constipation was of course due to fibrous anal stenosis.

Menstrual Disturbances

Miss J. R., an unmarried 18-year-old student complained of several months of cutting anal pain followed by four months of menstrual irregularity and three months of amenorrhea. She was nervous and irritable and cried at the slightest provocation.

Examination revealed a chronic posterior anal ulcer and subacute papillocryptitis. These structures were removed the following day. Since operation her menstrual periods have been regular and all nervousness has disappeared.

Miss G. M. whose case history was outlined under general nervousness, has had no menstrual irregularity since her surgery although her periods had been irregular for four years. In her case also, there was a posterior anal ulcer and associated cryptitis.

The menstrual disturbances were reflex in nature through the common sympathetic and parasympathetic innervation of the rectum, uterus and ovaries.

Urinary Disturbances

We are reminded of the role which rectal disease may play in the production of urinary symptoms, by the rather frequent bladder dysfunction following anorectal surgery.

The mode of production of these urinary symptoms is explained by the fact that the bladder represents the anterior division of the hindgut, caused by the descent of the cloacal septum at about the fourteenth week of fetal life, and that the bladder and the rectum have the same innervation through the second, third and fourth sacral nerves.

Symptoms of urinary frequency and urgency are so common as to preclude the necessity for case histories. All well-trained urologists recognize the fact that when urologic examination is negative, these patients should by all means be referred to a competent proctologist for proctologic evaluation.

Neuromuscular Symptoms

Aching across the sacrum and/or down the backs of the legs and in the region of the coccyx is not uncommon. Sacral aching with radiation down the course of the sciatic nerve or upward into the superior gluteal region has been found to be due to piriformis muscle spasm; and pain in the region of the coccyx (coccygodynia) has been found to be due to spasm of the levator ani muscles. These symptom complexes, secondary to anorectal disease, have been thoroughly discussed in several separate papers, and are referred to as the Thiele syndrome.

Bibliography

LANGWORTHY, O. O.: General Principles of Autonomic Innervation. Arch. Neurol. Psychiat. **50**, 590 (1943).

REID, L. C.: Fundamental Concepts of Autonomic Function. N.Y. St. J. Med. **50**, 1797–1801 (1950).

LYONS, R. H., and F. S. CALIVA: The Clinical Manifestations of Autonomic Dysfunction. N.Y. St. J. Med. **50**, 1801–1809 (1950).

Christopher, F.: Textbook of Surgery. 5th ed. Philadelphia: W. B. Saunders Co. 1949.

Thiele, G. H.: The Referred Symptoms of Anorectal Disease. J. Mo. med. Ass. **31**, 20–24 (1934).

Alvarez, W. C.: A Simple Explanation for Cardiospasm and Hirschsprung's Disease. Gastroenterology **13**, 422 (1949).

Lendrum, F. C.: Anatomic Features of the Cardiac Orfice of the Stomach, with Special Reference to Cardiospasm. Arch. intern. Med. **59**, 474 (1937).

Thiele, G. H.: The Genito-urinary Symptoms of Anorectal Disease. Sth. med. J. **39**, 166–172 (1946).

Smithwick, R. H., and J. C. White: The Autonomic Nervous System: Anatomy, Physiology, and Surgical Application. New York: The Macmillian Company 1948.

Thiele, G. H.: Coccygodynia: The Mechanism of its Production and its Relationship to Anorectal Disease. Amer. J. Surg. **69**, 110–116 (1950).

— Tonic Spasm of the Levator Ani, Coccygeus and Piriformis Muscles. Trans. Amer. proctol. Soc. (1936).

— Coccygodynia and Pain in the Superior Gluteal Region and Down the Back of the Thigh. J.A.M.A. **109**, 1271–1274 (1937).

— Coccygodynia: Cause and Treatment. Dis. Colon Rect. Vol. 6, No. 6, Nov.-Dec., (1963).

Rectal Anatomy with Clinical Significance

E. Levy, Bronx, N.Y., USA

The choice by the Ancients of the word to describe the perineum as the pudendum, "that of which I am ashamed" – is a comprehensive concept of the function of the structures here completely justified by intensive anatomic study. Great skill has, on rare occasions, been achieved by some in the management of these parts without detailed anatomic knowledge. However, such skill is rarely transmitted. Intensive study has now established knowledge which is transmissible. In this paper, information will be offered which is abundantly documented, and for the past twenty years has been used with excellent results.

Rectal columns are formed by the distal fibers of the conjoined longitudinal muscle accompanied by small arteries and veins. In hemorrhoidal disease, the direction of the surgical removal of the vascular tumor is carried out in a longitudinal direction. In fissures, margins are excised parallel to longitudinal fibers. In fistula a critical problem is the management of the curvature of the anal canal. The fistula is excised in two segments: 1. first, the abscessed external portion is excised, then 2. the probe enters the fistulous tract from the excised area and the tract with its enclosed probe is excised superficially. Again the longitudinal position of a parallel with the muscle fibers is respected. This consideration causes the least distortion of the mucosal wall.

Abscess formation about the rectum is localized by the spaces that result from the structural arrangement. Most usual in the perineum are the infralevator and the posterior triangular spaces. These appear with greatest regularity. Their localization is brought about by the septa of the conjoined longitudinal muscle which act as carriers of and barriers to infection.

The rectum in the pelvis is vulnerable to penetrating wounds of the buttock because of the incomplete protection by the pelvic bony girdle. Such an injury would demand immediate colostomy.

The levator musculature from their origin in the pelvis distribute their fibers in the wall of the rectum partly by insertion into the sacrococcygeal vertebrae. The portion that goes to the wall partly unites with the longitudinal muscle of the rectum forming the conjoined longitudinal muscle and the part of the levator that is left free forms the puborectalis muscle. The conjoined longitudinal muscle descends through the muscle mass of the external sphincter ani and terminates in strong fibro-elastic fibers in the deep layer of the skin; posteriorly the skin over the coccyx, and anteriorly, as it meets the posterior borders of the deep transverse perineal muscle meet and attach there and continue on to terminate in the skin anterior to the anus, along the line of the superficial transverse perineal muscle, fusing there with the posterior attachment of Colles fascia. The fusion of the anterior conjoined longitudinal muscle with the Colles fascia effectively divides the perineum into an anterior perineal-urogenital and posterior rectal area. The puborectalis muscle is that portion of the levator which is completely in the perineum. It is attached by a thick broad strap of condensed fibroelastic tissue to the tip of the coccyx and is free alongside the rectum. It is applied against the posterior wall of the rectum. The puborectalis is extrinsic to the rectal wall.

The septa of the conjoined longitudinal muscles, as they penetrate the sphincter ani muscle mass, carry with them the longitudinal fibers of the submucous coat. The penetrating septa, on achieving their destination, have cut off a substantial mass of sphincter fibers which remain free on the rectal wall and form the deep sphincter ani. The deep sphincter ani, free from the wall, is extrinsic to the wall of the rectum. Within the confines of the septa are two segments of the sphincter ani. The one closest to the internal lining of the canal is the subcutaneous sphincter ani which is completely circular and corresponds in position to the deep sphincter ani. This is the muscle mistakenly called the internal sphincter ani. The second and more superficial one, which is called the superficialis, is composed of two distinct sets of fibers: one set completely circular with an equal number of fibers (I have counted them) that run anteriorly becoming fused with the triangular ligament and posteriorly inserting into the fascia covering the coccygeal vertebrae. The septa faithfully go along the muscle to the insertion. The septa on the way to their termination establish a continuous attachment to the overlying skin. The longitudinal fibers of the superficialis come from each side of the muscle mass and form a base equal to the posterior margin and, joining, terminate in a narrow insertion. This explains the triangular shape of the posterior triangular space.

The deep sphincter, likewise, is composed of circular and longitudinal fibers but has no septa and is free in the rectum as an extrinsic component. The deep sphincter is felt in the anterior anal canal as the highest margin of circular muscle; here the puborectalis is absent.

The anterior palpated margin is the guide for the intersphincteric skin incision, which leaves the circular fibers of the urethral sphincter and the anal sphincter muscles untouched: a guide for the separation of the anorectal wall from the prostata and its urethra is thus established.

With the establishment of the extrinsic portion of puborectalis muscle each muscle group is then held in Allis clamps brought together and the muscles sutured to each other; an additional sphincter results.

Saggital sections of the pelvis through the rectum show quite plainly the direction of the canal from the outside in. Frame of reference is 1. sacrococcygeal vertebrae posteriorly, 2. symphysis pubis anteriorly, 3. sacral hollow posteriorly. The anal canal is entered from the posterior curvature with the exploring finger or examining instrument pointing to the pubis. Position is now changed 90 degrees, pointing to the hollow of the sacrum. The ampulla is checked. From here on we carry on under direct vision with the illuminated instrument. At the rectosigmoid region, the upper limit of the rectum, the patient is asked to cough, breathe hard, while we observe the physiologic intussusception.

Non-Radical vs. Radical Anorectal Surgery

F. Moran, Scranton, Pa., USA

To define non-radical anorectal surgery, the term implies the excision of the minimal amount of adjacent normal mucous membrane, anoderm and perianal skin in hemorrhoidal fistula, and fissure pathology, while performing adequate curative surgery. The result of this type of surgery has a great bearing on lessening pain and discomfort and decreasing the healing time and period of disability.

In the standard hemorrhoidectomy technic as described in books and performed by many proctologic surgeons, a considerable amount of skin and mucous membrane is removed with the individual hemorrhoidal mass. The external and internal hemorrhoids are grasped with clamps, Allis or Kelly, and incisions carried along the lateral borders to the apex of the latter. In placing the clamp, healthy, normal, uninvolved tissue is included, and then removed with the pathological tissue. The resulting constriction of the lower rectum resulting from suture of the mucosal edges, or from the granulation tissue if suture approximation is not used, results in varying degrees of pain, discomfort, and narrowing in the immediate and later postoperative stages. Insofar as the external elliptical skin wound, left when the external hemorrhoid has been removed is concerned, there is marked pain and soreness as well as delayed healing, depending upon the superficial infection present, as well as the degree of restorative response by adjacent tissue.

In almost every case of hemorrhoidal disease, there is little or no involvement of the skin covering except for various degrees of inflammatory reaction. The primary pathology is subcutaneous. In the low rectum, it is submucosal. The involvement is in the external and internal hemorrhoidal plexus, and in the typical uncomplicated case, further extension of surgical excision is not necessary. How often is too much surgery performed! While the rule in surgery to remove all the pathology is stressed, there is not much emphasis on the use of good sound judgment to preserve as much healthy, uninvolved tissue as possible. As we examine externally and internally, do we make a careful decision to remove only that localized area of pathology? How often would areas of insignificant anorectal inflammatory pathology provide no physical discomfort and heal spontaneously; yet during operative procedures everything must be excised in spite of the loss of a considerable amount of normal, healthy tissue. We all realize there are occasional exceptions, so that discussion is not considered necessary.

In fissure and fistula pathology, there is so little localized pathology present that simple incision with minimal saucerization of the edges is usually all that is required. In the former, the incision includes a portion of the internal and external sphincter muscle, as well as slight overstretching. A minimum of catgut is recommended, using the fulgeration current whenever possible, after a short period or manual or clamp pressure. In fissure cases with stenosis, adequate divulsion is suggested. The mobilized edge of incised mucous membrane is attached high on the inner border of the external sphincter muscle. The base or floor of the fissure is curretted of all granulation tissue and the skin edges mobilized and saucerized. A simple incision extends a short distance outward from the distal point of the fissure.

In fistula procedures, the incision exposes the tract adequately, the curling sides are saucerized, and the base curretted of all granulation tissue from the internal to the external sphincter.

If incision through the sphincter is necessary following currettement, the internal cryptic opening is removed and, following repair of the muscle, the mucosal edge is brought down and sutured to the muscle distal to the repair suture. A furacin wick gauze is left in the fistulotomy wounds.

I might add that bowel sterilization is used on practically all cases beginning the day prior to surgery until the sixth to tenth postoperative day.

The procedure of hemorrhoidectomy is discussed last because of the wide variation in the types and pattern of hemorrhoidal pathology.

I shall present the technic used in the three most common types of hemorrhoids seen by the proctologist.

Where the three primary hemorrhoidal masses are present individually with no intervening secondary hemorrhoids. Each hemorrhoid – external and corresponding internal – is removed with the following technic: with the operating speculum in place and positioned to reveal the full extent of the internal hemorrhoid, the incisions are carried through the skin from the dentate line outward along the lateral margins of the external hemorrhoid to the distal end. The incisions are joined at the inner margin, i. e., dentate border, and by sharp dissection, the external hemorrhoid is dissected from within outward, using Babcock clamps for elevation. The dissection is carried over the sphincter muscles and outward over the deep perianal areolar tissue to the distal margin of the hemorrhoid.

With the hemorrhoid thus elevated, the left index finger presses the central area of the mass inward, resulting in a flattened surface. The hemorrhoidal pathology is quickly excised from the inner skin surface by dissection with small Metzenbaum scissors. Electric cauterization is used to control the bleeding. The reflected skin is left free and the corresponding internal hemorrhoid is removed in a similar manner. Frequently, ligation with triple 0 plain catgut is used to control bleeding encountered with this phase. The skin edge is drawn into the anal canal and approximated with a mattress type suture to the free edge of mucosa. The suture is placed to secure a bite of the internal sphincter muscle. Care is taken to avoid excessive suture tension. Loose, redundant external skin may be trimmed away.

Each of the other two primary hemorrhoids are similarly removed. A small wick of thin vaseline gauze is placed over each incision extending into the anal canal as far as the mucocutaneous line.

In the second type of hemorrhoidal case in which there is a large hemorrhoid involving one side or the entire anal opening, similar to the doughnut ring, the following technic is used: at the beginning of the operation, 2 to 4 cc. of 1% xylocaine with epinephrine are injected subcutaneously into the hemorrhoidal mass, resulting in slight distention. This does two things – it controls considerably the usually encountered milder bleeding and oozing during dissection, and it creates a more defined line of cleavage between the skin and underlying hemorrhoidal tissue. With the operating retractor in place and lateral skin traction attained by use of towel clips, incisions are made along the hemorrhoidal mass, in the anterolateral and posterolateral areas from the dentate line outward to the outermost pole of the hemorrhoid. If the entire anal ring is involved there will be four incisions, the two anterior, and two posterior, close together on either side of the midline.

By sharp dissection, the hemorrhoidal mass is elevated from within outward and the hemorrhoidal tissue totally excised from the lower skin surface. The inward pressure exerted by the left index finger greatly facilitates the complete removal of the pathological tissue.

The skin is left free and the internal hemorrhoid removed as described above. Because of the large extent of mucosal and skin edges, two to three mattress sutures are used for approximation, again with a small bite of the internal sphincter muscle. A running stitch is not used because of the eventual constricting effect on the anal circumference. If hemorrhoidal tissue is present under the thin remaining strip of skin and mucous membrane anteriorly and posteriorly, they are each elevated and the underlying pathological tissue excised from the side.

In the third case where, in addition to the primary hemorrhoids, there are one or more secondary hemorrhoids, an incision is made over the dome, the skin edges retracted, and the hemorrhoidal tissue enucleated as with an acute thrombotic hemorrhoid. A suture may be used to approximate the incision over the internal hemorrhoid.

Conclusion

In conclusion, the results have been so impressive that the "open wound procedures" have been practically entirely discontinued on our services.

Surgical Management of Strangulated, Thrombosed Hemorrhoids as an Emergency Procedure

D. A. Zambouras, A. I. Trampaklos and S. Tsilividis, Athens, Greece

It is well known that thrombosed, incarcerated, bleeding and ulcerated hemorrhoids have been a controversial subject from the standpoint of immediate (or late) surgical management. The most acceptable typical management is conservative treatment, that is, reduction of the hemorrhoids, bed rest, local cleansing and administration of therapeutic agents against the inflammation. These patients go to surgery at a later time when the acute stage has passed.

However, the reduction of the hemorrhoids in the acute stage can be very difficult, and prolapse of the rectal mucosa can very easily recur in spite of conservative measures. Spontaneous disappearance of the hemorrhoids after the acute stage is rather seldom, however. The only treatment which irradicates the hemorrhoids is the surgical one.

In this paper we present our experience from 1962 to 1967 where 53 cases with exacerbation of the hemorrhoids were admitted for treatment in our hospital. Of these 53 cases, 42 had immediate surgery in the acute stage (Table 1).

Table 1

			Incarcerated hemorrhoids 1962–1967			
			Males	30	Age	32–75
			Females	23	Age	26–64
Operative Management on 42 cases			No. of cases	53		
Hemorrhoidectomy	12	9				
		3				
Hemorrhoidectomy	15	13				
Sphincterotomy		2				
Hemorrhoidectomy						
Anal fissure excision	15	6				
Sphincterotomy		9				
Polypectomy						

Preoperative management: It approximates that of an elective hemorrhoidectomy:

1. Local cleansing (soap baths, sit baths),
2. Antiseptic solutions for local application,
3. Decongestive agents (enzymes) q 12 h.,
4. Analgesics, spasmolysics and sedative drugs.

Anesthesia: 27 patients were operated upon under endotracheal general anesthesia, 15 patients under low spinal or caudal anesthesia.

Procedure: An open hemorrhoidectomy by MILLIGAN and MORGAN was performed on 12 cases; on 15 cases where there was a very tight internal sphincter an open hemorroidectomy plus sphincterotomy was carried out. On the remaining number of cases (15) the hemorrhoidectomy was combined with anal fissure excision or polypectomy or sphincterotomy (Table 2). Special care was taken to preserve good skin flaps between the hemorrhoidal clusters. In the few cases where good skin flaps could not be preserved, hemorrhoids were left behind to be excised at a later time (two-stage hemorrhoidectomy). This was observed in cases of huge secondary internal hemorrhoids.

Table 2

Type of Procedure	No. of Cases	Anal Pathology
Simple Hemorrhoidectomy	12	Incarcerated hemor. Thrombosis Ulceration
Hemorrhoidectomy Sphincterotomy	15	Incarcerated hemor. Thrombosis Ulceration Spastic Sphincter Pectinosis
Hemorrhoidectomy Sphincterotomy Fissure excision-Polypectomy	15	Incarcerated hemor. Anal fissure Polyps

Postoperative management: The postoperative management was the same as in conventional hemorrhoidectomies, that is, Demerol 50 mg. q 6 h, analgesics, spasmolysics and sedatives in between and decongestive drugs q 12 h. If the patient had surgery in the morning, he could take fluids by mouth in the afternoon. Full house diet was started on the first postoperative day. If a patient was unable to urinate, 12 hours after surgery, the bladder was catheterized. The patient was allowed out of bed the following morning and the loose intrarectal pack with ointment (xylocaine 5% and antibiotic) which had been left in at the time of surgery was removed. The patients were taken off pain medication slowly and a mild laxative was administered on the second postoperative day. We recommend sit baths immediately after each bowel movement.

Sphincter dilatations after surgery were avoided and have not been a problem in our experience, especially in cases where a sphincterotomy had been performed. In post-bowel movement pain, we used an ointment containing cortisone; this is also helpful in post-bowel movement rectal itching. If the above symptoms were associated with tenesmus, we administered spasmolytics as they were necessary. Depending on the patient's special psyche, a sedative was administered for 10 to 15 days.

The results with this sort of treatment have been satisfactory. The postoperative course of the patients was similar to those who underwent elective hemorrhoidectomies. All the patients returned to their occupation in eight to fifteen days from the time of surgery. They were seen in the outpatient department every second day until a complete healing of the traumatic rectal area had occurred, usually in 25 to 41 days after surgery. In 9 cases, a second stage of hemorrhoidectomy was necessary because of hemorrhoids left behind for the sake of skin flaps.

Discussion

The objections to operating in the acute stage of hemorrhoids come from the fear of complications such as pylophlebitis, septic emboli, fulminating local flare up with extensive necrosis. However, these complications have appeared even in elective hemorrhoidectomy cases. In recent years, histologic study of the hemorrhoid has shown that thrombosis and inflammation occur in the incarcerated part of the hemorrhoid and none in its vascular pedicle. These histological findings were observed in our cases also.

On the basis of our 42 cases, we think that an emergency hemorrhoidectomy means no more risk than an elective hemorrhoidectomy. This procedure seems to be surgically sound if one is selects the cases. Extensive local infiltration or gangrene, of course, precludes the emergency hemorrhoidectomy. An open hemorrhoidectomy in the acute stage can help in free local drainage and decongestion of the anal area. Finally, the fears of a local flareup of the infection are groundless if one considers the local immunity of the anal area due to repeated infections. A strong example of this is the low incidence of wound infection after colostomy closure.

Bibliography

Ackland, E.: Brit. J. Surg. **54,** 141 (1967).
Gabriel, W.: The Principles of Rectal Surgery. 5th Edition, pp. 123, 124.
Morgan, C. N.: Surg. Clin. N. Amer. **1457,** 35, 5 (1955).
—, and Thomson: Ann. roy. Coll. Surg. Engl. **114,** 19 (1956).
Parks, A. G.: Surg. Clin. N. Amer. **1305,** 45, 5 (1965).
Turell, R.: Amer. J. Surg. **105,** 649 (1963).

Cataclysmic Rectorrhagia of Unusual Cause: the Myeloma

J. Lentini, E. Fornells and R. Ortiz, Barcelona, Spain

Very few are the communications about anorectal complications in blood dyscrasias, even though we believe that they are more frequent than is generally believed.

In the anorectum, five types of fundamental complications may be produced alone or associated with others disorders including hematological disorders:

1. Non-specific inflammatory reaction;
2. Infection (focal or disseminate);
3. Ulceration;
4. Vascular alterations (as thrombosis and hemorrhages);
5. Infiltration (neoplastic or granulomatous).

The reduction of the organic resistance to infection, the defects in coagulation even the subclinical ones, the capillary dilatation and the circulatory extasis among other causes, are to be found in the disorders characterized by leucopenia, hypogammaglobulinemia, thrombopenia, polycythemia, notably an increase in the possibility of the appearance of complications in the anorectal region, especially if the patient was previously already prone to diseases in this area.

In multiple myeloma, there are lower levels of useful gammaglobulins. Just as in chronic lymphatic leukemia, there can be high levels of gamma or beta abnormal fractions in multiple myeloma but these proteins do not act as antibodies. Thus, patients with these diseases do not suffer a myelopathy alone, but are especially prone to infections during the course of their disease, the first indication of a severe leucopenic or leukemic process may be the ulceration and infection of a mucosal membrane even though the mouth is the most frequent site of said lesions, the anorectal zone may also show itself to be extremely sensitive.

The first good observations in Spain were published by Dr. F. Palma. He reported several cases of leukemia where first symptoms occurred in the anorectal region. Personally we have several cases, some of them very singular. Many cases have been reported in the world literature, among them a very extraordinary one of amyloidosis of the rectum. There is also one of multiple myeloma. However the history which we present now, seems to us to be of a certain interest.

1962. – J. C. Male – 62 years old. – Landowner – Slight rectorrhagias on isolated occasions and some epistaxis.

No other antecedents of interest. While taking a walk through his land 3 days ago, the patient noticed weakness in his legs and a slight fainting. He recovered but had a bowel movement nearly exclusively composed of blood clots. In three days, this occurred five times. His physician, immediately called us for consultation.

On physical examination he was very pale but very quiet; tachycardia; hepatomegaly (1 finger width); at the rectal examination only some voluminous hemorrhoids. After a short cleansing enema, rectoscopy was performed. This showed a pale mucosa but normal up to 25 cms. with a sigmoid free of blood. There were only some ulcerated and bleeding hemorrhoids and slight vascular hyperemia. A blood count examination was urgently asked for which showed the presence of 1,200,000 erythrocytes. Because of this the patient was admitted to a clinic and a transfusion of 500 cc. is given. Local anticlotting measures. The complete analysis was now asked for with the following results.

Leucocytes – 4,800 with some plasmocytes; B.S.R. 1 hour = 112; 2 hours = 116; plaquettopenia: 60,000; Bence-Jones proteinuria, slightly positive; hyperproteinemia with hypergammaglobulinemia.

In view of these results, a sternal puncture is performed, *which is diagnosed at the first examination as lymphoid leukemia*. Later on this is rectified to be a myeloma. A radiographic examination of the thorax and skull is made (Fig. 1 and 2) which shows a slight decalcification and two cranial osteolytic lesions in the vault.

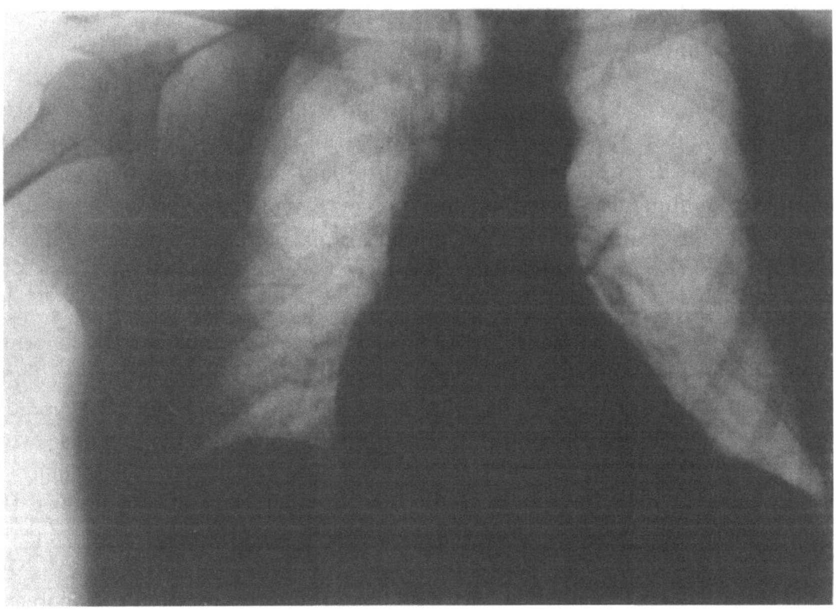

Fig. 1

At this time the patient passes into the care of hematologist who begins general treatment. We limit ourselves only to the treatment of the hemorrhoids.

During this period, the patient received several transfusions, the last one of which produced a very intense reaction. After the first transfusion the rectorrhagias stopped, even though the epistaxis persisted for some days.

In view of the amelioration of the clinical picture, we made the decision to sclerose the hemorrhoids by injections of chlorhydrate of quinine and urea. During the fifteen days of his stay in the clinic, the patient received two injections of 5 cc. and daily underwent an anuscopy. He shows good tolerance of the treatment; the hemorrhoids are still ulcerated and bleeding at the last contact.

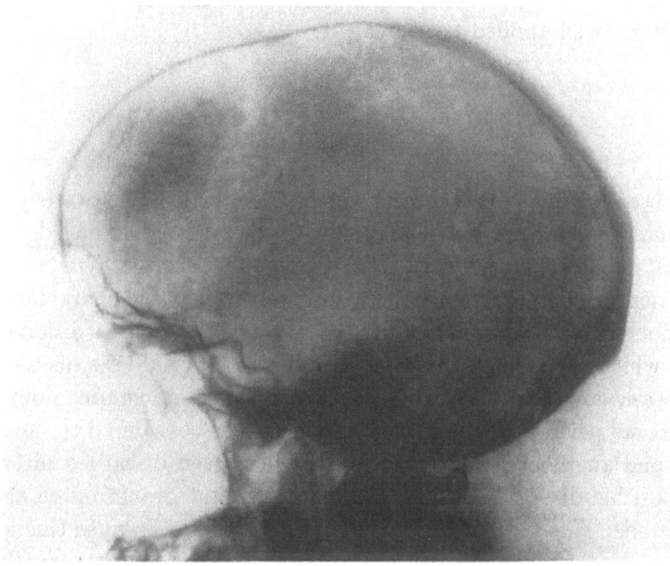

Fig. 2

Fifteen days later, the patient is in an ameliorated general condition with nearly three million erythrocytes and hundred thousand plaquettes. Against the opinion of the hematologist, the patient undertakes an inspection on his land. Upon arrival there, he suffers a new rectorrhagia which lasts all night. In the morning he receives a transfusion, but during the same, he dies, due to acute anemia, as it seems.

Comment

1. We have not found any other case of cataclysmic rectorrhagia due to multiple myeloma in the world literature.

2. *A sclerosing treatment*, under these conditions must always be practised under very strict control in order to avoid any eschar which might prove to be fatal. The sclerotherapy should always be practised with the patient in a clinic and daily an anuscopy must be preformed to control the evolution of the treatment in order to be able to effect the opportune treatment should the production of an eschar begin.

The basic treatment of the disease by the specialist, is obvious. We do not believe the intervention to be indicated. Even though we may see a good evolution of the blood picture and of the sclerotherapy, the patient must not escape our control at least until three weeks after having the last injection.

3. We have seen similar hemorrhages in cirrhotic patients with portal hypertension, in which very painful giant fissures are frequently also found. The whole picture fits very well to the sclerosis.

4. Possibly, the fatal denouement could have been avoided if the patient had not left the city travelling at such a prenature moment of his treatment. In cirrhotic patients, in which a rectorrhagica has ocurred and who have been treated by means of sclerosis, we have never seen the repetition of these hemorrhages, after a well applied treatment.

Diagnosis

In 1964, we were in a period during which the specialized laboratory studies did not exist but this does not mean that now, in our present knowledge we do not intend to catalogue it.

This patient undoubtedly suffered a disease whose basic characteristics were: hyperproteinemia with gammaglobulinemia. Nowadays, three different diseases are known which give this proteic picture. These are Kahler's disease, Waldenström's disease and Franklin's disease. The increase of gammaglobulin in the period where we performed the proteinogramme was considered to be an increase of α 2, β 1 and augment β 2. Nowadays, this has been discarded already. From the three possible diseases, Kahler, Waldenström and Franklin, we are going to discard this one. This patient did not suffer a Franklin, because this is a disease whose fundamental characteristics are: adenopathies, hepatomegaly, splenomegaly, practically no bone disturbance, no pain, since it is a biological discovery.

There remains the Kahler, and the Waldenström's disease and I believe that it will be possible for us to classify it in one or in the other. Nowadays, the myeloma is of Kahler, but at that time both were called myeloma. Now we can classify it with a classical Kahler, or with a Waldenström which is a macroglobulinemia, because the differences are clinical and are also marked by the laboratory findings.

It cannot be differentiated by the proteinogramme. But clinically, the most important symptoms of what may be called Kahler's disease are: osseous pains, geodes and the cells which are increased are plasmocytes, more or less normal or tumor cells. However, in Waldenström's disease, the symptoms which predominate are: hemorrhages due to plaquettopenias, a generalized decalcification of the skeleton without geodes, and the predominating cells are of lymphocytic origin. So perhaps this case fits more to the Waldenström which is a more unusual disease than the myeloma. In every 100 cases of myeloma, 98 are of Kahler and 2 of Waldenström; of Franklin, only 5 cases have been described in all the world literature.

The gammaglobulins, which we now call immunoglobulins, is where the greatest number of immunological reaction have their site and are precisely the globulins affected by these diseases. The gammaglobulin is formed by four fractions which are: the gamma A, the gamma G, the gamma M, and another more recently described, the gamma D. The denomination of the gammaglobulins is based on three capital letters: the I, which means immune; the G globulin, and the third letter the A, the M or the G.

The M means macroglobulin, which is of very high molecular weight. When it multiplies it gives rise to a Waldenström or macroglobulinemia; the G is the most important fraction of the gamma, that is, nearly all the gamma is G. The increase in the I.G.G., in myeloma, is nearly a 70–75% of the cases; the increase in I.G.A. is perhaps a 30% of the cases, and the increase in I.G.D. is very rare. This globulin has been described for a very special case of myeloma. Thus, among the hyperglobulinemias there are two types: myeloma in which one of these three (G. A. D.) is increased and the macroglobulinemia (increase in M). This differentiation is thus important because the macroglobulinemia is different and gives rise to a completely different syndrome. In this case, it can very well be Waldenström's considering the clinical findings since the laboratory findings at that time could not clearly differentiated. The puncture was described at the beginning as a lymphoid leukemia which leads us to think that it was a Waldenström. However, this is not so mathematical that plasmocytes mean a Waldenström, and lymphoid cells indicate a myeloma.

Moreover, the patient had no pain, because it was a rectorrhagia which led to the discovery of the disease; he never had osseous pains which probably he would have suffered if it had been a typical myeloma; instead, he suffered hemorrhages which are classical of Waldenström's. Moreover, he did not present large goedes but only small decalcifications. Furthermore the laboratory findings were of a very high monoclonal gamma, an anemia of one or two millions and a hemorrhagic syndrome with plaquettopenia of 60, 70 and 80 thousand.

In this patient also, the proteinuria of Bence-Jones was slightly positive as in Waldenström's; the same in the myeloma is always very positive. The immunoglobulins are formed by polypeptide components and have two kinds of chains, very long ones and heavy which are the H and others light, which may be the K and the L. All the immunoglobulins have two heavy and two light chains. The immunological characteristics are usually given by the light chain. The protein of Bence-Jones is nothing more than the light chain of protein unfolded and as it is of very little molecular weight it passes into the urine in greater quantity in Kahler's disease than in Waldenström's. The perfect differentiation of the three diseases as can be now obtained in the laboratory, could not be obtained in the period (the Franklin's disease was described in 1963) as there were no laboratory means in Spain for this differentiation.

For the proctologist it is of less importance that the patient be diagnosed as a Kahler or as a Waldenström. Even though at the moment in which the observation of the patient was done we did not have of the laboratory means to obtain an exact differential diagnosis, our collaborators of that time, want to explain in this chapter on "Diagnosis", their observations about same and comments which, at present suggest, to them a revision of the data obtained in 1962.

Discussion

A plaquettopenia of less than 100,000, is already sufficient to produce a hemorrhage in a feeble or delicate mucosa. In the anorectal region where the varicose complex sometimes develops with such exaggeration, it is natural that it is one of the most sensitive sites to the lack of the hemostatic factors.

A localized infection in the vascular wall and thrombosis is produced until the rupture, which is only a very limited hemorrhage in a normal patient, may on occasion become an important hemorrhage which is fatal. In truth it may be difficult to discover which is the deficient factor, and we must always carry out all known tests to try to reach a conclusion, for which we strongly advise that our efforts be added to those of hematologist. Even though this is not the case, we want to show that, in spite of the advances in the field of clotting, there still exist many cases in which the tests performed give normal results. We still know with certainty that some important factor escapes us. The complete blood transfusion continues to be our best and sometimes only means of treatment.

If an absolute complete recuperation of the original ailment is obtained, or at least a stabilization with an acceptable coagulation or clotting, some of the anorectal diseases may be treated with the greatest caution. But generally, it is most judicious to limit ourselves to the least manipulations. The sclerosis in the afore mentioned condition is a good measure to be undertaken. For purulent collections, there is no other way than to drain them and in some cases, paradoxically, a good improvement of the local wound is seen, while the general condition of the patient gets worse.

However, we believe that it is most important that the internist, the surgeon and the proctologist, be aware of the relative frequency of the association of the rectal processes with hematological ones. It is important to discover this disorder in time, as it necessitates treatment of the basic disease, before a surgical procedure. We insist that a hematological examination must be performed before undertaking any surgical intervention in the anorectal region.

Bibliography

BIRNBAUM, W., and R. AHLIQUIST: "Rectal infections and ulcerations associated with blood Dyscrasias". Amer. J. Surg **90**, 367 (1955).

BLANK, W. A.: "Anorectal Complications in leukemia". Amer. J. Surg. **90**, 738 (1955).

BLUEFARB, S. M.: "Anorectal Complications of Acute Leukemia Simulating Lymphopathia Venerum". Quart. Bull. Northw. Univ. med. Sch. **31**, 198 (1957).

CURRIE, O. J., and J. C. LUKE: "Giant Follicular Hyperplasia of the Rectum Showing Malignant Degeneration". Canad. med. Ass. J. **63**, 150 (1950).

GRANET, E., M. B. KAGAN, and C. SOLOMON: "Lymphomas of the Anorectum". Amer. H. Surg. **80**, 311 (1950).

HOROWITCH, S., y L. R. WASSERMAN: "Enfermedades del ano y recto asociades con alteraciones hematologicas". Ano, recto y colon. Buenos Aires: Beta edit. (1962).

MARKS, M. M.: "Monocytic Leukemia with Oral and Anorectal Complications". J. Intern. Coll. Surg. **20**, 750 (1953).

PALMA, F.: "Afecciones anorrectales y hemopatías". Rev. Clin. Esp. **90**, 102 (1963).

PESSEL, J. V., E. B. BEARSTO, J. S. WISE, M. H. ECWARDS, G. SCARAVELLI, and T. K. RATHMELL: "Unusual Causes of Gastrointestinal Hemorrhage". Gastroenterology **31**, 538 (1956)

SPEARE, G. S.: "Anorectal Disease in the Community". New Engl. J. Med. **255**, 377 (1956)

A Method for the Adequate Preparation of Rectoscopic Examinations

Á. ALFÖLDY and M. FEHÉR, Budapest, Hungary

Rectoscopy is of especial importance for the examination of the anal region. It involves hardly any risks and, being a routine method of examination, requires no special preparatory measures.

Rectoscopy is invariably preceded by digital examination of the rectum and an enema which is often painful; besides, the introduction of the enema tube, the examiner's finger or the rectoscope may encounter some obstacle, an impediment which is fortunately due in most cases to functional factors.

Periodic proctospastic and paroxysmal rectal pains may arise owing to proctalgia fugax or rectalgia nervosa, coccygodynia, neuralgia and tabetic crisis.

Inflammatory processes, haemorrhoidal disturbances, stenosis, pectenosis, or rupture, as also benign or malignant neoplastic growths may impede and even make impossible the carrying out of digital and rectoscopic examinations.

Rectoscopy requires no therapeutic sedation. By way of therapeutic preparation it is usual to administer opium tincture in order to reduce peristaltic movements. Swabs saturated with pantocaine or lidocaine solution are applied to the anal canal prior to examination if the patient complains of painfulness and if the sphincter is impaired.

This is not invariably successful, and the mechanical action or a possible allergic effect may render the situation still worse.

The anal canal, 3 cm long and richly provided with sensory nerves, is encircled by the striated muscles of the sphincter ani externus, while the muscles of the sphincter ani internus and the rectal columns are smooth. The anal canal and perianal area receive their nervous supply from the sacral part of the spinal cord, whereas the rectum is innervated by the fibres of the autonomic nervous system. It is thus natural that the area situated above the anorectal line is but slightly sensitive, while the anal canal and the perianal area, through which the finger of the examiner, the rectal tube of the enema and the relevant instruments have to be passed, show a high degree of sensitivity.

In the normal course of voluntary defecation the contraction of the diaphragm and the muscles of the abdominal wall exert a pressure which results in the relaxation of the external sphincter. With a view to facilitating the introduction of the rectoscope, the patient is invited to imitate normal evacuatory efforts. It has, of course, to be borne in mind that an unnatural knee-elbow or knee-chest position may impede the normal effect of the abdominal muscular pressure.

Taking into account the given anatomical conditions (muscles, nerves), the patients' unnatural posture during the examination as also the resulting inadequacy of the abdominal pressure, further, the inevitable stress caused by the examination as well as the pathologico-anatomic conditions to be expected, we have elaborated a new preparatory method which is described here.

The method prevents pain, eliminates the possibility of proctospasms, and ensures a smooth course of the examination even under pathological conditions. It goes without saying that an a-limine existing narrowness of the 3 cm-long anal canal or its pathologic constriction, whether functional or organic, may make the introduction of any type of rectoscope difficult if not impossible, even in paediatric cases.

Spasms supervening during examination may cause its repeated interruption. Hitherto it was necessary to await the spontaneous cessation of such attacks. Existing impediments must not be overcome by force. Spasmodic pains frequently arise when the rectoscope reaches the lower portion of the sigmoid colon. Stronger insufflation of air may give rise to intensive pressure-like pains and should therefore not be performed. Such insufflations in patients of advanced age may produce inflammation, oedema and even perforation. The abandonment of unnecessary insufflations and a steady visual control of the introduction and removal of the examining instruments prevent any complaints in connection with the preparatory measures described in this communication.

This is of especial importance because some 75 per cent of the cancers of the large intestine are in its lower segment of 25 cm, so that a rectoscopic inspection of the cancerous areas encounters no difficulty.

A cleansing camomile enema is applied if inflammatory or ulcerative phenomena are suspected. Flos chamomillae has, moreover, a spasmolytic and antiphlogistic effect. The tip of the rectal tube used for the irrigation must not be used more than once so as to prevent helminthiasis, bacterial and other infections. Micralax (Pharmacia, Uppsala) is employed in other cases. Simplicity, the saving of time, elimination of mucosal irritation and reduced physical stress recommend this method of preparation for routine employment.

In addition to the therapeutic preparatory measures to be described below, rectoscopic examinations can be prepared by the micralax method also in cases of haemorrhoidal prolapse, haemorrhoidal thrombosis and anal fissure.

The patients are given 2×2 Scutamil-C tablets and 2×2 tablets of papaverine hydrochloride an hour before and an hour after the camomile infusion, and it is only thereafter that the examination begins. These drugs are perorally administered two hours and one hour before the employment of micralax.

That the examination elicits no complaint whatever from the patients is due to the muscle-relaxing and moderately analgesic action of carisosprodol and the analgesia-potentiating effect of paracetamol. They relax the muscles of the external sphincter and have, thus, a proctospasmolytic effect. The combined effect of paracetamol and carisosprodol allays the painful irritation of the anal canal and the adjacent tissues. Papaverine hydrochloride, administered at the same time, produces spasmolysis of the smooth muscles and reduces their tone. Moreover, it stops the spasm of smooth muscles in the intestine between the sphincter and the lower part of the sigmoid colon, an effect which considerably facilitates painless insertion of the rectoscope.

We want to add that in some of our kinetic examinations the administration of Scutamil-C yielded satisfactory results, among other reasons because it helped the patients in assuming the required posture without inconvenience.

The above-described methods of preparation make it possible to obtain a clear picture of the mucous membrane, relax the sphincters and render the examination painless. Examiners, provided with up-to-date instruments, possessing adequate manual skill and the appropriate clinico-pathologic training, will be able to make correct diagnoses by employing the methods of preparation outlined above·

Bibliography

STRAUSS, H.: Die Prokto-Sigmoskopie. 2nd ed. Thieme, Leipzig 1930. Report on Scutamil-C submitted to the United Works for the Manufacture of Pharmaceutical and Dietetic Products, Budapest.

FEHÉR, M.: Magyar Belorv. Arch. Suppl. 2, 30 1969. Symposium of the Clinical Evaluation of a New Disposable Microenema. New Brunswick – New Jersey, June 1963.

MIX
Papier aus verantwortungsvollen Quellen
Paper from responsible sources
FSC® C105338

If you have any concerns about our products,
you can contact us on
ProductSafety@springernature.com

In case Publisher is established outside the EU,
the EU authorized representative is:
Springer Nature Customer Service Center GmbH
Europaplatz 3, 69115 Heidelberg, Germany

Printed by Libri Plureos GmbH
in Hamburg, Germany